Practical Issues in Bariatric Surgery

Edited by Livia Palmieri and Eleonora Rapanotti

Published in London, United Kingdom

Practical Issues in Bariatric Surgery
http://dx.doi.org/10.5772/intechopen.1003447
Edited by Livia Palmieri and Eleonora Rapanotti

Contributors
Abdullah Hasan, Ahmed Elfaioumy, Ahmed Mostafa Abdel-Hameed, Alanoud Alobaidly, Alberto Rodríguez Gallardo, Alessandro M. Paganini, Alessandro Troisi, Alexander A. Rogut, Alexander G. Khitarian, Amr Ashour, Amr Rashwan, Anıl Ergin, Arut V. Mezhunts, Arutyun A. Abovian, Asad Ullah, Belal Khalil, Bonifacio García Ramos, Bruno Sander, César David Quiróz Guadarrama, Denis A. Melnikova, Edgar Alejandro Ibáñez Cruz, Eleonora Rapanotti, Federica Rizzo, Germana Ginevra Perrone, Halil Buluç, İksan Taşdelen, Isabelle Debergh, Jimi Izaques Bifi Scarparo, Johar Jamil, José Antonio Angulo Trejo, Kamil S. Veliev, Koninica Sanyal, Livia Palmieri, Marta Celiento, Mohamed Eshmandi, Mohamed Hussein, Mohamed Mohamed, Monica Angulo Trejo, Muhammad Jamil, Mustafa Karaagac, Mónica Angulo Trejo, Nicola Perrotta, Pasquale Campagna, Roberta Russo, Sameh Abdel-Khalek Ahmed, Sedat Carkit, Silvia Quaresima, Tarek Abdel-Hay Mostafa, Victor García Ramos, Víctor García Ramos

First published in London, United Kingdom, 2025 by IntechOpen
IntechOpen is the global imprint of INTECHOPEN LIMITED, registered in England and Wales, registration number: 11086078, 167-169 Great Portland Street, London, W1W 5PF, United Kingdom

For EU product safety concerns: IN TECH d.o.o., Prolaz Marije Krucifikse Kozulić 3, 51000 Rijeka, Croatia, info@intechopen.com or visit our website at intechopen.com.

British Library Cataloguing-in-Publication Data
A catalogue record for this book is available from the British Library

Practical Issues in Bariatric Surgery
Edited by Livia Palmieri and Eleonora Rapanotti
p. cm.
Print ISBN 978-0-85466-416-0
Online ISBN 978-0-85466-415-3
eBook (PDF) ISBN 978-0-85466-417-7

If disposing of this product, please recycle the paper responsibly.

Meet the editors

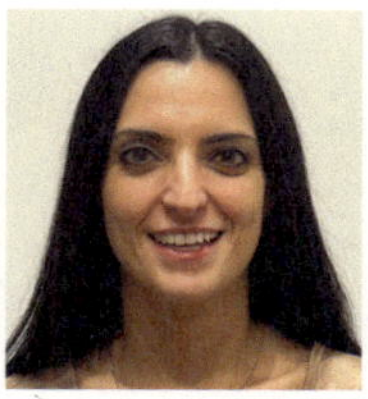

Livia Palmieri earned her Master's Degree in Medicine and Surgery from the University of Bari in 2015. She then moved to the Sapienza University of Rome, where she completed her Specialization Degree in General Surgery with cum laude honors in 2021. She is also pursuing a Ph.D. in "Experimental and Clinical Hepato-Gastroenterology" within the Physiopathology Surgery curriculum. After specialization, she obtained a one-year research grant in *Bariatric and Mini-invasive Surgery* at the Sapienza University of Rome, in Policlinico Umberto I. Later, she moved to Policlinico Universitario Agostino Gemelli, also in Rome, to become a Physician Consultant in Endocrine and Metabolic Surgery. She currently serves as a Physician Consultant in Endocrine Surgery at the Azienda Ospedaliera Santa Maria in Terni at the University of Perugia. Dr. Palmieri is the author or co-author of numerous scientific articles published in national and international journals; she participated as a speaker and faculty in numerous national and international conferences and is a member of multiple scientific societies. She was the winner of grants for various national and international research projects in the field of General Surgery, especially regarding endocrine and bariatric surgery. She has fervent clinical and research activities in general, laparoscopic, bariatric and endocrine surgery.

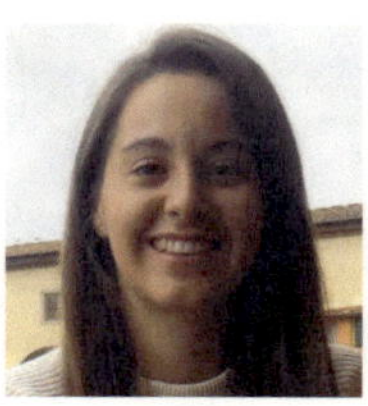

Eleonora Rapanotti earned her Master's degree in Medicine and Surgery from Sacred Heart Catholic University of Rome in 2021. She is currently in the penultimate year of her General Surgery Specialization at Sapienza University of Rome. Eleonora has actively participated in numerous national conferences as both a participant and a speaker. Her primary interests include minimally invasive, general, and endocrine surgery.

Contents

Preface

In the last 30 years, obesity and its associated disorders have been reaching epidemic proportions worldwide. Today, obesity represents the most common chronic disorder in industrialized societies, and increasing attention has been given to this health problem, with the involvement of most physicians. Therefore, obesity is becoming a major point in the healthcare planning system. Bariatric surgery is the only effective treatment for obesity and its comorbidities, acknowledged by the International Federation for the Surgery of Obesity and Metabolic Disorders (IFSO) and by the American Society for Metabolic and Bariatric Surgery (ASMBS).

The advent of video laparoscopic instrumentation, critical care advancements and modern stapling devices have significantly transformed the field of bariatric surgery during the past three decades. Before the 2000s, the annual number of bariatric surgeries conducted in Europe ranged between 10000 and 12000, accompanied by elevated morbidity and mortality rates. However, this number has expanded significantly today, reaching over 140000 operations per year. This expansion is closely linked to the evolution and shift from open surgery to laparoscopy, particularly in performing Roux-en-Y gastric bypass. Additionally, the endorsement of the laparoscopic adjustable gastric band significantly increased the volume of bariatric surgeries. More recently, laparoscopic sleeve gastrectomy has emerged as a viable bariatric surgical alternative, with a risk and benefit profile intermediate to that of laparoscopic gastric bypass and laparoscopic adjustable gastric banding. Finally, bariatric endoscopy has been developed as a minimally invasive alternative to bridge the gap between conservative and conventional surgical therapies in the last few years.

As the global obesity pandemic continues to grow, bariatric surgery has gained prominence, becoming a widely recognized term. This volume aims to be an accessible and pragmatic resource for a broad range of personnel, including the extensive medical support staff within a bariatric center, as well as bariatric surgeons, anesthesiologists, nurses, and, crucially, general surgeons who may not specialize in bariatrics.

This book addresses most of the practical issues in bariatric surgery, especially in patient selection, preoperative management, different bariatric surgical and endoscopic procedures, the advent of new technologies, anaesthetic reflections, and complication management. Each chapter in this book is written by experts in their field, and the editors are grateful to every author who dedicated time and effort to share their knowledge in concise and easy-to-read language.

Livia Palmieri
General and Endocrine Surgery Unit,
Santa Maria Hospital,
Terni, Italy

Eleonora Rapanotti
Department of General Surgery and Surgical Specialties,
Sapienza University of Rome,
Rome, Italy

Section 1

Preoperative Management of Bariatric Surgery

Chapter 1

Bariatric Surgery: Can It Perform Benefits or Risks?

Tarek Abdel-Hay Mostafa, Ahmed Mostafa Abdel-Hameed and Sameh Abdel-Khalek Ahmed

Abstract

Obesity is associated with an increased incidence of heart failure (HF), myocardial infarction (MI), stroke, and death. Weight loss has become a standard recommendation for all patients with cardiovascular disease (CVD) and coexisting obesity. Bariatric surgery has been shown to reduce cardiovascular risk factors significantly; however, whether surgery can reduce major adverse cardiovascular events (MACE), especially in patients with established cardiovascular disease. Bariatric surgery has been associated with a significant reduction in daily insulin requirement and a considerable reduction in body mass index, resulting in long-term results. Furthermore, studies suggest that bariatric surgery for type 1 diabetes results in the improvement of comorbidities related to obesity including hypertension and dyslipidemia. Obesity is thought to be the strongest risk factor for the development of type 2 diabetes. Bariatric surgery has emerged as the single most effective treatment option for type 2 diabetes and obesity. The individuals who underwent bariatric surgery compared with medical/lifestyle intervention had superior glycemic control with less diabetes medication use and higher rates of diabetes remission. Obesity is a pro-inflammatory condition in which some cytokines such as leptin, a pro-inflammatory protein, are elevated and adiponectin, an anti-inflammatory protein, is decreased. In patients undergoing weight reduction surgeries, these hormone levels behave paradoxically. It is not known whether bariatric surgery protects against the development of autoinflammatory or autoimmune conditions; nevertheless, changes occurring in the immune system are incompletely understood. Patients undergoing bariatric surgery show immunological changes which might eventually lead to developing an autoimmune disease.

Keywords: bariatric surgery, cardiovascular disease, thyroid disease, hyperparathyroidism, malnutrition

1. Introduction

Obesity is linked to substantial morbidity and death, making it one of the largest healthcare issues of our day. As of 2016, obesity was linked to four million annual fatalities [1, 2]. Increased adipose tissue, or "adiposopathy," is linked to obesity and may have detrimental effects on the cardiovascular (CV) system through several processes. First, the development of risk factors may lead to the systemic effects of adipose tissue, which might result in CV disease. Second, the heart and blood arteries may be directly or locally affected by adipose tissue through perivascular and epicardial actions [3, 4]. Third, the buildup of fat tissue may result in the compression of an organ, which can induce obstructive sleep apnea, hypertension, and renal failure [5]. Diabetes and hypertension are the two most prevalent CV risk factors linked to obesity. Their prevalences typically range from 30 to 40% of patients and rise with the degree of obesity. In addition, dyslipidemia and heightened inflammation are prevalent in obese individuals (20–40%). Atrial fibrillation (AF), heart failure (HF), coronary artery disease/myocardial infarction, and stroke are cardiovascular disorders that are linked to obesity. The hazard ratio (HR) for developing various CV illnesses is at least 1.5–2.0, but in cases of extreme obesity (defined as a BMI of $\geq$40 kg/m^2), it rises noticeably to 6.0 [6–8]. Although there are far fewer studies on this subject, obesity is also a well-known risk factor for stroke and has been linked to an increased incidence of aortic valve stenosis [9, 10].

1.1 Effect on all-cause and cardiovascular mortality

A total of 28 studies looked at how bariatric surgery affected both CV and all-cause mortality. All-cause mortality after bariatric surgery ranged from 0.0 to 23.7%, while for controls it ranged from 1.4 to 28.2%, with follow-up lasting between 2 and 24 years. The van Veldhuisen, et al.'s meta-analysis was appropriate since 21 papers that looked at all-cause mortality and provided adjusted HRs were included in the study. In these 21 trials, there were 263,478 obese controls and 133,524 patients who had undergone bariatric surgery. In comparison to obese participants in the control group, patients who had undergone surgery had a pooled HR of all-cause mortality of 0.55, according to the van Veldhuisen, et al.'s meta-analysis. CV mortality was the subject of seven research, with rates ranging from 0.2–8.3% in bariatric patients to 0.5–12.9% in controls. According to the findings of the meta-analysis by van Veldhuisen, et al., bariatric surgery also decreased CV mortality.

The incidence of AF decreased non-significantly following bariatric surgery compared to controls, according to the van Veldhuisen, et al.'s meta-analysis. When compared to controls, bariatric surgery was linked to a reduced risk of myocardial infarction. The frequency of all strokes was decreased by the bariatric procedure [11].

Atrial fibrillation (AF) and myocardial infarction (heart attack) are significantly impacted by weight reduction.

1. Atrial fibrillation (AF):

- Connection to Obesity: AF and obesity are intimately associated. Compared to healthy people, AF sufferers have a greater prevalence of obesity.

Mechanisms: Several processes link AF and obesity, including:

- Hypertension: The development of AF is influenced by hypertension associated with obesity.

- Diabetes: Being obese raises the chance of developing diabetes, which is linked to AF.

- Obstructive Sleep Apnea: AF is associated with obesity-related sleep apnea.
- Epicardial Fat: Obesity-related increases in epicardial fat can cause electrical irregularities and atrial hypertrophy.
- Obesity increases the risk of atrial fibrillation (AF) by inducing systemic inflammation and oxidative stress.

  1. Effect of Weight Loss: Losing weight helps with AF:

     Anti-inflammation and fibrosis: Losing weight improves the prognosis for AF by reducing inflammation and fibrosis. Weight Fluctuations: However, weight fluctuations might counteract the advantages of losing weight [12].

2. Myocardial Infarction:

   - Obesity and Risk: Obesity raises the possibility of myocardial infarction.
   - Benefits of Losing Weight: Losing weight provides several heart-healthy advantages.
   - Reduced Risk: A heart attack is less likely when weight is lost.
   - Reduced Cardiac Strain: Losing weight lessens the workload on the heart and enhances cardiac function.
   - Metabolic Gains: Reducing weight improves insulin sensitivity, blood pressure, and cholesterol.
   - Exercise and Weight Loss: Losing weight and engaging in regular exercise improve heart health and lower the chance of a heart attack [13].

2. Bariatric surgery and hypertension

Even if bariatric surgery (BS) has been shown to alleviate comorbidity, there may be other underlying variables that are equally significant. The causes for the improvement in blood pressure following bariatric surgery are likely complex and yet up for discussion [14]. It has been hypothesized that normalizing blood pressure levels might result from a reduction in arterial stiffness and salt reabsorption as well as an improvement in insulin resistance. The renin-angiotensin-aldosterone system is known to be more activated in patients with central obesity; this system may also return to normal following surgery [15]. A rise in gastrointestinal gut hormones, such as glucagon-like peptide-1 (GLP-1) and peptide YY (PYY), may also be significant because of their effects on the gastrointestinal tract in addition to their diuretic and natriuretic effects on the kidney [16]. Additionally, a potential impact of GLP-1 on the sympathetic nervous system has been reported, which might contribute to the decrease of blood pressure following BS [17]. Additionally, ghrelin may help return blood pressure to normal, while the surgical process may cause its levels to rise, decline, or stay the same following BS [18]. Moreover, adipokines and other inflammatory cytokines seem to have a role in HTN recuperation. In this regard, earlier research found that adiponectin concentrations increased in conjunction with a decrease in leptin levels from 1 week to 1 year following BS [19]. Furthermore, C-reactive protein and interleukin-6 levels fall with increased insulin sensitivity, reducing adipocyte inflammation and averting vascular constriction. Lastly, the resolution of other obesity comorbidities, including obstructive sleep apnea, which shares pathophysiologic pathways with hypertension, may also contribute to an improvement in blood pressure [20, 21].

It has been hypothesized that normalizing blood pressure levels might result from a reduction in arterial stiffness and salt reabsorption as well as an improvement in insulin resistance. Renin-angiotensin-aldosterone system activation is known to be higher in patients with central obesity, and it may return to normal following surgery [15]. Furthermore, because these gastrointestinal gut hormones have a diuretic and natriuretic effect on the kidney in addition to their effects on the gastrointestinal tract, a rise in peptide YY (PYY) and glucagon-like peptide-1 (GLP-1) may also be essential [16]. Additionally, a potential impact of GLP-1 on the sympathetic nervous system has been reported, which might contribute to the decrease of blood pressure following BS. Ghrelin may also help return blood pressure to normal, albeit depending on the surgical technique used after BS, its levels may rise, reduce, or stay the same [18].

Moreover, adipokines and other inflammatory cytokines seem to have a role in HTN recuperation. In this regard, earlier research found that adiponectin concentrations increased in tandem with a decrease in leptin levels from 1 week to 1 year following BS. Furthermore, C-reactive protein and interleukin-6 levels fall with increased insulin sensitivity, reducing adipocyte inflammation and averting vascular constriction [19]. In this regard, prior research discovered that 1 week following GB, there were notable reductions in both the systolic (9 mm Hg) and diastolic (7 mm Hg) blood pressure, and these were sustained 1 year following surgery. Given that the two surgical techniques are distinct, it is known that GLP-1 and PYY rise following both; however, the increase following GB is more pronounced, which might explain the better outcomes following this treatment [22].

In terms of heart modifications, a number of studies documented morphologic and functional abnormalities in obese individuals' echocardiograms. The primary changes included left ventricular (LV) hypertrophy and decreased LV diastolic performance; LV systolic dysfunction was less frequent, and as a result, there were conflicting findings on the ejection fraction in obese individuals [23]. Patients with morbid obesity have been shown to have morphologic abnormalities in their left ventricle (LV), with a meta-analysis of 22 studies involving 5486 obese participants reporting 56% of LV hypertrophy. Numerous of these alterations are signs of more obvious cardiac dysfunction and heart failure [24]. Obesity does, in fact, appear to raise the risk of myocardial infarction, atrial fibrillation, heart failure, and unexpected death [25].

In addition to the results of observational epidemiology, Larsson et al. discovered evidence linking an increased risk of aortic stenosis, heart failure, deep venous thrombosis, hypertension, peripheral artery disease, coronary artery disease, atrial fibrillation, and pulmonary embolism (estimates ranging from 6 to 13% higher risk) to a genetically instrumented 1 kg/m^2 higher body mass index. Regarding fat mass, the results were mostly in agreement. In particular, there is a documented higher correlation between obesity and heart failure than there is for other subtypes of cardiovascular disease, and this correlation cannot be well explained by conventional risk factors [26, 27]. Regarding the mechanisms underlying the improvement of the heart following bariatric surgery, a number of authors agree that the effects of weight-loss surgery on cardiac morphology and function are either centrally or hormonally regulated, most likely involving the renin-angiotensin-aldosterone axis, leptin, and other adipokines [28]. Crucially, weight reduction techniques like BS have demonstrated the ability to reverse these changes in cardiovascular structure and function, hence reducing the risk of cardiovascular disease. The effects of BS on cardiac anatomy and function were examined in a meta-analysis and systematic review of 23 studies. The findings demonstrated that BS significantly reduced absolute LV mass and relative wall thickness (RWT), two reliable indicators of LV hypertrophy and LV geometry that have been demonstrated to predict cardiovascular outcomes, in obese patients with preserved LV systolic function. Additionally, that meta-analysis demonstrated reductions in left atrial size, which is an indirect indicator of persistently high LV filling pressure and diastolic dysfunction, as well as improvements in LV diastolic function, as demonstrated by a definite increase in the mitral flow ratio of the early (E) to late (A) ventricular filling velocities (E/A ratio) [29]. Owan et al. observed comparable findings on LV hypertrophy and RWT 2 years following BS. The authors discovered that there was a correlation between the reduction in body mass index and the reductions in LV mass index and RWT but not with changes in blood pressure [30].

The development of arterial stiffness (AS) is one of the primary signs of vascular change. The reduced capacity of an artery to expand and contract in response to a given pressure change is regarded as an independent cardiovascular risk factor [31]. Over the past 20 years, it has been discovered that being overweight is linked to increased aortic stiffness in both younger and older persons. Therefore, obesity may increase cardiovascular risk independently of established risk factors, and one mechanism by which this may happen is higher AS. Regardless of the presence of HTN, it is linked to an elevated risk of cardiovascular disease [32]. In obese people, AS may occur before increases in incident hypertension and systolic blood pressure. Regarding how BS affects AS, several studies found that many months following BS, there was a considerable drop in the AS indicators, the augmentation index, and pulse wave velocity. More significantly than higher blood pressure, increased heart volume and output in obese people were also identified as potential mediators of AS [33–35].

Regardless of diabetes and high blood pressure, which are both predominantly caused by obesity, obesity is a risk factor for kidney disease on its own. Renal lipotoxicity, inflammatory cytokines, and hemodynamic variables are the key hypothesized reasons underlying the link between obesity-associated kidney failure and hyperfiltration [36]. In terms of hemodynamic parameters, before nephron damage, being overweight first results in functional renal vasodilation, as well as increases in renal blood flow and glomerular hyperfiltration. Declines in renal blood flow and the glomerular filtration rate (GFR) due to kidney damage and the progressive loss of nephrons occur after these changes. The increase in tubular sodium reabsorption linked to obesity leads to an increase in the amount of extracellular fluid. This might be because of the increased renal sympathetic nerve activity and the raised levels of anti-natriuretic hormones like angiotensin II and aldosterone that result from renal compression caused by visceral, perirenal, and renal sinus fat [37].

The observed afferent arteriola vasodilation may be explained by the changed tubule-glomerular feedback, or macula densa feedback, which may involve these and other factors. Even with increased sodium chloride reabsorption in the loop of Henle, compensatory increases in GFR and blood pressure rise can restore sodium balance. Moreover, renal vasodilation may also be facilitated by the activation of the mineralocorticoid receptor (MR). Aldosterone activates MR expressed on macula densa cells, boosting their nitric oxide generation and causing glomerular hyperfiltration and renal vasodilation [38].

This rise in glomerular hydrostatic pressure most likely plays a major role in the renal damage seen in obesity, even if glomerular hyperfiltration has an adaptive role in counteracting renal salt reabsorption. Additionally, an unhealthy adipocytokine pattern that is typified by an excess of angiotensinogen and angiotensin II and an increase in pro-inflammatory cytokines including interleukin-6, C-reactive protein, and tumor necrosis factor-α is promoted by obesity. Experimental models demonstrate the induction of renal fibrosis by these substances through the transforming growth factor-β (TGF-β) pathway and oxidative stress [38].

Furthermore, it is well known that obese people have elevated serum leptin levels and increased leptin receptor expression in the kidney, which in turn promotes cellular proliferation and the release of the prosclerotic TGF-β1 cytokine, which is linked to the early onset of scarring in renal failure. Lastly, decreased levels of adiponectin, another adipokine, have been linked to renal impairment associated with obesity by damaging podocytes and causing albuminuria. Long-term hyperfiltration can cause pathologic alterations such as the onset of glomerulomegaly and focal segmental glomerulosclerosis-related kidney lesions, which can result in glomerulopathy linked to obesity [39].

Li et al.'s study included a systematic review and meta-analysis of 32 trials that showed substantial decreases in albuminuria, proteinuria, and hyperfiltration (as evaluated by GFR, eGFR, and creatinine clearance with and without body surface area adjustment) following BS. When examined as a binary variable following surgery, they discovered statistically significant decreases in hyperfiltration as well. Additionally, following BS, there were decreases in the frequencies of proteinuria and albuminuria of 58 and 69%, respectively [40].

Data comparing patients receiving BS and controls followed up for a median of 18 years in the Swedish Obese Subjects study, which included 4047 patients, revealed a decreased incidence of chronic kidney disease (CKD) stages 4 and 5 among patients in the surgery group. Similar findings were found by O'Brien et al. in a retrospective analysis, wherein a cohort of 4000 diabetic patients receiving BS saw a 59% reduced incidence of nephropathy after 5 years when compared to 11,000 matched patients who did not get surgical treatment [41, 42].

Friedman et al. examined 2144 obese patients who had BS and discovered that, throughout a 7-year follow-up period, a significant percentage of patients had improved in CKD risk categories. They stated that those with high baseline risk had the greatest reduction in risk [43]. Regarding renal protective variables, Favre et al. found that in highly obese patients receiving BS, kidney protection was predicted by low C-reactive protein levels, high-fat mass, absence of HTN, and young age [36].

The glomerular function may be associated with the return of normal insulin signaling in glomerular podocytes, the reduction of hyperfiltration, and the restoration of renin-angiotensin system equilibrium through improved renal perfusion. Furthermore, decreases in the pro-inflammatory state associated with obesity as indicated by urine monocyte-chemoattractant protein-1/creatinine ratios may potentially be a contributing factor to this improvement. Recent research has demonstrated that intestinal endocrine L cells generate the incretin hormone glucagon-like peptide 1 (GLP-1), which inhibits tubular reabsorption of sodium and has reno-protective effects. After BS, these effects intensify, indicating a potential contribution to the improvement in glomerular function. Regarding the remission of albuminuria, one important cellular event that may contribute to the advantages of BS, at least in obese diabetics, is the restoration of podocyte health [44]. According to Lieske et al., the chance of developing new kidney stone events increased in these patients compared to obese controls who had not had surgery, and up to 50% of these patients may remain hyperoxaluric a year following surgery. However, for the majority of individuals, the overall impact on long-term renal health may be favorable [45].

For individuals with obesity-associated hypertension, BS has shown to be a very successful therapy, leading to HTN remission in over 50% of cases. Nevertheless, achieving total HTN remission may be hampered by a higher need for antihypertensive medication before BS and a lower rate of weight reduction during follow-up. Furthermore, in morbidly obese people, BS has also been associated with a decrease in cardiovascular morbidity and death. These positive findings of cardiovascular outcomes might be mediated by a number of mechanisms other than weight loss, one of which could be decreased target organ damage and better blood pressure levels.

3. Bariatric surgery and type 1 DM

A tiny percentage of individuals undergoing bariatric surgery have Type 1 diabetes, but because of their underlying condition, they need specialized care. Patients with type 1 DM are impacted by this sharp rise in the frequency of overweight and obesity since they are more susceptible to being overweight. Accordingly, compared to T1D patients who are slim, elevated BMI is linked to a higher risk of cardiometabolic disease and an increased likelihood of developing chronic problems. Conversely, insulin resistance increases the need for insulin and makes it more difficult to control blood sugar levels and lose weight [46].

Six months following bariatric surgery, the present group showed notable reductions in weight and BMI.

After 2 years, the mean BMI dropped from 39.5 to 27.5 kg/m^2, a difference of 12 units, marking the most weight loss. The mean BMI at the end of the follow-up was 9 units lower than the mean BMI before surgery, although BMI climbed in the third year following surgery; 8/15 (65%) were classified as normal weight or overweight. In contrast, obese individuals with type 1 diabetes treated at the same clinics but without surgery saw a little rise in BMI throughout the same period. There is broad consensus that bariatric surgery is a successful weight loss solution for people with type 1 diabetes, despite variations in follow-up time [47–50].

Parallel to the significant weight loss in the first 6 months following surgery, a decline in the mean HbA1c level was noted. This decrease in HbA1c is most likely the result of rigorous postoperative calorie restriction. However, HbA1c levels did not alter substantially from baseline or from those who did not have surgery between the 12-month follow-up period and the conclusion of the follow-up period. The absence of a reduction in HbA1c following bariatric surgery is not associated with weight; rather, it is a reflection of behavioral problems and challenges in adhering to diabetes treatment plans.

Psychosocial variables that include depressed symptoms, limited social support, low self-esteem, and a negative body image have been linked to both poorer BMI and poorer glycemic control. Bariatric surgery is one way to address obesity, but it does not always address the psychological problems associated with it. Notably, during the follow-up period, the non-surgery group's mean HbA1c level progressively rose. This trend was only marginally significant, but it could indicate that people with type 1 DM and obesity are losing their ability to manage their blood sugar with time [51].

In addition to the improvement in insulin sensitivity during weight loss, which necessitates a suitable decrease in the amount of exogenous insulin administered, the alteration in glucose kinetics and the intake and absorption of nutrients may promote hypoglycemia episodes. In relation to this, hypoglycemia is encouraged by food aversion, vomiting following bariatric surgery, and the discrepancy between the insulin peak following subcutaneous injection and the larger and earlier postprandial glucose excursion brought on by the quick transport of carbohydrates to the jejunum. It follows that a higher risk would be anticipated following mixed and malabsorptive procedures [52].

Life-threatening diabetic ketoacidosis (DKA) occurs in 6.2–25% of type 1 DM patients undergoing BS, according to a series of studies [53]. After RYGB surgery, there was a greater incidence of major hyperglycemic episodes in the countrywide Swedish cohort as compared to controls. DKA was linked to inadequate peri-operative glucose management as well as missing or not taking recommended insulin doses. Notably, the Swedish study discovered that having surgery dramatically increased the likelihood of alcohol and drug dependence, which has also been seen in other bariatric series [54, 55].

According to the findings of the Landau et al. study, bariatric surgery helped people with Type 1 DM and obesity lose a considerable amount of weight over time and improved their lipid profile and blood pressure. The adverse events that were reported included a significant risk of diabetic ketoacidosis (DKA), severe hypoglycemia episodes that necessitated hospitalization, and a two-fold increase in hospitalizations in comparison to those with Type 1 diabetes who did not have surgery. Nevertheless, the glycemic control did not improve. Patients with Type 1 DM who undergo bariatric surgery should take several precautions into account, such as careful selection, preparation, and discussion of realistic expectations; pre- and post-operative consultation with a diabetologist; frequent follow-up visits to diabetes clinics to adjust insulin dose and prevent hypoglycemic episodes; and attention to psychological concerns [56].

The Vilarrasa N, et al.'s trial demonstrated improvements in various cardiovascular risk variables, namely hypertension, dyslipidemia, and obstructive sleep apnea, as well as a substantial decrease in body weight and weight-adjusted insulin needs. Nonetheless, little and temporary improvements in glycemic control have been observed, with the majority of these advantages happening in the first year following bariatric surgery [57].

Recent studies have demonstrated a substantial reduction in cardiovascular disease and mortality among Type 1 DM patients who are severely obese and who have undergone bariatric surgery. This procedure has also been effective in lowering weight and insulin dosage, as well as in relieving related comorbidities. The advantages far outweigh the side effects, which include a higher chance of hypoglycemia and DKA. However, close observation of these patients by a multidisciplinary team is essential to provide diabetes education and care as well as a customized, adjustable insulin regimen at all stages of therapy. In this case, new diabetes technology like real-time monitoring might be quite beneficial.

4. Bariatric surgery and type 2 DM

Up to 25% of the patient's total body weight is lost after bariatric surgery, which is more than they would lose with conventional weight-loss techniques. Additionally, 87% of people with type 2 diabetes obtain improved glucose control and require fewer anti-diabetic medications1. On average, 78% of people with type 2 diabetes achieve normal glycemic control without using any anti-diabetic drugs [58, 59]. However, not every bariatric treatment has the same impact on diabetes and weight; some surgeries have a bigger impact. Gastric restriction operations and intestinal bypass surgeries are the two main categories. Initially, the categorization was founded on the assumed mechanism of weight reduction. By reducing stomach capacity and causing fullness, gastric restriction surgeries (such as vertical gastroplasty, sleeve gastrectomy, and laparoscopic adjustable gastric banding) decrease the amount of calories consumed. Patients then lose between 10 and 20% of their entire body weight. Furthermore, laparoscopic adjustable gastric banding has been demonstrated to remit type 2 diabetes in several investigations, including a randomized controlled study, although traditional medication treatment has not. Improved insulin sensitivity and weight reduction, which happen many months after surgery, are the main factors mediating the impact [60, 61].

Similar to gastric banding and vertical gastroplasty, intestinal bypass surgeries (Roux-en-Y gastric bypass, biliopancreatic diversion) limit the number of calories consumed. Nevertheless, they also have an additional factor of malabsorption of fat and nutrients due to the shortening of the small intestine. Following gastric restriction surgeries, a greater number of patients (82–99%) experience remission of type 2 diabetes, including those with longer-term illness and those using insulin. Therefore, the effects of various operations on diabetes vary. There are differences in the rate of remission between restrictive and malabsorptive methods for type 2 diabetes. Even before the patient has lost a significant amount of weight, diabetes remits after a Roux-en-Y gastric bypass with biliopancreatic diversion within a few days. Following gastric restriction operations, this does not occur [58, 62].

Losing weight makes one more sensitive to insulin. Insulin resistance is decreased by weight loss following bariatric surgery, enforced calorie restriction, and negative energy balance. Because they do not have to make as much insulin, the beta cells may relax. Following both gastric bypass and gastric restriction operations, these effects have been noted [61].

By decreasing "lipotoxicity," a disorder linked to dysregulated fatty acid flow, lipid metabolites in tissues, and the direct and indirect effects of hormones released by adipocytes, bariatric surgery reduces insulin resistance. Bikman et al.'s discovery that insulin sensitivity rose following Roux-en-Y surgery more than would be predicted from weight loss alone provides the best support for this idea. After a year after surgery, the patient's insulin sensitivity levels were comparable to those of a control group of lean individuals (BMI < 25 kg/m^2), even though they were still anthropometrically obese (BMI > 30 kg/m^2). Within a week following intestinal bypass surgery, insulin sensitivity starts to increase, indicating that the operations are accomplishing more than just imposing calorie restriction on weight reduction, as stomach-restrictive treatments do [63, 64].

The most plausible idea probably has to do with the many hormones the stomach secretes in reaction to meals. The duodenum is surgically excluded in the Roux-en-Y technique, and the duodenum and jejunum are surgically excluded in biliopancreatic diversion, which results in changed locations of absorption of fat and carbohydrates, or at least altered relative distribution. According to the "hindgut hypothesis" proposed by Cummings et al., the reversal of hyperglycemia and obesity is explained by increased production of insulinotropic and appetite-controlling substances as a result of the accelerated transit of concentrated nutrients, especially glucose, to the distal intestine. Bypassing the duodenum would rectify this deficiency, according to the "foregut hypothesis" put out by Rubino et al., which contends that nutritional interactions in the duodenum are diabetogenic [65, 66].

According to recent research by Zhou X, et al., bariatric surgery is superior to non-surgical therapy for achieving diabetes remission and blood glucose control in type 2 diabetes patients with a BMI of less than 35 kg/m^2. After bariatric surgery, weight reduction is evident for individuals whose baseline BMI is greater than 30 kg/m^2. However, for those whose BMI is less than 30, weight loss is less evident, but effective glycemic control can still be attained. Although further research is needed to determine the precise mechanism, it could be pertinent to bariatric surgery that directly impacts glucose metabolism [67].

5. Bariatric surgery and thyroid functions

Obesity and hypothyroidism are two clinical disorders that are frequently correlated. Due to low thyroid hormone levels, hypothyroidism is an endocrine ailment that can cause weight gain. This condition is characterized by a decrease in energy expenditure, thermogenesis, and metabolic rate in the body. However as evidenced by the increased frequency of overt and subclinical hypothyroidism (SH) in obese people compared to normal-weight persons, obesity itself induces thyroid dysfunction. Thyroid-stimulating hormone (TSH) levels and obesity (body mass index [BMI] > 30 kg/m) have been linked in several studies, with serum TSH positively connected with weight increase [68, 69].

Globally, bariatric procedures have been increasingly popular during the last 20 years. It is noteworthy to note that clinical trials have demonstrated a 29.6% weight loss in 6 months after bariatric surgery [70]. Furthermore, it significantly contributes to the improvement and resolution of obesity-related comorbidities, including hypertension, dyslipidemia, obstructive sleep apnea, and type 2 diabetes. Still, not much research has been done on SH and much less on hypothyroidism. The results of these investigations on changes in thyroid hormone levels after bariatric surgery-induced weight reduction were inconsistent. Differences in the preoperative thyroid function status or the kind of operation might account for the variation in the results. For instance, some research assessed malabsorptive procedures (biliary pancreatic diversion), others employed restrictive surgeries (sleeve gastrectomy, adjustable gastric bands), and yet others examined both kinds of surgery [71, 72].

The rising prevalence of obesity and its associated endocrine comorbidities, such as thyroid dysfunction, have become worldwide health concerns. Thyroid hormones interact with body weight because they are crucial for controlling food intake and energy expenditure [73, 74]. Thyroid function has been linked to body weight, and obesity has been linked to an increased risk of overt or subclinical hypothyroidism. On the other hand, losing weight might help to protect the thyroid gland, lessen the body's inflammatory condition, and improve irregularities in blood sugar and cholesterol levels [75, 76].

The most popular bariatric surgery techniques are sleeve gastrectomy (SG) and Roux-en-Y gastric bypass (RYGB), which are successful and long-lasting weight loss strategies [77, 78]. Previous research has linked bariatric surgery to the treatment of thyroid dysfunction, including overt and subclinical hypothyroidism, and to a decrease in the requirement for thyroid hormone-lowering medications [79, 80]. These results might be explained by post-operative decreases in blood levels of ghrelin, adipokines, and leptin [81, 82].

Nonetheless, the effects of bariatric surgery on thyroid-stimulating hormone (TSH) differed greatly throughout studies. Most studies including individuals with overt or subclinical hypothyroidism revealed that TSH levels decreased dramatically after bariatric surgery [83, 84]. Numerous studies examining people with normal thyroid function have shown similar outcomes [85–87]. However, a 2-year follow-up research by MacCuish et al. with 55 euthyroid individuals following RYGB discovered that TSH levels had not changed [88]. In a retrospective analysis of 258 euthyroid individuals who had gastric banding, Dall'Asta et al. were unable to detect a statistically significant alteration in TSH after surgery [89].

It is yet unclear how bariatric surgery affects blood levels of free thyroxine (FT4) and free triiodothyronine (FT3). Previous investigations have revealed either high, unchanged or lowered FT3 and FT4 levels after a variety of surgical operations performed on patients from different nations [87, 90, 91]. After bariatric surgery, FT3 fell while FT4 stayed the same in euthyroid people, according to a 2017 meta-analysis. Thus, it is still debatable how weight loss after bariatric surgery affects thyroid function in euthyroid people who are obese [92].

Changes in thyroid hormone levels after bariatric surgery are inconsistent. In some investigations, it was shown that levels of free thyroxine (FT4) increased without influencing TSH levels; in other studies, the converse was seen. This uncertainty explains the rising interest in understanding how hormones are affected by weight loss after bariatric surgery [88, 93].

Optimizing levothyroxine medication dosages is critical since individuals who underwent LSG while on treatment had altered thyroid function tests after surgery. The Demirpolat et al. research showed a significant reduction in the weekly weight-adjusted dosage and total weekly dose of levothyroxine during the 6th postoperative month [94]. TSH levels were decreased, FT4 levels significantly increased, while FT3 levels stayed the same in the 6th month. According to the findings of the Demirpolat et al. study, LSG may lower the weight-adjusted dosage of levothyroxine in postoperative patients; as a result, patients should be closely watched for potential weight-loss-related levothyroxine dose readjustments. Increased follow-up frequency may be required in LSG patients with hypothyroidism because levothyroxine dosage modification may be required throughout the postoperative period.

The inadequate signal of iodothyronines within the target tissues is known as hypothyroidism. After ruling out uncommon illnesses, clinical practitioners can evaluate three primary causes of hypothyroidism: (1) thyroidectomy (complete or partial), (2) autoimmune thyroiditis (AIT), and (3) radioiodine therapy. No matter what causes hypothyroidism, long-term sodium levothyroxine (LT4) medication is often used to treat hypothyroid patients [95]. The most common and conventional LT4 formulation is the tablet. The LT4 pill is taken orally when fasting, half an hour before breakfast, and it dissolves and disintegrates in the stomach lumen. Significantly, the later stage is essential for achieving the active principle's best activation and full absorption in the small intestine [96, 97].

Unfortunately, there are a number of things that can obstruct the LT4 tablet route. First off, because to their widespread worldwide distribution, gastrointestinal illnesses (such as *Helicobacter pylori* gastritis, atrophic gastritis, celiac disease, and lactose malabsorption/intolerance) might have an impact on LT4 absorption and play a significant role in clinical practice [98, 99]. Second, LT4 bioavailability may be decreased by a number of medications (such as phosphate binders, aluminum-containing antacids, calcium carbonate, ferrous sulfate, sucralfate, raloxifene, bile acid sequestrants, and coffee), as well as by certain meals and drinks. Apart from the aforementioned variables, several studies have proposed that bariatric surgery might be an additional cause of decreased LT4 effectiveness in maintaining the ideal balance of hypothyroidism. Although there are alternative surgical techniques such as biliopancreatic diversion, gastric banding, and jejunoileal bypass, the most popular bariatric procedures are sleeve gastrectomy (SG) and Roux-en-Y gastric bypass (RYGB) [100, 101].

RYGB and SG are the most well-studied bariatric operations as possible variables influencing LT4 since they are the most dispersed. Bypassing the stomach, duodenum, and proximal jejunum, RYGB involves the creation of a tiny gastric pouch that is connected to the small intestine immediately distal to the gastroesophageal junction. A small gastric tube is formed along the smaller stomach curvature with SG.

Gadiraju et al. conducted a comprehensive analysis that comprised 10 trials that assessed how bariatric surgery affected LT4 needs. These trials included individuals who had undergone various surgical procedures and discovered that the LT4 dosage varied following SG, rose following JIB, and had variable results following other surgical alternatives (such as RYGB). A more recent systematic study and meta-analysis examined the connection between bariatric surgery and thyroid function [81, 102].

The Trimboli P, et al. research states that the current data permit the following conclusions to be drawn 1 year following bariatric surgery: (1) the daily LT4 dosage does not change, and (2) even with a large weight loss, the LT4 dose per weight rises. The majority of results pertain to LT4 tablets, and further research is necessary to determine how well LT4 caps work [103].

6. Bariatric surgery and secondary hyperparathyroidism

The number of people receiving obesity diagnoses and the number of bariatric surgeries performed are increasing at the same time. The most common of these surgeries are the sleeve gastrectomy (SG) and the Roux-en-Y gastric bypass (RYGB). In addition to helping people lose weight, better their chances of developing obesity-related disorders, and have numerous metabolic and cardiovascular advantages, both bariatric surgeries come with a number of dietary deficiencies. Over time, vitamin D insufficiency has drawn more attention [104]. A recognized cause of secondary hyperparathyroidism (hPTH) and consequent osteopenia is vitamin D insufficiency, as it plays a crucial role in maintaining calcium homeostasis. There is a fear that people who have bariatric surgery may then be susceptible to fragility fractures and secondary hPTH. Research has revealed that bariatric patients are more likely to break bones [105, 106].

Regarding the best supplements to take and the right amount of vitamin D to take following bariatric surgery, there is no consensus. Scandinavian guidelines now suggest lifetime treatment with 800 IU of cholecalciferol and 500 mg of calcium daily for individuals undergoing RYGB. According to guidelines from Scandinavia, bariatric patients should also have annual follow-ups, which should include blood test analysis for calcium, parathyroid hormone (PTH), and vitamin D levels, with an optimal 25-hydroxy vitamin D (25-OHD) level of 0.75 nmol/L [107].

By far the largest study comparing PTH and 25-OH-D levels before and 5 years after bariatric surgery has been conducted [108]. The findings show a relationship between PTH levels and time since surgery, type of bariatric procedure, and 25-OH-D levels. Two-thirds of patients had inadequate 25-OH-D levels (0,75 nmol/L) postoperatively, and a consistent increase in PTH was seen, in spite of supplement instructions. Regardless of the operation type, vitamin D levels rose throughout the first year following surgery, which is consistent with numerous previous research [109, 110]. It is unclear if the initial weight reduction or taking the vitamin pills consistently is to blame for this, but it is probably a mix of the two. However, during the second postoperative year, vitamin D levels started to fall, with a modest increase in PTH levels corresponding to a growing percentage of patients with 25-OH-D levels of 75 nmol/L. In comparison to SG, the RYGB operation results in more severe postoperative levels of PTH and 25-OH-D, despite similar trends. Following bariatric surgery, a new meta-analysis suggests taking 2000 IU of cholecalciferol daily as a supplement [111].

The operations are different because SG does not change the intestinal structure, while RYGB involves bypassing the proximal jejunum and duodenum. In light of the findings of this study and the fact that the proximal small intestine contains calcium channels that are reliant on vitamin D, it is probable that the architecture following an RYGB results in decreased calcium absorption and the inability to use vitamin D-dependent pathways. Significant reductions in fractional calcium absorption occur both with RYGB and even following SG [108, 112]. Reduced stomach acid levels, quicker gastric emptying, and enhanced intestinal motility have all been proposed as causes for decreased fractional calcium absorption in SG patients [113].

Regardless of postoperative blood 25OHD and calcium consumption, the de Holanda NCP et al. study reported a significant incidence of SHPT following bariatric surgery, particularly in individuals who received RYGB compared to SG. Similarly, after 5 years, we observed significant bone loss at the femur's total length and femoral neck in the RYGB group as opposed to the SG group. Multivariate linear regression analysis revealed that the length of time after surgery had no effect on the different bone metrics, despite the fact that the mean follow-up after surgery was longer in the RYGB. Compared to the SG group, RYGB patients had a higher risk of developing SHPT even with comparable blood 25OHD and calcium levels [114]. In comparison to the SG group, the RYGB group had greater blood phosphorus and PTH levels and lower levels of serum calcium and 25OHD, according to a recent meta-analysis of 13 observational studies. In addition, serum calcium by itself might not be a reliable indicator of calcium absorption. It would be more accurate to include fractionally labeled calcium assays or urine calcium readings instead [115].

Significant bone loss at the femoral neck was seen in the patients receiving bariatric surgery, as well as long-lasting elevations in bone remodeling indicators, according to the various investigations. When comparing patients undergoing RYGB to those receiving non-surgical control, these studies found a progressive decrease in bone marrow density (BMD) in both central and peripheral sites over a 2-year follow-up period. This was linked to a persistent increase in serum levels of P1NP and C-telopeptide (CTX) 6 months after surgery, even though weight loss stabilized and serum levels of calcium, PTH, and 25OHD were normal [114, 116–118].

Notably, de Holanda NCP et al. reported a substantial and progressive loss of bone at all sites based on the percentage of TWL, with a greater loss in patients who reached 20–40% compared to those who only reached 20% of TWL, and no difference in SG and RYGB, indicating that weight loss influences the amount of bone loss [114]. Aside from that, some data associate's various obesity phenotypes with distinct cardiovascular risk factors based on physical and behavioral characteristics. This might lead to distinct phenotypes concerning bone health after bariatric surgery [119].

7. Bariatric surgery and autoimmune diseases

For obese individuals, bariatric surgeries are a useful means of achieving weight loss and managing concomitant conditions including insulin resistance, hypertension, and dyslipidemia. Bariatric surgery has been linked to a number of consequences, the most prevalent of which are nutritional imbalances and illnesses that are directly related to the surgery (fistulas, infections, etc.) [120, 121]. Since adiponectin is an anti-inflammatory protein and leptin is a pro-inflammatory protein, obesity is thought to be a pro-inflammatory condition. Hormone levels in people having weight reduction surgery exhibit contradictory behavior. Although the effects of bariatric surgery on the development of autoimmune or autoinflammatory diseases are unknown, our understanding of the alterations in the immune system remains limited. The impact of weight reduction, particularly rapid and significant weight loss, on the immune system is still up for debate [122, 123].

Generally speaking, obesity is a long-term, low-grade inflammatory condition. Following bariatric surgery, the obesity-related proinflammatory state is altered. CCL2, resistin, adiponectin, leptin, and other cytokines and chemokines are among those that are aberrantly expressed in obese individuals. Adipocytes secrete adipocytokines, such as resistin and leptin, which trigger the release of TNF-x alpha, IL-6, and IL-12. This results in chemotaxis, which in turn triggers the activation of natural killer cells and macrophages [124, 125]. Additionally, resistin promotes cell migration to inflammatory areas by upregulating VCAM-1 and ICAM-1. Within the adaptive immune system, leptin promotes T cell lymphopoiesis, survival, and proliferation. However, adiponectin functions as an anti-inflammatory regulator in the innate immune system through the production of adhesion molecules, activation of the transcription factor nuclear factor κB, and a decrease in TNF-α, IL-6, and interferon-γ levels as well as phagocytosis [121, 125]. Additionally, it boosts the synthesis of regulatory cytokines including IL-10. Adiponectin inhibits T-cell responsiveness and B-cell lymphopoiesis in the adaptive immune system [122]. These results might all help to explain the positive effects of weight loss on insulin resistance, hyperlipidemia, and inflammatory components in obese individuals receiving this kind of surgery [126].

Adipocytokines alter during bariatric surgery in a number of ways, most notably an inversion of the blood levels of adiponectin and leptin. On the other hand, the rapid weight loss that some patients have experienced might compromise immunological homeostasis and ultimately lead to the onset of autoimmune disorders [127]. Furthermore, especially when weight loss is significant and occurs more quickly than anticipated, the immune system's reaction to weight reduction is not fully understood. There have been some documented reports of autoimmune disorders emerging following bariatric surgery. Following a jejunoileal bypass, Jewell et al. reported the onset of rheumatoid arthritis in two instances and systemic lupus erythematosus in two more [128]. Furthermore, it is widely acknowledged that bariatric surgery can result in postoperative arthropathy, and there have been documented instances of spondylarthritis developing following bariatric surgery [129]. These instances displayed varying periods, distinct joint involvement, and unequal distribution of incidence rates. Although a longer period has been reported, arthritis often appears during the first 2 years following the operation [130].

A persistent inflammation of the excluded bowel with bacterial overgrowth, cytokine generation, and immune complex deposition are some of the hypothesized processes. The disrupted gut homeostasis that results in the development of an autoimmune disease may be caused by additional processes, such as changes in the balance of T regulatory cells and the effects of IgA on the intestinal mucosa [131, 132].

In the study by Illan-Gomez et al., patients undergoing bariatric surgery showed improvements in their inflammatory patterns, as evidenced by decreased levels of C-reactive protein and IL-6 and high levels of adiponectin compared to baseline values up to a year after surgery [133]. According to South Korean research by Kyoung Kim et al., following bariatric surgery, blood levels of several significant adipokines, including BMP-4 (bone morphogenetic protein 4) and PAI-1 (plasminogen activator inhibitor-1) fell, indicating a change to an anti-inflammatory state. According to all of these data, bariatric surgery may be helpful for inflammatory conditions and may even prevent the onset of autoimmune disorders [134]. The results of Tobón GJ, et al., however, are inconsistent since they first demonstrate that certain people may experience autoimmune illnesses following weight loss, and then they also demonstrate that several immunological alterations take place. Following bariatric surgery, obese people experience immune alterations. While the onset or absence of autoimmune illnesses is unpredictable, it is essential to be aware of this risk [135].

8. Bariatric surgery and malnutrition

Regretfully, bariatric surgery has emerged as a global solution to the obesity pandemic. Following bariatric surgery, iron, vitamin B12, calcium, vitamin D, folate, copper, and zinc deficits are the most prevalent. The kind of bariatric surgery that is done has a significant impact on the malabsorption mechanism [136].

1. Purely restrictive treatments, including laparoscopic adjustable gastric banding (LAGB), might produce micronutrient deficits due to the early postoperative period's low nutrient intake and avoidance of nutrient-rich foods. This could also happen later on as a result of severe band constriction. For the majority of these people, foods including meat, fibrous fresh fruits, and vegetables are poorly tolerated. 2. Another strictly restricted treatment that includes removing the stomach's larger curvature is the vertical sleeve gastrectomy (VSG). Reduced acid production and mechanical digestion following stomach resection impede the absorption and digestion of iron, vitamin B12, and other protein-bound nutrients. Furthermore, there is a decrease in the production of intrinsic factors, which leads to an even greater impairment in the absorption of vitamin B12. The removal of the gastric fundus causes a neurohumoral shift that ultimately leads to poor nutrient intake and appetite suppression due to decreased production of Ghrelin, the hormone that stimulates hunger and is generated by the gastric fundus.

Malabsorption of macronutrients (up to 25% of protein and 72% of fat) combined with concurrent malabsorption of micronutrients is the main cause of weight loss resulting from malabsorptive treatments like BPDS. Reduced gastrointestinal transit time leading to secondary malabsorption of micronutrients is another potential cause. This may be due to avoiding the jejunum and duodenum or to restricted brush border contact as a result of a short common limb. In addition to the deficiencies in other micronutrients including iron, calcium, vitamin B12, and folate, there is a significant impairment in the absorption of fat-soluble vitamins like zinc, vitamins D, A, E, and K.

Following a Roux-en-Y gastric bypass (RYGB), dietary insufficiency or primary or secondary malabsorption may lead to nutrient deficits. Following the operation, malabsorption is increased when the roux limb is extended. How much of this is caused by the malabsorption of micronutrients as opposed to calories is unclear, though. In the sections that follow, the specific processes behind deficits in each micronutrient are covered in depth. The locations of micronutrient absorption and RYGB's impact on metabolism, nutritional deficiencies are greatly variable and are influenced by dietary as well as host-related (achlorhydria, malabsorption, systemic diseases such as type 2 DM and use of medications, e.g. PPI and metformin use causes vitamin B12 malabsorption) factors [137].

8.1 Protein status in post-bariatric surgery

Protein deficiency is the most serious macronutrient problem linked to bariatric surgery techniques. The majority of reports of it come from BPDS, where it affects 3–21% of patients, according to estimates [138, 139]. Depending on the length of the Roux-limb, an incidence of up to 13% has been reported after RYGB [138, 140]. Poor results are linked to complications resulting from protein deficiency, which causes 1% of hospitalizations annually following malabsorptive treatments [141, 142]. After bariatric surgery, many patients experience impaired protein digestion and absorption due to variables such as smaller stomachs, changed gut structure, and altered bilio-pancreatic function. These changes might cause an aversion to foods high in protein. Most patients are restricted to a liquid diet in the early postoperative period and are not allowed to eat a lot, which can sometimes be made worse by prolonged vomiting. Post-bariatric individuals are at a heightened risk of developing protein malnutrition due to these variables, which lead to inadequate protein intake and absorption.

8.2 Vitamin D status in post-bariatric surgery patients

Among candidates undergoing bariatric surgery, vitamin D deficiency can affect up to 100% of them. After malabsorptive bariatric surgeries, it has been demonstrated that by the end of 2 and 4 years, about 10–25% and 25–48% of patients, respectively, suffer calcium shortage, whereas 17–52% and 50–63% develop vitamin D deficiency during the same time period [143, 144]. Food and supplements combine with pancreatic enzymes and bile in bypass treatments only after the intestines unite in the downstream common channel. Because of this changed architecture, it is less possible for fat-soluble vitamins—like vitamin D—that depend on bile acids and other digestive enzymes to be absorbed [145].

Reduced intestinal mucosal contact time during VSG may potentially impair nutrition absorption. Even among postoperative patients with vitamin D levels ≥30 ng/mL, there is a notable occurrence of secondary hyperparathyroidism, indicating selective calcium malabsorption [146]. In low-intake situations, the duodenum may absorb up to 80–100% of the calcium in food through a transcellular active transport process reliant on vitamin D. In the absence of the duodenum and jejunum, the remaining section of the small intestine absorbs calcium less effectively, absorbing just 20% of the calcium that is consumed by food. The duodenum and jejunum are the preferred locations for calcium absorption, and procedures like RYGB and BPDS avoid them, increasing the risk of hypocalcemia. Over time, increased calcium resorption from the bone can lead to osteopenia, osteoporosis, and osteomalacia if calcium and vitamin D insufficiency and the ensuing secondary hyperparathyroidism are ignored [147].

Compared to other operations, RYGB is more likely to result in problems in bone mineralization. Prolonged surveillance and cautious supplementation are crucial in averting the aftermath of secondary hyperparathyroidism. It is deemed suitable to maintain 25-hydroxyvitamin D levels over 30 ng/mL. However, the efficacy of vitamin D supplementation is dubious since the paracellular absorption of calcium in the distal jejunum and ileum is less dependent on vitamin D.

8.3 Vitamin B1 status in post-bariatric surgery patients

There have been several reports of non-alcoholic individuals following bariatric surgery experiencing Wernicke's encephalopathy. Following both restrictive and malabsorptive operations, cases of beriberi have been reported. Peripheral neuropathy and Wernicke Korsakoff syndrome (WKS) have been recorded after vertical banded gastroplasty and documented cases of WKS have been associated with AGB, RYGB, and BPDS. The frequency of thiamine deficit among post-bariatric patients is found to vary from deficiency, depending on the surgery type and time period taken into consideration [148]. For this reason, it is advised that patients undergo screening for thiamine deficiency before any bariatric surgery and that they take thiamine supplements following the treatment [149, 150].

8.4 Vitamin B12 status in post-bariatric surgery patients

When patients having combination procedures, like RYGB, do not receive particular supplements, more than one-third of them experience postoperative vitamin B12 insufficiency [151]. The primary cause is linked to decreased intrinsic factor production as a result of the gastrectomy-induced loss of mucosa-containing parietal cells, which impairs the absorption of vitamin B12. Additional reasons include lower dietary intake of B12 owing to aversion to foods like milk and meat, and achlorhydria, which hinders the conversion of pepsinogen to pepsin, which is essential for the release of vitamin B12 from its protein-bound dietary form [152]. On the other hand, purely restrictive procedures like gastric banding do not result in a substantial folate or vitamin B12 deficit. In postoperative bariatric surgery patients, folate insufficiency is not commonly observed in recent research, despite the possibility. The majority of the time, multivitamin supplements are sufficient to cover the needs, and deficiencies are assumed to arise when dietary consumption is reduced and multivitamin pills are not taken as directed. Serum folate levels in RYGB patients have been shown to range from 6–65% low [153].

8.5 Iron status in post-bariatric surgery patients

After bariatric surgery, the incidence of iron deficiency is thought to be between 30 and 60%. Nonetheless, these studies' criteria of ID differ, depending on whether serum ferritin levels or transferrin saturations are employed. Due to hypochlorhydria and skipping important iron absorption sites including the duodenum and proximal jejunum, bariatric surgical operations decrease the absorption of dietary iron [154]. Due to general appetite decline and the emergence of food intolerances, including a drop in meat consumption, there is also a decrease in the amount of iron consumed orally. Research has indicated an almost 50% daily decline in meat intake, indicating a lowered capacity to tolerate red meats [155]. In addition, chronic gastrointestinal blood loss and *H. pylori* infection, which are more common in individuals who have undergone bariatric surgery, may possibly be contributing factors. The enhanced response to iron treatment is seen following *H. pylori* eradication provides more evidence for the function of *H. pylori* in the development of refractory iron deficiency. It has been demonstrated that 185 patients who get anemia after surgery had a twofold increased risk of hospitalization and length of stay [156, 157].

8.6 Zinc status in post-bariatric surgery patients

Compared to preoperative levels, several studies have shown a considerable decrease in blood zinc concentrations following bariatric surgeries. Compared to patients undergoing other operations like RYGB (15–21%) or LSG (11–14%), the prevalence of zinc insufficiency is much greater among BPDS patients (45–91%) [158]. The main cause of deficiency is poor intestinal absorption since zinc is mostly absorbed in the duodenum through the Divalent Metal Transporter-1 (DMT-1) and to a lesser degree in the proximal jejunum. Deficiency is likely to occur early following bariatric surgeries due to the absence of functional reserves [159]. Remember that iron, copper, and zinc may all affect one another's absorption. Long-term oral zinc supplementation can also cause shortages in copper and iron as well as a reduction in intestinal absorption of zinc [160, 161].

8.7 Copper status in post-bariatric surgery patients

The most prevalent cause of acquired copper deficit is malabsorption following bariatric surgery. An analysis of Roux-en-Y patients who underwent surgery and were followed up longitudinally for 24 months revealed that the incidence and prevalence of postoperative copper insufficiency were 18.8 and 9.6%, respectively. The duodenum is the primary organ for absorbing copper, which makes patients undergoing intestinal resection as a component of malabsorptive treatments susceptible [162, 163]. Additionally, stomach acid releases copper bonded to ligands and chemical complexes, which enhances the bioavailability of dietary copper. However, it could take a few years following surgery for symptoms to appear for the body to run out of copper. Extended total parenteral feeding without sufficient copper supplements might potentially result in copper insufficiency. For adult TPN patients, the estimated daily need for copper is 0.3 mg [164]. Since copper insufficiency is not common in the US population as a whole, copper levels are seldom checked by doctors and copper is occasionally left out of vitamin-mineral supplements. While the hematological problems recover with sufficient supplementation, the neurological symptoms can be severe and frequently permanent, hence raising awareness and facilitating early identification are crucial. Given that greater dosages of zinc supplementation are known to cause copper depletion, care should be exercised when prescribing zinc supplements. A surplus of zinc stimulates the synthesis of metallothionine, a heavy metal binding protein that binds to copper more strongly and facilitates its excretion via the gastrointestinal system [165].

DOI: http://dx.doi.org/10.5772/intechopen.1006090

Author details

Tarek Abdel-Hay Mostafa[1]*, Ahmed Mostafa Abdel-Hameed[2]
and Sameh Abdel-Khalek Ahmed[1]

1 Anaesthesiology, Critical Care and Pain Medicine Department, Faculty of Medicine-Tanta University, Egypt

2 Critical Care Department, Faculty of Medicine - Benha University, Egypt

*Address all correspondence to: dr.tarek311@yahoo.com

References

[1] Afshin A, Forouzanfar MH, Reitsma MB, Sur P, Estep K, Lee A, et al. Health effects of overweight and obesity in 195 countries over 25 years. The New England Journal of Medicine. 2017;**377**(1):13-27

[2] Lassale C, Tzoulaki I, Moons KGM, Sweeting M, Boer J, Johnson L, et al. Separate and combined associations of obesity and metabolic health with coronary heart disease: A pan-European case-cohort analysis. European Heart Journal. 2018;**39**(5):397-406

[3] Bays HE. Adiposopathy is "sick fat" a cardiovascular disease? Journal of the American College of Cardiology. 2011;**57**(25):2461-2473

[4] Packer M. The epicardial adipose inflammatory triad: Coronary atherosclerosis, atrial fibrillation, and heart failure with a preserved ejection fraction. European Journal of Heart Failure. 2018;**20**(11):1567-1569

[5] Ashrafian H, Toma T, Rowland SP, Harling L, Tan A, Efthimiou E, et al. Bariatric surgery or non-surgical weight loss for obstructive sleep apnoea? A systematic review and comparison of meta-analyses. Obesity Surgery. 2015;**25**(7):1239-1250

[6] Nguyen NT, Magno CP, Lane KT, Hinojosa MW, Lane JS. Association of hypertension, diabetes, dyslipidemia, and metabolic syndrome with obesity: Findings from the National Health and nutrition examination survey, 1999 to 2004. Journal of the American College of Surgeons. 2008;**207**(6):928-934

[7] Aune D, Sen A, Schlesinger S, Norat T, Janszky I, Romundstad P, et al. Body mass index, abdominal fatness, fat mass and the risk of atrial fibrillation: A systematic review and dose-response meta-analysis of prospective studies. European Journal of Epidemiology. 2017;**32**(3):181-192

[8] Rosengren A, Åberg M, Robertson J, Waern M, Schaufelberger M, Kuhn G, et al. Body weight in adolescence and long-term risk of early heart failure in adulthood among men in Sweden. European Heart Journal. 2017;**38**(24):1926-1933

[9] Larsson SC, Wolk A, Håkansson N, Bäck M. Overall and abdominal obesity and incident aortic valve stenosis: Two prospective cohort studies. European Heart Journal. 2017;**38**(28):2192-2197

[10] Twig G, Yaniv G, Levine H, Leiba A, Goldberger N, Derazne E, et al. Body-mass index in 2.3 million adolescents and cardiovascular death in adulthood. The New England Journal of Medicine. 2016;**374**(25):2430-2440

[11] van Veldhuisen SL, Gorter TM, van Woerden G, de Boer RA, Rienstra M, Hazebroek EJ, et al. Bariatric surgery and cardiovascular disease: A systematic review and meta-analysis. European Heart Journal. 2022;**43**(20):1955-1969

[12] Feng T, Vegard M, Strand LB, Laugsand LE, Mørkedal B, Aune D, et al. Weight and weight change and risk of atrial fibrillation: The HUNT study. European Heart Journal. 2019;**40**(34):2859-2866

[13] Lopez-Jimenez F, Wu CO, Tian X, O'Connor C, Rich MW, Burg MM, et al. Weight change after myocardial infarction—The enhancing recovery in coronary heart disease patients (ENRICHD) experience. American heart journal. 2008;**155**(3):478-484

[14] Schiavon CA, Drager LF, Bortolotto LA, Amodeo C, Ikeoka D, Berwanger O, et al. The role of metabolic surgery on blood pressure control. Current Atherosclerosis Reports. 2016;**18**(8):50

[15] Bueter M, Ahmed A, Ashrafian H, le Roux CW. Bariatric surgery and hypertension. Surgery for Obesity and Related Diseases. 2009;**5**(5):615-620

[16] le Roux CW, Welbourn R, Werling M, Osborne A, Kokkinos A, Laurenius A, et al. Gut hormones as mediators of appetite and weight loss after Roux-en-Y gastric bypass. Annals of Surgery. 2007;**246**(5):780-785

[17] Yamamoto H, Kishi T, Lee CE, Choi BJ, Fang H, Hollenberg AN, et al. Glucagon-like peptide-1-responsive catecholamine neurons in the area postrema link peripheral glucagon-like peptide-1 with central autonomic control sites. The Journal of Neuroscience. 2003;**23**(7):2939-2946

[18] Virdis A, Lerman LO, Regoli F, Ghiadoni L, Lerman A, Taddei S. Human ghrelin: A gastric hormone with cardiovascular properties. Current Pharmaceutical Design. 2016;**22**(1):52-58

[19] Woelnerhanssen B, Peterli R, Steinert RE, Peters T, Borbély Y, Beglinger C. Effects of postbariatric surgery weight loss on adipokines and metabolic parameters: Comparison of laparoscopic Roux-en-Y gastric bypass and laparoscopic sleeve gastrectomy–A prospective randomized trial. Surgery for Obesity and Related Diseases. 2011;**7**(5):561-568

[20] Kopp HP, Kopp CW, Festa A, Krzyzanowska K, Kriwanek S, Minar E, et al. Impact of weight loss on inflammatory proteins and their association with the insulin resistance syndrome in morbidly obese patients. Arteriosclerosis, Thrombosis, and Vascular Biology. 2003;**23**(6):1042-1047

[21] Gottlieb DJ, Punjabi NM, Mehra R, Patel SR, Quan SF, Babineau DC, et al. CPAP versus oxygen in obstructive sleep apnea. The New England Journal of Medicine. 2014;**370**(24):2276-2285

[22] Ramón JM, Salvans S, Crous X, Puig S, Goday A, Benaiges D, et al. Effect of Roux-en-Y gastric bypass vs sleeve gastrectomy on glucose and gut hormones: A prospective randomised trial. Journal of Gastrointestinal Surgery. 2012;**16**(6):1116-1122

[23] Alpert MA, Omran J, Bostick BP. Effects of obesity on cardiovascular Hemodynamics, cardiac morphology, and ventricular function. Current Obesity Reports. 2016;**5**(4):424-434

[24] Cuspidi C, Rescaldani M, Sala C, Grassi G. Left-ventricular hypertrophy and obesity: A systematic review and meta-analysis of echocardiographic studies. Journal of Hypertension. 2014;**32**(1):16-25

[25] Kotsis V, Jordan J, Micic D, Finer N, Leitner DR, Toplak H, et al. Obesity and cardiovascular risk: A call for action from the European Society of Hypertension Working Group of obesity, diabetes and the high-risk patient and European Association for the Study of obesity: Part A: Mechanisms of obesity induced hypertension, diabetes and dyslipidemia and practice guidelines for treatment. Journal of Hypertension. 2018;**36**(7):1427-1440

[26] Larsson SC, Bäck M, Rees JMB, Mason AM, Burgess S. Body mass index and body composition in relation to 14 cardiovascular conditions in UK biobank: A Mendelian randomization study. European Heart Journal. 2020;**41**(2):221-226

[27] Ndumele CE, Matsushita K, Lazo M, Bello N, Blumenthal RS, Gerstenblith G, et al. Obesity and subtypes of incident cardiovascular disease. Journal of the American Heart Association. 2016;**5**(8):e003921

[28] Oliveras A, Molina L, Goday A, Sans L, Riera M, Vazquez S, et al. Effect of bariatric surgery on cardiac structure and function in obese patients: Role of the renin-angiotensin system. Journal of Clinical Hypertension (Greenwich, Conn.). 2021;**23**(1):181-192

[29] Cuspidi C, Rescaldani M, Tadic M, Sala C, Grassi G. Effects of bariatric surgery on cardiac structure and function: A systematic review and meta-analysis. American Journal of Hypertension. 2014;**27**(2):146-156

[30] Owan T, Avelar E, Morley K, Jiji R, Hall N, Krezowski J, et al. Favorable changes in cardiac geometry and function following gastric bypass surgery: 2-year follow-up in the Utah obesity study. Journal of the American College of Cardiology. 2011;**57**(6):732-739

[31] Safar ME. Arterial stiffness as a risk factor for clinical hypertension. Nature Reviews. Cardiology. 2018;**15**(2):97-105

[32] Niiranen TJ, Kalesan B, Hamburg NM, Benjamin EJ, Mitchell GF, Vasan RS. Relative contributions of arterial stiffness and hypertension to cardiovascular disease: The Framingham heart study. Journal of the American Heart Association. 2016;**5**(11):e004271

[33] Samaras K, Viardot A, Lee PN, Jenkins A, Botelho NK, Bakopanos A, et al. Reduced arterial stiffness after weight loss in obese type 2 diabetes and impaired glucose tolerance: The role of immune cell activation and insulin resistance. Diabetes & Vascular Disease Research. 2013;**10**(1):40-48

[34] Petersen KS, Blanch N, Keogh JB, Clifton PM. Effect of weight loss on pulse wave velocity: Systematic review and meta-analysis. Arteriosclerosis, Thrombosis, and Vascular Biology. 2015;**35**(1):243-252

[35] Ikonomidis I, Mazarakis A, Papadopoulos C, Patsouras N, Kalfarentzos F, Lekakis J, et al. Weight loss after bariatric surgery improves aortic elastic properties and left ventricular function in individuals with morbid obesity: A 3-year follow-up study. Journal of Hypertension. 2007;**25**(2):439-447

[36] Favre G, Anty R, Canivet C, Clément G, Ben-Amor I, Tran A, et al. Determinants associated with the correction of glomerular hyper-filtration one year after bariatric surgery. Surgery for Obesity and Related Diseases. 2017;**13**(10):1760-1766

[37] Hall JE, do Carmo JM, da Silva AA, Wang Z, Hall ME. Obesity, kidney dysfunction and hypertension: Mechanistic links. Nature Reviews. Nephrology. 2019;**15**(6):367-385

[38] Climent E, Oliveras A, Pedro-Botet J, Goday A, Benaiges D. Bariatric surgery and hypertension. Journal of Clinical Medicine. 2021;**10**(18):4049

[39] Rosenstock JL, Pommier M, Stoffels G, Patel S, Michelis MF. Prevalence of proteinuria and albuminuria in an obese population and associated risk factors. Frontiers in Medicine (Lausanne). 2018;**5**:122

[40] Li K, Zou J, Ye Z, Di J, Han X, Zhang H, et al. Effects of Bariatric surgery on renal function in obese patients: A systematic review and meta analysis. PLoS One. 2016;**11**(10):e0163907

[41] Shulman A, Peltonen M, Sjöström CD, Andersson-Assarsson JC, Taube M, Sjöholm K, et al. Incidence of end-stage renal disease following bariatric surgery in the Swedish obese subjects study. International Journal of Obesity. 2018;**42**(5):964-973

[42] O'Brien R, Johnson E, Haneuse S, Coleman KJ, O'Connor PJ, Fisher DP, et al. Microvascular outcomes in patients with diabetes after Bariatric surgery versus usual care: A matched cohort study. Annals of Internal Medicine. 2018;**169**(5):300-310

[43] Friedman AN, Wahed AS, Wang J, Courcoulas AP, Dakin G, Hinojosa MW, et al. Effect of Bariatric surgery on CKD risk. Journal of the American Society of Nephrology : JASN. 2018;**29**(4):1289-1300

[44] Tham JC, le Roux CW, Docherty NG. Cardiovascular, renal and overall health outcomes after bariatric surgery. Current Cardiology Reports. 2015;**17**(5):34

[45] Lieske JC. Bariatric surgery and kidney health. Journal of the American Society of Nephrology : JASN. 2018;**29**(4):1085-1086

[46] Corbin KD, Driscoll KA, Pratley RE, Smith SR, Maahs DM, Mayer-Davis EJ, et al. Obesity in type 1 diabetes: Pathophysiology, clinical impact, and mechanisms. Endocrine Reviews. 2018;**39**(5):629-663

[47] Brethauer SA, Aminian A, Rosenthal RJ, Kirwan JP, Kashyap SR, Schauer PR. Bariatric surgery improves the metabolic profile of morbidly obese patients with type 1 diabetes. Diabetes Care. 2014;**37**(3):e51-ee2

[48] Maraka S, Kudva YC, Kellogg TA, Collazo-Clavell ML, Mundi MS. Bariatric surgery and diabetes: Implications of type 1 versus insulin-requiring type 2. Obesity. 2015;**23**(3):552-557

[49] Kirwan JP, Aminian A, Kashyap SR, Burguera B, Brethauer SA, Schauer PR. Bariatric surgery in obese patients with type 1 diabetes. Diabetes Care. 2016;**39**(6):941-948

[50] Robert M, Belanger P, Hould FS, Marceau S, Tchernof A, Biertho L. Should metabolic surgery be offered in morbidly obese patients with type I diabetes? Surgery for Obesity and Related Diseases. 2015;**11**(4):798-805

[51] Driscoll KA, Corbin KD, Maahs DM, Pratley R, Bishop FK, Kahkoska A, et al. Biopsychosocial aspects of weight management in type 1 diabetes: A review and next steps. Current Diabetes Reports. 2017;**17**:1-9

[52] Hanaire H, Bertrand M, Guerci B, Anduze Y, Guillaume E, Ritz P. High glycemic variability assessed by continuous glucose monitoring after surgical treatment of obesity by gastric bypass. Diabetes Technology & Therapeutics. 2011;**13**(6):625-630

[53] Vilarrasa N, Rubio MA, Miñambres I, Flores L, Caixàs A, Ciudin A, et al. Long-term outcomes in patients with morbid obesity and type 1 diabetes undergoing Bariatric surgery. Obesity Surgery. 2017;**27**(4):856-863

[54] Liakopoulos V, Franzén S, Svensson AM, Miftaraj M, Ottosson J, Näslund I, et al. Pros and cons of gastric bypass surgery in individuals with obesity and type 2 diabetes: Nationwide, matched, observational cohort study. BMJ Open. 2019;**9**(1):e023882

[55] Höskuldsdóttir G, Ekelund J, Miftaraj M, Wallenius V, Ottosson J, Näslund I, et al. Potential benefits and harms of gastric bypass surgery in

obese individuals with type 1 diabetes: A nationwide, matched, observational cohort study. Diabetes Care. 2020;**43**(12):3079-3085

[56] Landau Z, Kowen-Sandbank G, Jakubowicz D, Raziel A, Sakran N, Zaslavsky-Paltiel I, et al. Bariatric surgery in patients with type 1 diabetes: Special considerations are warranted. Therapeutic Advances in Endocrinology and Metabolism. 2019;**10**:2042018818822207

[57] Vilarrasa N, San Jose P, Rubio MÁ, Lecube A. Obesity in patients with type 1 diabetes: Links, risks and management challenges. Diabetes, Metabolic Syndrome and Obesity. 2021;**14**:2807-2827

[58] Buchwald H, Estok R, Fahrbach K, Banel D, Jensen MD, Pories WJ, et al. Weight and type 2 diabetes after bariatric surgery: Systematic review and meta-analysis. The American Journal of Medicine. 2009;**122**(3):248-256 e5

[59] Buchwald H, Avidor Y, Braunwald E, Bariatric surgery. A systematic review and meta-analysis. ACC Current Journal Review. 2005;**1**(14):13

[60] Dixon JB, O'Brien PE, Playfair J, Chapman L, Schachter LM, Skinner S, et al. Adjustable gastric banding and conventional therapy for type 2 diabetes: A randomized controlled trial. Journal of the American Medical Association. 2008;**299**(3):316-323

[61] Kashyap SR, Gatmaitan P, Brethauer S, Schauer P. Bariatric surgery for type 2 diabetes: Weighing the impact for obese patients. Cleveland Clinic Journal of Medicine. 2010;**77**(7):468

[62] Kashyap SR, Daud S, Kelly KR, Gastaldelli A, Win H, Brethauer S, et al. Acute effects of gastric bypass versus gastric restrictive surgery on beta-cell function and insulinotropic hormones in severely obese patients with type 2 diabetes. International Journal of Obesity. 2010;**34**(3):462-471

[63] Bikman BT, Zheng D, Pories WJ, Chapman W, Pender JR, Bowden RC, et al. Mechanism for improved insulin sensitivity after gastric bypass surgery. The Journal of Clinical Endocrinology & Metabolism. 2008;**93**(12):4656-4663

[64] Guidone C, Manco M, Valera-Mora E, Iaconelli A, Gniuli D, Mari A, et al. Mechanisms of recovery from type 2 diabetes after malabsorptive bariatric surgery. Diabetes. 2006;**55**(7):2025-2031

[65] Cummings DE, Overduin J, Foster-Schubert KE. Gastric bypass for obesity: Mechanisms of weight loss and diabetes resolution. The Journal of Clinical Endocrinology & Metabolism. 2004;**89**(6):2608-2615

[66] Rubino F, Forgione A, Cummings DE, Vix M, Gnuli D, Mingrone G, et al. The mechanism of diabetes control after gastrointestinal bypass surgery reveals a role of the proximal small intestine in the pathophysiology of type 2 diabetes. Annals of Surgery. 2006;**244**(5):741-749

[67] Zhou X, Zeng C. Diabetes remission of bariatric surgery and nonsurgical treatments in type 2 diabetes patients who failure to meet the criteria for surgery: A systematic review and meta-analysis. BMC Endocrine Disorders. 2023;**23**(1):46

[68] Sanyal D, Raychaudhuri M. Hypothyroidism and obesity: An intriguing link. Indian Journal of Endocrinology and Metabolism. 2016;**20**(4):554-557

[69] Iacobellis G, Ribaudo MC, Zappaterreno A, Iannucci CV, Leonetti F.

Relationship of thyroid function with body mass index, leptin, insulin sensitivity and adiponectin in euthyroid obese women. Clinical Endocrinology. 2005;**62**(4):487-491

[70] Burguera B, Jesús Tur J, Escudero AJ, Alos M, Pagán A, Cortés B, et al. An intensive lifestyle intervention is an effective treatment of morbid obesity: The TRAMOMTANA study-a two-year randomized controlled clinical trial. International Journal of Endocrinology. 2015;**2015**:194696

[71] Al Khalifa K, Al Ansari A, Alsayed AR, Violato C. The impact of sleeve gastrectomy on hyperlipidemia: A systematic review. Journal of Obesity. 2013;**2013**:643530

[72] Schauer PR, Bhatt DL, Kirwan JP, Wolski K, Aminian A, Brethauer SA, et al. Bariatric surgery versus intensive medical therapy for diabetes - 5-year outcomes. The New England Journal of Medicine. 2017;**376**(7):641-651

[73] Laclaustra M, Moreno-Franco B, Lou-Bonafonte JM, Mateo-Gallego R, Casasnovas JA, Guallar-Castillon P, et al. Impaired sensitivity to thyroid hormones is associated with diabetes and metabolic syndrome. Diabetes Care. 2019;**42**(2):303-310

[74] Biondi B, Kahaly GJ, Robertson RP. Thyroid dysfunction and diabetes mellitus: Two closely associated disorders. Endocrine Reviews. 2019;**40**(3):789-824

[75] Babić, Leko M, Gunjača I, Pleić N, Zemunik T. Environmental factors affecting thyroid-stimulating hormone and thyroid hormone levels. International Journal of Molecular Sciences. 2021;**22**(12):6521

[76] Gajda SN, Kuryłowicz A, Żach M, Bednarczuk T, Wyleżoł M. Diagnosis and treatment of thyroid disorders in obese patients - what do we know? Endokrynologia Polska. 2019;**70**(3):271-276

[77] Wiggins T, Guidozzi N, Welbourn R, Ahmed AR, Markar SR. Association of bariatric surgery with all-cause mortality and incidence of obesity-related disease at a population level: A systematic review and meta-analysis. PLoS Medicine. 2020;**17**(7):e1003206

[78] Eisenberg D, Shikora SA, Aarts E, Aminian A, Angrisani L, Cohen RV, et al. 2022 American Society for Metabolic and Bariatric Surgery (ASMBS) and International Federation for the Surgery of obesity and metabolic disorders (IFSO): Indications for metabolic and Bariatric surgery. Surgery for Obesity and Related Diseases. 2022;**18**(12):1345-1356

[79] Abdelbaki TN, Elkeleny MR, Sharaan MA, Talha A, Bondok M. Impact of laparoscopic sleeve gastrectomy on obese patients with subclinical hypothyroidism. Journal of Laparoendoscopic & Advanced Surgical Techniques. Part A. 2020;**30**(3):236-240

[80] Richou M, Gilly O, Taillard V, Paul De Brauwere D, Donici I, Guedj AM. Levothyroxine dose adjustment in hypothyroid patients following gastric sleeve surgery. Annales d'endocrinologie. 2020;**81**(5):500-506

[81] Azran C, Hanhan-Shamshoum N, Irshied T, Ben-Shushan T, Dicker D, Dahan A, et al. Hypothyroidism and levothyroxine therapy following bariatric surgery: A systematic review, meta-analysis, network meta-analysis, and meta-regression. Surgery for Obesity and Related Diseases. 2021;**17**(6):1206-1217

[82] Aykota MR, Atabey M. Effect of sleeve gastrectomy on thyroid-stimulating hormone levels in morbidly

obese patients with normal thyroid function. European Review for Medical and Pharmacological Sciences. 2021;**25**(1):233-240

[83] Salman MA, Rabiee A, Salman A, Qassem MG, Ameen MA, Hassan AM, et al. Laparoscopic sleeve gastrectomy has a positive impact on subclinical hypothyroidism among obese patients: A prospective study. World Journal of Surgery. 2021;**45**(10):3130-3137

[84] Zendel A, Abu-Ghanem Y, Dux J, Mor E, Zippel D, Goitein D. The impact of Bariatric surgery on thyroid function and medication use in patients with hypothyroidism. Obesity Surgery. 2017;**27**(8):2000-2004

[85] Liu F, Di J, Yu H, Han J, Bao Y, Jia W. Effect of Roux-en-Y gastric bypass on thyroid function in euthyroid patients with obesity and type 2 diabetes. Surgery for Obesity and Related Diseases. 2017;**13**(10):1701-1707

[86] Yang J, Gao Z, Yang W, Zhou X, Lee S, Wang C. Effect of sleeve gastrectomy on thyroid function in Chinese Euthyroid obese patients. Surgical Laparoscopy, Endoscopy & Percutaneous Techniques. 2017;**27**(4):e66-ee8

[87] Gokosmanoglu F, Aksoy E, Onmez A, Ergenç H, Topkaya S. Thyroid homeostasis after Bariatric surgery in obese cases. Obesity Surgery. 2020;**30**(1):274-278

[88] MacCuish A, Razvi S, Syed AA. Effect of weight loss after gastric bypass surgery on thyroid function in euthyroid people with morbid obesity. Clinical Obesity. 2012;**2**(1-2):25-28

[89] Dall'Asta C, Paganelli M, Morabito A, Vedani P, Barbieri M, Paolisso G, et al. Weight loss through gastric banding: Effects on TSH and thyroid hormones in obese subjects with normal thyroid function. Obesity (Silver Spring). 2010;**18**(4):854-857

[90] Yu H, Li Q, Zhang M, Liu F, Pan J, Tu Y, et al. Decreased leptin is associated with alterations in thyroid-stimulating hormone levels after Roux-en-Y gastric bypass surgery in obese Euthyroid patients with type 2 diabetes. Obesity Facts. 2019;**12**(3):272-280

[91] Chen Y, Zhang W, Pan Y, Chen W, Wang C, Yang W. Thyroid function before and after laparoscopic sleeve gastrectomy in patients with obesity. Obesity Surgery. 2022;**32**(6):1954-1961

[92] Guan B, Chen Y, Yang J, Yang W, Wang C. Effect of Bariatric surgery on thyroid function in obese patients: A systematic review and meta-analysis. Obesity Surgery. 2017;**27**(12):3292-3305

[93] Chikunguwo S, Brethauer S, Nirujogi V, Pitt T, Udomsawaengsup S, Chand B, et al. Influence of obesity and surgical weight loss on thyroid hormone levels. Surgery for Obesity and Related Diseases. 2007;**3**(6):631-635. discussion 5-6

[94] Demirpolat MT, Sisik A. Effect of laparoscopic sleeve gastrectomy on thyroid function tests and levothyroxine doses in people with obesity. Cureus. 2024;**16**(3):e56219

[95] Jonklaas J, Bianco AC, Bauer AJ, Burman KD, Cappola AR, Celi FS, et al. Guidelines for the treatment of hypothyroidism: Prepared by the american thyroid association task force on thyroid hormone replacement. Thyroid. 2014;**24**(12):1670-1751

[96] Kitamori N, Iga K. Dissolution profiles of drugs from tablets. Journal of Pharmaceutical Sciences. 1978;**67**(10):1436-1439

[97] Hays MT. Localization of human thyroxine absorption. Thyroid. 1991;**1**(3):241-248

[98] Virili C, Antonelli A, Santaguida MG, Benvenga S, Centanni M. Gastrointestinal malabsorption of thyroxine. Endocrine Reviews. 2019;**40**(1):118-136

[99] Castellana M, Castellana C, Giovanella L, Trimboli P. Prevalence of gastrointestinal disorders having an impact on tablet levothyroxine absorption: Should this formulation still be considered as the first-line therapy? Endocrine. 2020;**67**(2):281-290

[100] Welbourn R, Hollyman M, Kinsman R, Dixon J, Liem R, Ottosson J, et al. Bariatric surgery worldwide: Baseline demographic description and one-year outcomes from the fourth IFSO global registry report 2018. Obesity Surgery. 2019;**29**(3):782-795

[101] Bray GA, Heisel WE, Afshin A, Jensen MD, Dietz WH, Long M, et al. The science of obesity management: An Endocrine Society scientific statement. Endocrine Reviews. 2018;**39**(2):79-132

[102] Gadiraju S, Lee CJ, Cooper DS. Levothyroxine dosing following Bariatric surgery. Obesity Surgery. 2016;**26**(10):2538-2542

[103] Trimboli P, Ossola N, Torre A, Mongelli F, Quarenghi M, Camponovo C, et al. The performance of levothyroxine tablet is impaired by bariatric surgery. Endocrine. 2023;**80**(3):563-569

[104] Sundbom M, Hedberg J, Marsk R, Boman L, Bylund A, Hedenbro J, et al. Substantial decrease in comorbidity 5 years after gastric bypass: A population-based study from the Scandinavian obesity surgery registry. Annals of Surgery. 2017;**265**(6):1166-1171

[105] Saad RK, Ghezzawi M, Habli D, Alami RS, Chakhtoura M. Fracture risk following bariatric surgery: A systematic review and meta-analysis. Osteoporosis International. 2022;**33**(3):511-526

[106] Blom-Høgestøl IK, Hewitt S, Chahal-Kummen M, Brunborg C, Gulseth HL, Kristinsson JA, et al. Bone metabolism, bone mineral density and low-energy fractures 10 years after Roux-en-Y gastric bypass. Bone. 2019;**127**:436-445

[107] Laurenius A, Näslund I, Sandvik J, Videhult P, Wirén M. Läkartidningen. Monitorering och supplementering med vitaminer och mineraler. Lakartidningen. 9 Jan 2018;**115**:ETD7

[108] Stevens K, Hultin H, Sundbom M. Hypovitaminosis D and hyperparathyroidism: A 5-year postoperative follow-up of 30,458 gastric bypass and sleeve gastrectomy patients. Surgery for Obesity and Related Diseases. 2024:S1550-7289(24)00076-5

[109] Dos Santos EM, de Lima DS, Padilha BM, Cabral PC, do Nascimento LC, Feitosa PH, et al. Vitamin D in the preoperative and postoperative periods of bariatric surgery. Obesity Surgery. 2021;**31**:2723-2728

[110] Musella M, Berardi G, Vitiello A, Dayan D, Schiavone V, Franzese A, et al. Vitamin D deficiency in patients with morbid obesity before and after metabolic Bariatric surgery. Nutrients. 2022;**14**(16):3319

[111] Giustina A, di Filippo L, Facciorusso A, Adler RA, Binkley N, Bollerslev J, et al. Vitamin D status and supplementation before and after Bariatric surgery: Recommendations based on a systematic review and meta-analysis. Reviews in

Endocrine & Metabolic Disorders. 2023;**24**(6):1011-1029

[112] Schafer AL, Weaver CM, Black DM, Wheeler AL, Chang H, Szefc GV, et al. Intestinal calcium absorption decreases dramatically after gastric bypass surgery despite optimization of vitamin D status. Journal of Bone and Mineral Research. 2015;**30**(8):1377-1385

[113] Wu KC, Cao S, Weaver CM, King NJ, Patel S, Kim TY, et al. Intestinal calcium absorption decreases after laparoscopic sleeve gastrectomy despite optimization of vitamin D status. The Journal of Clinical Endocrinology and Metabolism. 2023;**108**(2):351-360

[114] de Holanda NCP, Baad VMA, Bezerra LR, de Lima SKM, Filho JM, de Holanda Limeira CC, et al. Secondary hyperparathyroidism, bone density, and bone turnover after Bariatric surgery: Differences between Roux-en-Y gastric bypass and sleeve gastrectomy. Obesity Surgery. 2021;**31**(12):5367-5375

[115] Tian Z, Fan XT, Li SZ, Zhai T, Dong J. Changes in bone metabolism after sleeve gastrectomy versus gastric bypass: A meta-analysis. Obesity Surgery. 2020;**30**(1):77-86

[116] Yu EW, Bouxsein ML, Putman MS, Monis EL, Roy AE, Pratt JS, et al. Two-year changes in bone density after Roux-en-Y gastric bypass surgery. The Journal of Clinical Endocrinology and Metabolism. 2015;**100**(4):1452-1459

[117] Grethen E, Hill KM, Jones R, Cacucci BM, Gupta CE, Acton A, et al. Serum leptin, parathyroid hormone, 1,25-dihydroxyvitamin D, fibroblast growth factor 23, bone alkaline phosphatase, and sclerostin relationships in obesity. The Journal of Clinical Endocrinology and Metabolism. 2012;**97**(5):1655-1662

[118] Maghrabi AH, Wolski K, Abood B, Licata A, Pothier C, Bhatt DL, et al. Two-year outcomes on bone density and fracture incidence in patients with T2DM randomized to bariatric surgery versus intensive medical therapy. Obesity (Silver Spring). 2015;**23**(12):2344-2348

[119] Vecchié A, Dallegri F, Carbone F, Bonaventura A, Liberale L, Portincasa P, et al. Obesity phenotypes and their paradoxical association with cardiovascular diseases. European Journal of Internal Medicine. 2018;**48**:6-17

[120] Long SD, O'Brien K, MacDonald KG Jr, Leggett-Frazier N, Swanson MS, Pories WJ, et al. Weight loss in severely obese subjects prevents the progression of impaired glucose tolerance to type II diabetes. A longitudinal interventional study. Diabetes Care. 1994;**17**(5):372-375

[121] Pories WJ. Bariatric surgery: Risks and rewards. The Journal of Clinical Endocrinology and Metabolism. 2008;**93**(11 Suppl. 1):S89-S96

[122] Tilg H, Moschen AR. Adipocytokines: Mediators linking adipose tissue, inflammation and immunity. Nature Reviews. Immunology. 2006;**6**(10):772-783

[123] Manco M, Fernandez-Real JM, Equitani F, Vendrell J, Valera Mora ME, Nanni G, et al. Effect of massive weight loss on inflammatory adipocytokines and the innate immune system in morbidly obese women. The Journal of Clinical Endocrinology and Metabolism. 2007;**92**(2):483-490

[124] Maachi M, Piéroni L, Bruckert E, Jardel C, Fellahi S, Hainque B, et al. Systemic low-grade inflammation is related to both circulating and adipose tissue TNFalpha, leptin and IL-6 levels in obese women. International Journal of

Obesity and Related Metabolic Disorders. 2004;**28**(8):993-997

[125] Munoz M, Mazure R, Culebras J. Obesity and the immune system. Nutricion Hospitalaria. 2004;**19**(6):319-324

[126] Santos J, Salgado P, Santos C, Mendes P, Saavedra J, Baldaque P, et al. Effect of bariatric surgery on weight loss, inflammation, iron metabolism, and lipid profile. Scandinavian Journal of Surgery. 2014;**103**(1):21-25

[127] Moschen AR, Molnar C, Wolf AM, Weiss H, Graziadei I, Kaser S, et al. Effects of weight loss induced by bariatric surgery on hepatic adipocytokine expression. Journal of Hepatology. 2009;**51**(4):765-777

[128] Jewell WR, Hermreck AS, Hardin CA. Complications of jejunoileal bypass for morbid obesity. Archives of Surgery. 1975;**110**(8):1039-1042

[129] Ribeiro DS, Fernandes JL, Rangel L, de Araújo NC, D'Almeida F, Moura CG, et al. Spondyloarthritis after bariatric surgery: Is there a link? Clinical Rheumatology. 2010;**29**(4):435-437

[130] Clegg DO, Zone JJ, Samuelson CO Jr, Ward JR. Circulating immune complexes containing secretory IgA in jejunoileal bypass disease. Annals of the Rheumatic Diseases. 1985;**44**(4):239-244

[131] Leff RD, Towles W, Aldo-Benson MA, Madura J, Biegel AA. A prospective analysis of the arthritis syndrome and immune function in jejunoileal bypass patients. The Journal of Rheumatology. 1983;**10**(4):612-618

[132] Heyn J, Hey H, Jans H, Baek L, Ullman S, Halberg P. Episodic arthritis, skin manifestations and immune complexes following intestinal by-pass operations for morbid obesity. Scandinavian Journal of Rheumatology. 1983;**12**(3):257-259

[133] Illán-Gómez F, Gonzálvez-Ortega M, Orea-Soler I, Alcaraz-Tafalla MS, Aragón-Alonso A, Pascual-Díaz M, et al. Obesity and inflammation: Change in adiponectin, C-reactive protein, tumour necrosis factor-alpha and interleukin-6 after bariatric surgery. Obesity Surgery. 2012;**22**(6):950-955

[134] Kim MK, Jang EH, Hong OK, Chun HJ, Yoo SJ, Baek KH, et al. Changes in serum levels of bone morphogenic protein 4 and inflammatory cytokines after bariatric surgery in severely obese korean patients with type 2 diabetes. International Journal of Endocrinology. 2013;**2013**:681205

[135] Tobón GJ, Ospina FE, Suso JP, Posso-Osorio I, Echeverri AF, Muñoz-Buitrón E, et al. Autoantibodies production and immunological abnormalities after bariatric surgery. Journal of Translational Autoimmunity. 2019;**2**:100024

[136] Mohapatra S, Gangadharan K, Pitchumoni CS. Malnutrition in obesity before and after bariatric surgery. Disease-a-Month. 2020;**66**(2):100866

[137] Lange J, Königsrainer A. Malnutrition as a complication of Bariatric surgery - a clear and present danger? Visceral Medicine. 2019;**35**(5):305-311

[138] Faintuch J, Matsuda M, Cruz ME, Silva MM, Teivelis MP, Garrido AB Jr, et al. Severe protein-calorie malnutrition after bariatric procedures. Obesity Surgery. 2004;**14**(2):175-181

[139] Heber D, Greenway FL, Kaplan LM, Livingston E, Salvador J, Still C.

Endocrine and nutritional management of the post-bariatric surgery patient: An Endocrine Society clinical practice guideline. The Journal of Clinical Endocrinology and Metabolism. 2010;**95**(11):4823-4843

[140] Brolin RE. Bariatric surgery and long-term control of morbid obesity. Journal of the American Medical Association. 2002;**288**(22):2793-2796

[141] Skroubis G, Sakellaropoulos G, Pouggouras K, Mead N, Nikiforidis G, Kalfarentzos F. Comparison of nutritional deficiencies after Roux-en-Y gastric bypass and after biliopancreatic diversion with Roux-en-Y gastric bypass. Obesity Surgery. 2002;**12**(4):551-558

[142] Stocker DJ. Management of the bariatric surgery patient. Endocrinology and Metabolism Clinics. 2003;**32**(2):437-457

[143] Hamoui N, Kim K, Anthone G, Crookes PF. The significance of elevated levels of parathyroid hormone in patients with morbid obesity before and after bariatric surgery. Archives of Surgery. 2003;**138**(8):891-897

[144] Newbury L, Dolan K, Hatzifotis M, Low N, Fielding G. Calcium and vitamin D depletion and elevated parathyroid hormone following biliopancreatic diversion. Obesity Surgery. 2003;**13**(6):893-895

[145] Van der Schueren B, Green N, Gorroochurn P, Teixeira J, Altiner S, Laferrère B. Low vitamin D in candidates for bariatric surgery: Are the Americans better off than the French? Obesity Surgery. 2011;**21**(7):948-949. author reply 50

[146] Johnson JM, Maher JW, DeMaria EJ, Downs RW, Wolfe LG, Kellum JM. The long-term effects of gastric bypass on vitamin D metabolism. Annals of Surgery. 2006;**243**(5):701-704. discussion 4-5

[147] De Prisco C, Levine SN. Metabolic bone disease after gastric bypass surgery for obesity. The American Journal of the Medical Sciences. 2005;**329**(2):57-61

[148] Seehra H, MacDermott N, Lascelles RG, Taylor TV. Wernicke's encephalopathy after vertical banded gastroplasty for morbid obesity. BMJ. 1996;**312**(7028):434

[149] Kazemi A, Frazier T, Cave M. Micronutrient-related neurologic complications following bariatric surgery. Current Gastroenterology Reports. 2010;**12**(4):288-295

[150] Koch TR, Finelli FC. Postoperative metabolic and nutritional complications of bariatric surgery. Gastroenterology Clinics of North America. 2010;**39**(1):109-124

[151] Vargas-Ruiz AG, Hernández-Rivera G, Herrera MF. Prevalence of iron, folate, and vitamin B12 deficiency anemia after laparoscopic Roux-en-Y gastric bypass. Obesity Surgery. 2008;**18**(3):288-293

[152] Ponsky TA, Brody F, Pucci E. Alterations in gastrointestinal physiology after Roux-en-Y gastric bypass. Journal of the American College of Surgeons. 2005;**201**(1):125-131

[153] Boylan LM, Sugerman HJ, Driskell JA. Vitamin E, vitamin B-6, vitamin B-12, and folate status of gastric bypass surgery patients. Journal of the American Dietetic Association. 1988;**88**(5):579-585

[154] Muñoz M, Botella-Romero F, Gómez-Ramírez S, Campos A, García-Erce JA. Iron deficiency

and anaemia in bariatric surgical patients: Causes, diagnosis and proper management. Nutrición Hospitalaria. 2009;**24**(6):640-654

[155] Ruz M, Carrasco F, Rojas P, Codoceo J, Inostroza J, Rebolledo A, et al. Iron absorption and iron status are reduced after Roux-en-Y gastric bypass. The American Journal of Clinical Nutrition. 2009;**90**(3):527-532

[156] Knight T, D'Sylva L, Moore B, Barish CF. Burden of iron deficiency Anemia in a Bariatric surgery population in the United States. Journal of Managed Care & Specialty Pharmacy. 2015;**21**(10):946-954

[157] Sabate JM, Coupaye M, Ledoux S, Castel B, Msika S, Coffin B, et al. Consequences of small intestinal bacterial overgrowth in obese patients before and after Bariatric surgery. Obesity Surgery. 2017;**27**(3):599-605

[158] Sallé A, Demarsy D, Poirier AL, Lelièvre B, Topart P, Guilloteau G, et al. Zinc deficiency: A frequent and underestimated complication after bariatric surgery. Obesity Surgery. 2010;**20**(12):1660-1670

[159] Saif T, Strain GW, Dakin G, Gagner M, Costa R, Pomp A. Evaluation of nutrient status after laparoscopic sleeve gastrectomy 1, 3, and 5 years after surgery. Surgery for Obesity and Related Diseases. 2012;**8**(5):542-547

[160] Troost FJ, Brummer RJ, Dainty JR, Hoogewerff JA, Bull VJ, Saris WH. Iron supplements inhibit zinc but not copper absorption in vivo in ileostomy subjects. The American Journal of Clinical Nutrition. 2003;**78**(5):1018-1023

[161] Olivares M, Pizarro F, Ruz M, de Romaña DL. Acute inhibition of iron bioavailability by zinc: Studies in humans. Biometals. 2012;**25**(4):657-664

[162] Kiela PR, Ghishan FK. Physiology of intestinal absorption and secretion. Best Practice & Research. Clinical Gastroenterology. 2016;**30**(2):145-159

[163] Gletsu-Miller N, Broderius M, Frediani JK, Zhao VM, Griffith DP, Davis SS Jr, et al. Incidence and prevalence of copper deficiency following roux-en-y gastric bypass surgery. International Journal of Obesity. 2012;**36**(3):328-335

[164] Shike M. Copper in parenteral nutrition. Gastroenterology. 2009;**137**(Suppl. 5):S13-S17

[165] Rowin J, Lewis SL. Copper deficiency myeloneuropathy and pancytopenia secondary to overuse of zinc supplementation. Journal of Neurology, Neurosurgery, and Psychiatry. 2005;**76**(5):750-751

Chapter 2

Perioperative Management: Successes and Challenges of a Multidisciplinary Team Approach in Bariatric Surgery

Alanoud Alobaidly and Abdullah Hasan

Abstract

A multidisciplinary team approach for the management of people with type 2 diabetes undergoing bariatric surgery was highly recommended by the International Diabetes Federation (IDF). The advantages of a multidisciplinary team when successfully operating would provide healthcare professionals with a clear management plan and defined roles for each of the team members. This understanding would contribute to providing patients with their treatment plan and enable them to actively manage their glucose levels, which would in return delay complications of obesity and type 2 diabetes. However, several perceived disadvantages of having a multidisciplinary team approach were mentioned by healthcare professionals, which could hinder the workflow and burden patients seeking treatment for their obesity. Having the right mindset of teamwork and respecting the different roles of the disciplines in a multidisciplinary team approach would yield effective management for patients with obesity.

Keywords: bariatric surgery, multidisciplinary team, obesity, success, challenges, type 2 diabetes, patient management

1. Introduction

As a nurse, I come across numerous patients who struggle with managing their glycaemic levels. Most of them were diagnosed with type 2 diabetes and were often being shuffled between departments due to unclear roles and lack of diabetes specialists. Later, a diabetes team was initiated where I became a diabetes educator. Here, I understood the difficulties patients were going through to have their diabetes managed, whether it was because of the lack of knowledge about diabetes, the incorrect technique of monitoring their blood glucose levels, or the overwhelming information they received from different specialities that were often in conflict.

For example, a physician would prescribe oral hypoglycaemic medication that would be replaced by the pharmacist due to its unavailability and then replaced again when the initial medication was available, which confused the patients on the type of medication they were taking. Another example was the nutritional guide that dietitians would provide the patient that included a piece of cake or a glass of juice, which made no sense to a person with diabetes because what they know is that sugar is not allowed in their diet.

This got me questioning why it was so difficult for these disciplines to communicate, why were patients confused about their diet, and why did patients have to be the ones searching for the correct information. In this chapter, I will be discussing the goals of having a multidisciplinary team approach, the benefits from having this approach, the challenges when implementing this approach, and its effectiveness when implemented on people with type 2 diabetes who are obese and eligible for bariatric surgery.

By studying this population, people with type 2 diabetes eligible for bariatric surgery, I was able to further understand their need of how the current service delivery is being managed, what might be the challenges faced by this population, and whether any improvements could be implemented for the betterment of type 2 diabetes and bariatric management. Interviews with healthcare professionals from different disciplines who are involved in the management of patients with type 2 diabetes and obesity were carried out. Patients with type 2 diabetes and obesity eligible for bariatric surgery also participated in the study following their consent [1]. In addition, I have observed these healthcare professionals and patients during their consultations to grasp a clear and detailed picture of the patient's management plan and treatment pathway.

2. Multidisciplinary team management

Multidisciplinary team management or interprofessional practice is described as a collaborative practice between healthcare professionals who work with people within their disciplines, with people from different disciplines, with patients and their families, and with communities to deliver health care. A multidisciplinary team in health care is defined as a group of healthcare professionals from different disciplines that collaborate, cooperate, and communicate together to determine a patient's treatment plan. Bear in mind that, for a multidisciplinary team to be effective, healthcare professionals' roles, targeted outcomes, and method of service delivery need to be defined clearly. The goal of a multidisciplinary team is to address the problems of access to health care and create a positive impact on the health outcomes of the patients and eventually the community.

The importance of a multidisciplinary team for the management of patients with type 2 diabetes and obesity was strongly endorsed by the International Federation of the Surgery of Obesity (IFSO) in their statement "only those who have worked or are working in a comprehensive team, which has demonstrated the ability to manage and provide the necessary resources to look after the morbidly obese patient, should be considered fully trained". This recognition has implications for bariatric surgeons in training, who are expected to develop skills in the coordination of multidisciplinary care for their patients.

Bariatric surgeries were found to be effective as treatment options for morbid obesity. With an increasing number of bariatric operations being performed, there has been an associated increase in demand for comprehensive and specialised medical and surgical services for these patients. People with morbid obesity may suffer from chronic and progressive disease associated with a variety of comorbid conditions.

Managing this complex multisystem disease requires coordinated input from a range of healthcare professionals. This specialisation of care has led to the evolution of the multidisciplinary team approach in bariatric surgery.

2.1 The importance of multidisciplinary team management and care

In the multidisciplinary diabetic care, an obesity expert evaluates the patient, even if he does not undergo surgery aiming at controlling weight gain from diabetic treatment. Different from the routine clinical consultations when a patient receives orientation about food and physical exercises, the obesity expert evaluates the behaviour of the patient in the face of food, and he can detect emotional dependence on food requesting psychiatric help if necessary. After surgery, an energy intake that is insufficient to maintain a normal body weight after weight loss achieves better control in other comorbidities, including diabetes. All patients who are candidates for metabolic surgery are obliged to pass through psychological tests to identify those who have therapeutic adherence or eating disorder. After surgery, psychiatric help for food disorder is essential in refractory cases. The association of a motivational psychology expert for continuous exercise with a group of non-surgical patients and with a group to begin and maintain physical activity in the postoperative phase contributes significantly. All the psychometric data obtained from the questionnaire handed out to the patients in the pre- and postoperative periods have the aim and are used as instruments to measure the success or not of the assistance given to the obese diabetic patients in the multiprofessional-surgical team. The final objective is to guarantee quality of life, return to social normalisation, and adherence to the multidisciplinary resources available.

Until recently, the treatment of diabetes was the responsibility of endocrinologists, as they are the experts in respect to endocrine metabolism. Several factors prompted the introduction of experts in obesity amongst the multidisciplinary approach of diabetes: association of diabetes paving the way to the development of obesity in the future generation; the direct effect of obesity on metabolic dysregulation; the incomplete diabetes control if associated with obesity; the fact that metabolic/gastric surgery is the treatment of choice in some stages of diabetes as it can cure it while reducing mortality and comorbidities.

3. Benefits of multidisciplinary teams

Where multidisciplinary care has been implemented, there is evidence to suggest improved patient outcomes. Though there are relatively few published studies on the impact of multidisciplinary care on the management of patients with severe and complicated obesity, there is evidence to suggest that a multidisciplinary approach is beneficial. A systematic review on the role of allied health professionals in weight management found consistent evidence in support of multidisciplinary treatment for obese patients, including improved weight loss, increased physical activity, and enhanced quality of life [2]. This was particularly the case in studies involving dietitians and physiotherapists. The greatest improvements were seen in studies with the strongest presence of non-physician health professionals.

There is a single discipline that coordinates the interactions between the healthcare professionals in multidisciplinary teams for the care and management of the patient. A nurse-led multidisciplinary team approach has been studied for its effectiveness and acceptance in numerous countries across the globe, such as the UK [3], the USA [4], China [5], and Iran [6]. This suggests that it is not simply the involvement of multiple specialists but a true multidisciplinary approach that is of most benefit to patients.

3.1 Improved patient outcomes

There is evidence to suggest that multidisciplinary teams are effective at improving the health of both individuals and the population as a whole, particularly in the context of chronic disease management. A multidisciplinary team that has a physician, endocrinologist, anaesthetist, intensivist, nutritionist, physiotherapist, psychologist, and bariatric coordinator is necessary to provide efficient care to people undergoing bariatric surgery. Nurse-led multidisciplinary teams have shown equality successful outcomes for patients with type 2 diabetes and obesity.

A recent study has shown that diabetes multidisciplinary teams are effective at improving glycaemic control and cardiovascular risk factors. This same study also highlighted the variability in multidisciplinary team's effectiveness, raising questions about what factors are necessary for a successful multidisciplinary team [7]. It is logical to assume that improved coordination and information sharing between healthcare professionals would cause an improvement in health outcomes, yet this has seldom been quantified. Another study analysed the roles of nurses in diabetes care and found that when nurses were given the chance to lead the management of diabetes care, the outcomes of their patients were improved, and adequate quality health care was achieved [8]. These studies give some indication that coordinated care by multidisciplinary teams can have a positive impact on health outcomes and that it is vital that these interventions are well defined and adhere to the key principles of effective multidisciplinary team working.

Healthcare professionals in a multidisciplinary team usually respond to the extent or degree in which their professional interest has been represented in client-care decision-making and often creates a type of quality indicator. The more actively the members of the nursing staff participate in decision-making, the greater the satisfaction with their influence, whereas dissatisfaction with influence on decision-making is one of the most important reasons physicians give for wanting to leave their present employment. The improvement in bariatric patient satisfaction represents a cornerstone of quality improvement efforts; patient satisfaction greatly influences the physician-patient relationship, the relationship amongst healthcare providers, and acts as an indirect measure of health outcomes. Findings relating to improved patient satisfaction have even revealed reduced long-term healthcare costs. Recommend that for settings such as bariatric care, which include long-term lifestyle changes and constant coping with complex comorbidities, patient satisfaction and the impact of care on quality of life should be utilised as a method for evaluation. There were suggestions that current healthcare providers in bariatric care should improve their knowledge on the impact of bariatric surgery on patient quality of life and design interventions that enhance the long-term effects. They have recommended the use of visual and verbal analogue scales and other qualitative methodology. Patient satisfaction can be measured indirectly by the health outcome. Recognise the importance of specialist teams measuring health outcome as a quality indicator for effective interventions with higher risk patients; however, failure to address patient satisfaction will often lead to disengagement from care.

3.2 Holistic approach to care

This approach has been supported by qualitative studies of bariatric patients. For example, by interviewing patients with diabetes who are eligible for bariatric surgery, Alobaidly found that patients needed to have a primary care provider who cared about them, to know more about what caused their weight problem and type 2 diabetes, and what could be done to solve these problems [1]. An approach that focuses on thorough assessment and education would have been the most ideal for these patients.

The holistic approach to care using a multidisciplinary team is of utmost importance in the management of bariatric patients. This is because these patients can have a range of complex issues which contributed to their obesity, and they often suffer from a range of comorbidities. These patients require thorough assessment and treatment of their medical, psychological, and social issues if they are to succeed in their long-term weight management. This is something which cannot be achieved in the standard 15-minute consultation with a medical doctor or by seeing a specialist who is not aware of the range of issues the patient has.

It is recommended that healthcare professionals share their tasks and responsibilities with other disciplines when providing type 2 diabetes care and management for patients eligible for bariatric surgery. Sharing management plans could also assist these healthcare professionals when planning their patients' management and referrals to other departments.

A holistic approach to patient care is the contemporary ideal and is accepted to result in the best treatment for patients. In recent years, the care of patients has moved towards evidence-based practice, considering the evidence in the treatment of patients. Because of this, a multidisciplinary team is the ideal as it allows the pooling of knowledge from the various specialties into one treatment plan. This is very beneficial to patients as it means they are receiving the best evidence-based treatment.

4. Challenges faced by multidisciplinary teams

Challenges usually come before benefits when it comes to asking multiple disciplines to work together. These barriers could be because of the disciplines' different perspectives, the different approaches they used, and the line of hierarchy that these disciplines have labelled themselves amongst one another. Status differences amongst health professionals, different professional dialects, conflicting work schedules, and geographic dispersion of team members were also other barriers mentioned when research was done on multidisciplinary approaches.

4.1 Power dynamics and role conflicts

The most agreed upon barrier amongst healthcare professionals is status difference. What I mean by this is when team members from different professions have different levels of power and status. Status differences lead to an increase in task and person conflicts as well as increased work strain. High-status professionals tend to use lower levels of communication with lower-status professionals and sometimes ignore them altogether. This can result in a decrease in decision-making quality and an increase in levels of role ambiguity for the lower-status professional. Finally, status differences have been shown to increase the levels of within-profession team member communication, which leads to professional subgrouping in teams and a loss of overall team cohesiveness.

Due to concerns over the safety and effectiveness of bariatric surgery, the American Society for Metabolic and Bariatric Surgery (ASMBS) and other international bodies have suggested that it would be best for surgery to be a 'last resort' and for patients with obesity to be managed in primary care and medical specialist settings. With this in mind, it is apparent that there is a preference towards a more conservative treatment approach for bariatric patients. This would be the case when healthcare teams treating bariatric patients could face power struggles, with bariatric medicine and generalist practitioners favouring non-surgical treatment options, while surgeons will be pushing towards surgical management. The aforementioned power struggles and role conflicts can create a lack of clear direction in team objectives and patient treatment pathways. This, in turn, can impede the coordination of care and potentially lead to marginalised patient groups who become caught between conflicting professional opinions.

Commonly found in healthcare organisations are professional groups with different values, beliefs, and norms. These differing professional identities result in varying conceptualisations of illness, which in turn can lead to conflicts concerning the aims of treatment. In the specific context of bariatric surgery, a study involving a diverse range of health professionals revealed that different professions held different perspectives on the causes of obesity and what the most appropriate treatment would be [9]. This led to the conclusion that to facilitate an integrated bariatric health service, it is necessary to resolve differences in role perceptions and treatment approaches. As certain specialties are more powerful than others in the healthcare hierarchy, it is likely that those in higher-status positions will use their influence to redirect decisions in a manner that is consistent with their own professional role. An interview-based study involving a range of healthcare providers identified concerns that physicians were generally given higher importance than other professionals on the bariatric healthcare team [1]. This had resulted in patients being encouraged towards surgical treatment, even in cases where it might not be the most appropriate option.

4.2 Resistance to change

Professional resistance is a natural response to change. It is a process where medical professionals oppose, overtly or covertly, the implementation of a new treatment. The resistance may range from aggressive undermining of the change to a passive lack of support. The reasons for resistance are complex and often interrelated. It is rarely due to a single factor. Fear of the unknown, threat to professional identity, poor timing of the change, and lack of conviction are some of the areas that resistance can manifest. It represents a political response to change where the medical professional is protecting the *status quo* or their professional position. Healthcare professionals by and large have had little formal management education or training, yet they are expected to be leaders of new programmes and champions of change. This expectation is often a source of inner conflict and personal resistance to change. Healthcare professionals often feel out of their depth in the leadership of change and can revert to professional autonomy as a defence mechanism. The challenge for change agents is to recognise and mobilise their strategies to overcome this resistance. Failure to do so can result in the change being abandoned or implemented in a compromised manner. This then impacts upon team effectiveness and ultimately patient care.

4.3 Communication and coordination

Communication in multidisciplinary teams has long been recognised as a critical issue. It involves the sharing of information using mutually understood signs and symbols. Effective communication is one of the most fundamental behaviours in teams and is an integral part of the majority of theories on team behaviour. Good communication has been linked to numerous positive team outcomes including member and leader satisfaction, decision quality, reduced team member role ambiguity, task and member cohesiveness, and lower levels of team conflict and work strain.

Ineffective communication between healthcare professionals has been highlighted as a potential barrier to coordinated care. This often results in fragmented care delivery, with each healthcare professional managing one aspect of the patient's health. Communication is a process by which information is clearly and accurately exchanged between team members, by means of a structured system (e.g. meetings, notes, and referral forms), resulting in shared understanding amongst team members, leading to more effective and safe patient care. Coordination, on the other hand, is the process of aligning actions of team members to ensure the achievement of a common goal. It involves task assignment and the allocation of resources between team members. High-quality coordination occurs when there is a shared mental model of what needs to be done, who is to do it, and when it is to be completed. An important outcome of effective coordination is the adaptation of team member behaviours in response to changes in the patient's needs or changes in the external team environment. High levels of communication and coordination have been linked to favourable patient outcomes in a variety of healthcare settings. Specifically, in the context of bariatric patients, better communication has been linked to improved psychosocial and physical functioning outcomes for the patient. And higher quality coordination has been shown to improve patient access to obesity services. High-quality communication and coordination are critical for multidisciplinary teams to maximise the effectiveness of their treatment for the complex and varied needs of bariatric patients.

5. Effective multidisciplinary teamwork

An effective team is formed by knowing the criteria of each team member, which are often based on their previous performances in team environments and their skills in interprofessional interaction. This is consistent with the team development stages model proposed by Tuckman [10], where essence of the progress of a team is the requirement of ability to work towards a common goal and an associated set of performance goals. This implies education of the team and shared mental models, specifically in the form of agreeing on what types of patients are suited for bariatric surgery and having subsequent criteria for acceptable outcomes.

Sources of poor team performance are neither hard to find nor difficult to comprehend. Ineffective team working, such as insufficient communication, coordination, cooperation, roles undefined, lack of cohesiveness, unclear leadership, lack of clear objectives, and poor decision-making, have been associated with performance deficits from simple tasks to more complex individual and collective responsibilities. To enhance the potential success of working in teams, strategies to improve poor team behaviours have been developed and include team leadership, membership selection, training, team building, and process consultation.

5.1 Clear communication channels

Communication and coordination are at the heart of any bariatric programme. For multidisciplinary teams, they are particularly crucial. Weight management is the quintessential example of a multifactorial health issue. Bariatric patients present with a diverse range of needs emanating from the physical, psychological, and social effects of obesity. Their care frequently spans acute and primary care services and health providers, and many bariatric patients will require ongoing treatment for a range of obesity comorbidities, such as type 2 diabetes, chronic heart diseases, and sleep apnoea. Effective team communication is posited as a critical determinant of patient outcomes across a variety of healthcare settings.

There were various communication issues identified on each day of observation involving all three teams. These issues ranged from a lack of dinner break for the ward nursing staff, poor communication between the surgical team and the physiotherapists regarding patient suitability for therapy programmes through to cancelling of the observed medical doctor's round during the final week as there were no patients suitable to discuss. This is indicative of a lack of good information exchange which is vital to make informed decisions and plans. A structured approach to information exchange is critical and can come in many forms, the key is that there is a pre-defined and understood method and purpose. The surgical team and the medical team would be better served with a formal discussion regarding patient therapy goals and the medical team needs to be able to access and understand surgical caseloads and outcomes when deciding on patient suitability.

Communication is a vital element in health care and without clear channels, the quality and safety of patient care may be compromised. Effective communication has been shown to be a foundation stone of patient safety, reducing the risk of adverse events and decreasing the length of hospital stay. It has been reported in complex and high-risk industries that effective communication can be the difference between life and death.

5.2 Defined roles and responsibilities

In order to define roles, there must be an ongoing dialogue between the team members where their role is constantly evaluated in comparison to what the intervention requires. Surgeons involved in a national survey-based research study assessed their roles and responsibilities within bariatric care [11]. They had noted that although they were enthusiastic to provide the interventions, they were not all adequately trained. This indicated a varied role between different surgeons and therefore they were not meeting as a team to define their roles on a constant basis. This blurred professionals' roles between each other, and the experts' opinion was that the patient was not getting the best possible treatment. This highlights that role definition requires communication and continuous evaluation in order to succeed in team treatment. This process should always be referred back to patient care, and it must be questioned whether a role meets the specific requirements of a certain intervention.

Several studies found that registered nurses who are actively involved in type 2 diabetes management by delivering patient education and undertaking leadership roles were efficient in optimising and improving delivery of service [12–14]. The roles and responsibilities of the team members must be clearly defined. This must be established during a team meeting so that all members are aware of what their role is and what is expected of them. Keynotes from these meetings can specify that professional boundaries must be kept and not be overstepped, senior members are not to dominate, and all members must have equal participation. The surgeons, anaesthetists, dietitians, psychologists, and specialist nurses play key roles in the assessment and management of the bariatric patient [15]. They are the individuals who deliver the interventions and therefore it is essential they are aware of what is expected of them. This will be varied depending on the discipline-specialist training and therefore must be clearly outlined.

The bariatric doctor, like the bariatric surgeon, is only one part of the specific treatment for obesity. They have a significant and important role in treating obesity and its comorbidities. As emphasised by the American Society for Metabolic and Bariatric Surgery (ASMBS) Bariatric Surgery Guidelines and Recommendations, the long-term success of bariatric surgery depends on the patient's physical, emotional, and behavioural abilities. These abilities include following dietary, supplement, drug, and behaviour-related restrictions, as well as maintaining or adjusting energy intake and physical activity. Other health professionals, such as registered nurses, physiotherapists, health educators, and social workers, are also needed to assist the patient and their family in supporting the success of bariatric surgery.

The surgical approach to severe and complex obesity should adhere to safety, benefits, and quality standards. These standards are part of a multidisciplinary approach that involves various professionals. In this book, readers will find a comprehensive exposition of the work done by these professionals, who are dedicated to achieving excellence in every step of the integrated treatment of the disease and its comorbidities. The professionals involved include anaesthesiologists, bariatric dietitians, endocrinologists, bariatric professionals, family physicians, personal trainers, image-diagnostic specialists, infectious disease specialists, nutritionists, podiatrists, pulmonary health professionals, psychologists, psychiatrists, and weight loss surgeons. Each of these professionals plays an important role within the team.

5.3 Regular team meetings and collaboration

Patients with physical and mental health problems need appropriate referral to multidiscipline specialists, including psychologists/psychiatrists, internists, neurologists, physiatrists, urologists, and caregivers. Family physicians are of great value as constant care coordinators, especially during the early post-discharge setting if well informed by immediate at-discharge comprehensive summary of the former patient's postsurgical limitations, needs, and expected adaptive behaviour profiles. Psychologists working for the Veterans Affairs Healthcare System in the United States identified the use of case reviews as a method to help integrate with healthcare providers and understand patient needs. This resulted in psychologists feeling more involved with patient care and becoming inclined to take on greater responsibilities with medical treatments. In addition, isolated programmes running group therapy for bariatric patients have demonstrated the benefits of regular collaboration with other health professionals to enhance patient management. Despite these examples, setting a time and date that allows all team members to attend regular meetings can be difficult and may require flexibility to accommodate different disciplines.

A coordinated approach to preoperative preparation and postoperative management of bariatric patients involving dietitians, psychologists, and exercise specialists is of paramount importance. Increased collaboration between health professionals will lead to a more effective management of patients and improved outcomes. This is supported by the Dietitians Association of Australia, whose guidelines for the management of bariatric patients state that dietitians should engage in regular communication and participate in multidisciplinary team meetings to discuss the nutritional management of patients. Regular collaboration between dietitians and other health professionals has been shown to identify and resolve behavioural and environmental factors that impact food choices, weight, and health. This can be achieved via numerous methods, including preoperative training in behaviour, monitoring and increasing physical activity, balance reducing proactive intake behaviour, help initiate and monitor postsurgical adaptive food behaviour, and observe changing nutrient intake adequacy. There are often a bariatric surgery nurse coordinator and a surgical room or office nurse who double as office weight loss counsellor or right-sized garb providers as well. Inpatient and immediate post-discharge nursing staff will often have or develop programmes to augment the supplied discharge follow-up information to recognise and treat hypo and dehydration, hyperemesis and dumping symptoms, and any residual nausea and early satiation symptoms. Despite medication or nutrient alleviated hunger not occurring post-surgery until achieving advanced weight loss, some obese patients might experience return or persistent self-medication of transient non-hunger flavours of oral intake or inappropriately snacking on ingested modified glucose beverage.

In addition to regular patient management, effective multidisciplinary teams need to meet regularly to discuss ongoing management problems, treatment plans, and programme evaluation. Busy schedules and differences in professional timings have been identified as common barriers to scheduling meetings. Despite evidence showing team meetings to be clinically cost-effective, the experience of the authors in setting up regular team meetings for bariatric patients has identified several challenges that require consideration.

When comprehensive care plans can be initiated, the best collaborative practice involves team members identifying both their overlapping and differential roles. The providers must develop close personal connections, learn to communicate efficiently using short-structured discussions, and share patient care records within the evolving Health Information Technology ecosystems. Patient care is labour intensive and frequent interruptions are the norm. The surgeon and the bariatric office team or the diabetologist and the clinic team engaged in providing care of diabetes/obesity must learn to establish boundaries about their key responsibilities, yet keep intersecting roles efficient enough to promote patient-centred beneficial communications. This core team is experienced-based with relationships made stronger by frequent direct communications and shared supportive roles.

6. Preoperative management of the obese patient

The motivation of a potential bariatric surgery patient and the patient's understanding and knowledge of the pre- and postoperative process and physical restrictions are critical to the patient's success. This member of the obesity surgery team should be the healthcare professional at the weight loss centre. The primary care physician refers the severely obese patient to the weight loss centre and should be a knowledgeable addition to this obesity surgery management team to help in the patient's journey. The candidate for surgery will usually have ongoing health issues of which the primary care physician is aware of and can manage and may have psychosocial issues such as the stress of a separation. The referral is the first step in the patient's total management.

Patients seeking bariatric surgery to induce weight loss do so to resolve health and/or social issues. The consumption of food plays a major role in all of these aspects of human nature. Severely obese patients who cannot control their weight by lifestyle modalities such as diet and are experiencing failing health are unable to functionally fulfil their roles in society or are experiencing depression will claim they have little choice but to seek bariatric surgery. The management of severely obese patients is often said to be difficult by physicians who may feel less empathy for these patients. Nevertheless, these patients must be given the same thorough evaluation as any other patient, perhaps with the addition of more tests and procedures as they do have unique medical, anatomical, functional, and psychological issues.

6.1 Medical assessment and screening

A careful examination is essential and should retain indications for the presence of acanthosis nigricans, hirsutism, joint enlargement, periodontitis, and skin changes. Besides the assessment of weight, waist-hip ratio, intertriginous areas, and ankle or knee oedema, an essential goal is the accurate and reliable estimation of body fat, muscle mass, weight, and robustness. Further exploration goes together with the gathering of objective evidence, such as orthopnoea or snoring (for sleep apnoea-hypopnoea) and the investigation of the lowest oxygen desaturation during sleep by pulse oximetry and the presence of any oedema norms for the Oswestry Disability Index (ODI) > 5, and a body mass index (BMI) chart categorising the severity of OSAHS (obstructive syndrome of obstructive sleep apnoea-hypopnoea). Based on the above data, it is very important to prepare the patient not only for bariatric surgery but also to predict his medical condition as much as possible by examining those criteria similar to chances for sexual satisfaction.

Preoperatively all patients should be in optimal medical condition before major surgery. A thorough history of related obesity- and diabetes-associated problems must be obtained. This involves inclusive drug history, the medical exploration of symptoms or signs for anxiety, statistical analysis of obesity, pain, dyspnoea, oedema, any indicator that reflects, for instance, cardiac failure or sleep apnoea-hypopnoea, and either respiratory or liver disorder. Patients with diabetes should be optimally controlled before bariatric surgery with HbA1c (glycosylated haemoglobin) < 6.5%, as higher HbA1c is associated with higher morbidity in non-diabetic obese patients. History of chronic pain, osteoporosis, and the history of previous bone fractures may indicate osteoporosis.

6.2 Nutritional counselling and support

Most patients undergoing surgical treatment are advised to lose weight prior to surgery in order to reduce the surgical risk. These patients are typically encouraged to follow a diet that is low in sugar, fat, complex carbohydrates, and gluten, while ensuring adequate protein intake. They are also encouraged to engage in mild physical activity. Therefore, an overly restrictive diet does not appear to be the most appropriate approach. However, once again, there is no consensus on this matter. Currently, in addition to nutritional guidelines, we have the option to offer patients an additional tool for weight management through endoscopic treatment several months before bariatric surgery in an outpatient setting. This option is available to patients who have not been able to lose weight through other means or who have experienced significant weight loss prior to surgery in a safe manner. The use of this treatment is more controlled, particularly for those who have undergone biliopancreatic diversion.

Morbidly obese patients suffer from micronutrient deficiencies, including a lack of intake of vitamins and minerals, as well as malabsorption syndromes due to concomitant medication use. Deficiencies in vitamin D, magnesium, zinc, and iron are highly prevalent in morbidly obese patients undergoing surgery, regardless of the technique used. These patients also typically have reduced levels of vitamins B12 and folate, as well as other micronutrients. There is no consensus on the recommended intake of vitamins and minerals for preoperative patients in order to address these deficiencies. In our institution, we often rely on the current recommendations for the general population. Additionally, there is no consensus on the type of multivitamin to prescribe, the dosage, or the form (liquid, chewable, or bolus). It is important that the formula be highly available and that the capsules be small, as a liquid or chewable formulation is preferred to reduce the risk of capsule-related stricture.

7. Postoperative care and follow-up

Postoperative care requires weight maintenance if remnant stomach and medications are not given per orally immediately after the intervention. In some procedures, peculiar food forms, such as filling, are recommended. Follow-up examinations should be done from the first day after the operation, not only in case of anaesthesia difficulties or unusual courses but according to national guidelines. In the Czech Republic, the first postoperative follow-up examination takes place 15 days following the intervention to remove staples; anti-thrombotic cover and proton pump inhibition are finished, normal stomach function is usually resumed, and patients start taking established diabetes medications there in the morning. Its introduction starts on the first day to be taken orally (except suture line leakage or other intra-abdominal infection risk) as trans-anastomotic glucose transport is re-established soon after the operation. Other novel diabetes medications should not be prescribed to be taken by mouth (per oral) before the consultation with the surgeon performed two weeks postoperatively. For other indications, the administration of these drugs needs to be postponed in some operations, for example, 10 weeks after a bypass because of the hazard of anastomosis dehiscence caused by profound hypoglycaemia following intranasal glucose intake. Blood glucose levels should be monitored for some time even in normoglycaemic individuals. Indication can be given by diabetic ketoacidosis at the time of the diabetes diagnosis on the field of established bacterial infection with severe hyperglycaemia in a patient with no medical history. Products containing glucose should be used for treatment.

Immediate postoperative care after digestive surgery presents several unique features. Not only is traditional surgical treatment of diabetes implemented in the form of surgery in obese individuals, but glucose metabolism is also modified by different mechanisms on the first day after the operation. Novel diabetes medications largely influence postoperative diabetes therapy. Undiagnosed diabetes may complicate postoperative care of other affected patients. Digestive surgery itself poses anaesthesia challenges. The timing and nature of carbohydrate repletion following bariatric procedures can be novel to anaesthesiologists. Incentive spirometry can be effective for reducing episodes of oxygen desaturation. Conversion from parenteral to oral nutrition can require longer hospital stays in morbidly obese patients. The use of altered anatomy-following procedures and residual obesity will result in frequent advice seeking by future anaesthesiologists. Therefore, interdisciplinary approaches should include movement close to the operating room, dietary, psychiatry, in addition to endocrinology and other internal medicine specialists, as usual.

7.1 Monitoring for complications

In the long term, as the comorbidities are resolved, direct patients to the complete blood analysis to semiannual, for the nutritional assessment of potential micronutrient deficits and the hepatic and renal analysis, in which the nephropathy marker should be included.

7.2 Lifestyle modification support

The proposed method of treating the obese and overweight patients with stage-preoperative preparation for the operation achieves complete preparation of metabolic function at a significantly lower level of excess weight. This method is also effective in achieving stable weight loss in the early postoperative and follow-up periods, especially in patients with a less pronounced feeling of postprandial restriction and reduced appetite, which is due to increased glucose and hormone dynamics after overcoming full-thickness skin graft. With a smooth beginning of the process of alimentary post-operative self-reconstruction, due to the booking of part of the surgical weight reduction effect for maintaining this effect, long-term total preserving the early return of the maximum lost weight in the early postoperative period, the appearance and delay of the ideal weight, sufficient reduction in weight, and ensuring the absence of weight during the whole period of long-term remission during the treatment in general.

Weight loss before bariatric surgery is very important in the treatment of obesity (BMI > 35). In addition, weight reduction, especially in patients for surgical treatment of diabetes, gives a significant positive effect. If necessary, such patients should be treated for years to achieve rapid and stable long-term remission. It is necessary to control the accompanying disease, type 2 diabetes, and its comorbid disorder-free genesis. It is also advisable to use the techniques for stage reducing and stretchability of a standard stomach for general bariatric patients because there is a direct relationship between weight reduction associated with these surgical parameters of the bariatric surgery and the degree of normalisation of all types of metabolism, lipid, and hormonal spectrum at different stages after surgery. This approach is proposed for the patients in whom the preoperative body mass index is more than 35 kg/m^2, and for the high-risk patients, actual guidelines are recommended.

8. Conclusion

The success of a multidisciplinary team, as perceived by the healthcare professionals from different disciplines in managing patients undergoing bariatric surgery holistically, included them being able to contribute to the management plan of these patients while focusing on the individual needs of each patient. The benefits of a multidisciplinary team would delay the known complications associated with obesity. However, power struggles, resistance to change, and communication were main concerns about using a multidisciplinary team approach for managing patients eligible for bariatric surgery. Clear communication, defined roles, and regular meetings were that solutions that would contribute to having an effective multidisciplinary team approach for people undergoing bariatric surgery.

Author details

Alanoud Alobaidly[1,2]* and Abdullah Hasan[1,3]

1 College of Nursing and Health Sciences, Flinders University, Australia

2 Healthy Cities Office, Ministry of Health, Sulaibikhat, Kuwait

3 College of Nursing, Public Authority for Applied Education and Training, Shuwaikh, Kuwait

*Address all correspondence to: alobaidly.84.a@gmail.com

References

[1] Alobaidly A, Abigail W, Hill P. Life post bariatric surgery: The experiences of people with type 2 diabetes mellitus. Current Research in Obesity and Diabetes Journal. 2020;**13**(2):0014-0021

[2] Marshall S, Mackay H, Matthews C, Maimone IR, Isenring E. Does intensive multidisciplinary intervention for adults who elect bariatric surgery improve post-operative weight loss, co-morbidities, and quality of life? A systematic review and meta-analysis. Obesity Review. 2020;**21**(7):e13012 n/a

[3] James J, Gosden C, Winocour P, Walton C, Nagi D, Turner B, et al. Diabetes specialist nurses and role evolvement: A survey by Diabetes UK and ABCD of specialist diabetes services 2007. Diabetic Medicine. 2009;**26**(5):560-565

[4] Naylor MD, Kurtzman ET. The role of nurse practitioners in reinventing primary care. Health Affairs. 2010;**29**(5):893-899

[5] Ni Y, Liu S, Li J, Dong T, Tao L, Yuan L, et al. The effects of nurse-led multidisciplinary team management on glycosylated Hemoglobin, quality of life, hospitalization, and help-seeking behavior of people with diabetes mellitus. Journal of Diabetes Research. 2019;**2019**:9325146-9325149

[6] Nayeri ND, Samadi N, Mehrnoush N, Allahyari I, Bezaatpour F, NaseriAsl M. Experiences of nurses within a nurse-led multidisciplinary approach in providing care for patients with diabetic foot ulcer. Journal of Family Medicine and Primary Care. 2020;**9**(6):3136

[7] Manders IG, Stoecklein K, Lubach CHC, Bijl-Oeldrich J, Nanayakkara PWB, Rauwerda JA, et al. Shift in responsibilities in diabetes care: The nurse-driven diabetes In-hospital treatment protocol (N-DIABIT). Diabetic Medicine. 2016;**33**(6):761-767

[8] Bockwoldt D, Clements JN, Grossman S, Isaacs D, Weidman-Evans E, Rodriguez K, et al. The role of the diabetes educator in diabetes formulary and Medcal device decisions. The Diabetes Educator. 2018;**44**(1):31-34

[9] Al-Alawi K, Al Mandhari A, Johansson H. Care providers' perceptions towards challenges and opportunities for service improvement at diabetes management clinics in public primary health care in Muscat, Oman: A qualitative study. BMC Health Services Research. 2019;**19**(1):18

[10] Tuckman BW, Jensen MAC. Stages of small-group development revisited. Group and Organization Studies. 1977;**2**(4):419-427

[11] Hirpara D, Cleghorn M, Kwong J, Saleh F, Sockalingam S, Quereshy F, et al. Perception and awareness of bariatric surgery in Canada: A National Survey of general surgeons. Obesity Surgery. 2016;**26**(8):1799-1805

[12] Balcha Hailu F, Hjortdahl P, Moen A. Effect of locally-contextualized nurse-led diabetes self-management education on psychosocial health and quality of life: A controlled before-after study. International Journal of Africa Nursing Sciences. 2021;**15**:100325

[13] Guo J, Wang H, Ge L, Valimaki M, Wiley J, Whittemore R. Effectiveness of a nurse-led mindfulness stress-reduction intervention on diabetes distress, diabetes self-management, and HbA1c

levels among people with type 2 diabetes: A pilot randomized controlled trial. Research in Nursing and Health. Feb 2022;**45**(1):46-58

[14] Krederdt-Araujo SL, Dominguez-Cancino KA, Jiménez-Cordova R, Paz-Villanueva MY, Fernandez JM, Leyva-Moral JM, et al. Spirituality, social support, and diabetes: A cross-sectional study of people enrolled in a nurse-led diabetes management program in Peru. Hispanic Health Care International. 2019;**17**(4):162-171

[15] Nithin Shah P. Role of MDT in bariatric practice. 6th global gastroenterologists meeting. Journal of Gastrointestinal and Digestive System. Aug 2016;**6**(4):56

Section 2

Anaesthetic Considerations for Bariatric Patients

Chapter 3

Anesthetic Considerations for Obese Patients Undergoing Surgeries

Belal Khalil, Koninica Sanyal, Mohamed Eshmandi, Ahmed Elfaioumy, Mohamed Mohamed, Amr Ashour, Amr Rashwan and Mohamed Hussein

Abstract

The authors will delve into the critical considerations necessary when administering anesthesia to obese patients, underscoring the unique challenges this demographic population presents. It will describe the necessity of individualized preoperative respiratory and cardiovascular assessments, using tools like spirometry and ECGs to tailor anesthesia plans. The text emphasizes the importance of respecting patient dignity and outlines perioperative strategies for managing altered pharmacokinetics and airway challenges in the obese population. They aim to highlight how obesity significantly alters the pharmacokinetics of various anesthetic agents, necessitating adjusted dosing and vigilant monitoring. Postoperative care focuses on respiratory function optimization and mobilization, highlighting the critical role of a multi-disciplinary team in improving outcomes for obese surgical patients. By reviewing the latest research and guidelines, this chapter will provide a thorough overview of anesthetic considerations for obese patients, emphasizing the necessity for tailored care plans to ensure both safety and efficacy.

Keywords: obesity and anesthesia, pharmacotherapy, anesthetic medications, preoperative evaluation, postoperative care

1. Introduction

Obesity is firmly established as one of the great epidemics of the twenty-first century. Affecting both adults and younger people worldwide: now there are 2.5 billion overweight adults and over 890 million obese adults and over 37 million children and 390 million adolescents aged 5–19 yo were overweight or obese in 2022, resulting in enormous social and economic impact due to obesity-related health concerns [1].

Obesity can be defined as a disease since it is a physiologic dysfunction of the human organism with environmental, genetic, and endocrinologic aetiologies [2].

Classification	BMI (Kg/m^2)	Risk of developing health problems	ASA grading
Underweight	<18.5	Increased	1
Normal weight	18.5–24.9	Least	1
Overweight	25–29.9	Increased	1
Obese			
Class 1	30–34.9	High	1
Class 2	35–39.9	Very high	2
Class 3	≥40	Extremely high	3

Table 1.
WHO classification of obesity.

Obesity most frequently develops when food caloric intake exceeds energy expenditure over a sustained period. Factors influencing obesity include either energy intake or energy expenditure, and are influenced by genetic, behavioral, cultural, and socioeconomic factors [3]. There are syndromes that are associated with obesity, including leptin deficiency, Prader-Willi syndrome, and Lawrence Moon-Biedl syndrome [4].

Metabolic factors play a pivotal role in energy regulation, involving a complex interplay of hormones, peptides, nutrients, uncoupling proteins, and neural regulatory substances originating from various sources such as the gut, liver, brain, and fat cells. However, the precise mechanisms underlying many of these factors remain poorly understood [5].

BMI is the most widely applied classification tool used to assess individual weight status (**Table 1**). The BMI is specifically defined as the patient's weight, measured in kilograms, divided by the square of the patient's height, measured in meters, yielding a measurement bearing units of kilograms per square meter (kg/m^2) [6].

Obesity is commonly related to multiple and specific diseases/comorbid states that include: resistance, type 2 diabetes mellitus, obstructive sleep apnoea (OSA), asthma, chronic obstructive pulmonary disease, hypoventilation, cardiovascular disease, hypertension, certain malignancies, and osteoarthritis. Virtually every organ system can be included in the extended list of health risks associated with having an abnormally elevated BMI. As a result, obesity is also associated with early death [7].

2. Preoperative evaluation of morbidly obese patients

2.1 Assessment of airway and respiratory system

Obesity can impact the respiratory system through different ways. The accumulation of fat in the chest wall, abdomen, and upper airway directly diminishes lung volumes, notably the expiratory reserve volume, and induces structural modifications that disrupt essential ventilatory mechanics [8]. It's essential to recognize that the risk of encountering difficult or failed intubation is significantly higher in obese patients. Additionally, adipose tissue functions as an endocrine and paracrine organ, generating numerous cytokines and pro-inflammatory agents, which are believed to heighten the likelihood of asthma among individuals with obesity [9].

Below, we delve into the effects of obesity on the respiratory system and explore different measures of respiratory function.

Given the alterations in respiratory function associated with obesity, it's crucial to select the most suitable respiratory function test when evaluating an obese patient undergoing surgery, especially when in presence of breathing difficulties. Healthcare professionals must discern whether dyspnoea and other symptoms stem from a pre-existing respiratory disease or are exacerbated by obesity. Thus, test selection should align with the patient's clinical presentation and history [10].

Spirometry remains relatively unaffected by obesity within the mild to moderate range, offering valuable insights into airway size and function in these cases [11]. Assessing bronchodilator responsiveness is essential due to the heightened risk of asthma in this population. Objective measures of airway reactivity, such as mannitol or methacholine challenges, may help confirm or rule out asthma, particularly in patients unresponsive to typical treatments [12, 13].

While total lung capacity is minimally influenced by obesity, significant abnormalities may indicate underlying pathophysiology unrelated to obesity [14, 15]. Conversely, reductions in functional residual capacity, associated with changes in expiratory reserve volume, are likely attributable to obesity itself [14].

In individuals with obesity, there is an elevation in airway resistance which increases the resistive load. This population also experiences reductions in both lung and chest wall compliance. The decrease in lung compliance is attributed to breathing at reduced lung volumes, which can induce microatelectasis, while the decline in chest wall compliance is due to the mechanical pressure exerted by adipose tissue on the rib cage's capacity for expansion [16–18]. As a result, there is an increase in elastic load due to decreased pulmonary compliance. Furthermore, positive end-expiratory pressure (PEEPi) is elevated in obese individuals, especially in the supine position, reflecting an enhanced threshold load [19]. This phenomenon is likely caused by expiratory flow limitation when supine, leading to gas trapping at the end of expiration and consequently, the generation of PEEPi [19]. Correcting for volume-related variations, such as specific airway conductance, may better elucidate airway mechanics in obese patients [20].

Gas exchange measures, like DLCO and PaO2, are generally unaffected by obesity. Abnormalities in these tests are unlikely to be solely due to obesity and may indicate conditions such as obesity hypoventilation syndrome [20].

Cardiopulmonary exercise testing can be invaluable in evaluating exertional dyspnoea in obese individuals, providing insights into both cardiac and respiratory function [20]. While obesity may have a minor impact on test results, significant physiological issues unrelated to obesity may be identified through this testing [21–23].

The effect of OSA on perioperative risk remains controversial, but most patients are screened for OSA using overnight oximetry using oxygen desaturation index or polysomnography, or both, if appropriate [24–26]. If identified with OSA and recommended for CPAP, then patients are encouraged to initiate therapy at home, and it should be continued throughout the perioperative period [27, 28].

An Apnoea Hypopnea Index (AHI) score exceeding 30 (**Table 2**), indicating severe sleep apnoea, serves as a cautionary marker and predicts rapid and severe desaturation during induction [28].

Another valuable aspect of the preoperative assessment involves reviewing the patient's history of previous surgeries, including any encountered anesthetic challenges such as difficulty securing the airway or obtaining intravenous access, as well

Apnoea severity	Apnoea-hypopnea index (events/hour of sleep)
Normal	<5
Mild	$5 \leq$ AHI <15
Moderate	$15 \leq$ AHI <30
Severe	≥ 30

Table 2.
Apnoea hypopnea severity index.

as the need for intensive care unit admission and surgical outcomes, along with the patient's weight at the time. This information can alleviate concerns or facilitate more comprehensive preparation for the forthcoming anesthesia care.

2.2 Cardiovascular assessment

The utilization of electrocardiograms (ECGs) plays a crucial role in cardiovascular evaluations, facilitating the detection of previously undiagnosed cardiac abnormalities, which is particularly vital for obese and overweight patients. These individuals are at higher risk of developing arrhythmias, notably atrial fibrillation and ventricular tachycardia, which can be identified through ECG monitoring. Various factors, including hypoxia and existing heart conditions, often precipitate cardiac arrhythmias in this population. Recent studies suggest a strong association between obesity and atrial fibrillation, with overweight and obese patients exhibiting a 50% increased risk. Mechanisms such as atrial remodeling, elevated blood volume, and neurohormonal factors significantly contribute to this risk. Hemodynamic alterations in obesity lead to structural and functional changes in the heart, predisposing to atrial fibrillation and other arrhythmias [29, 30].

Echocardiography has the capability to assess systolic and diastolic function as well as chamber dimensions, though obtaining clear images via the transthoracic method can be challenging. Chest X-rays, on the other hand, can be utilized to evaluate the cardiothoracic ratio and detect signs of cardiac failure [30].

Additionally, cardiopulmonary exercise testing serves as a valuable tool in predicting postoperative outcomes and lengths of hospital stay. Understanding various risk factors, including the type of surgery, history of cardiovascular diseases, and preoperative insulin use, aids in assessing the potential cardiovascular morbidities in obese patients undergoing surgery [31].

2.3 Risk assessment

The Obesity Surgery Mortality Risk Score (OS-MRS), as detailed in **Table 3**, can aid in forecasting risk. This score helps in strategizing postoperative care requirements; patients with a score between 4 and 5 are considered high-risk and may require post-operative critical care admission. While its validation is specific to bariatric surgery, its application can extend to patients undergoing non-bariatric procedures [32].

Recommended preoperative laboratory evaluations include fasting blood glucose, lipid profile, and serum chemistries (evaluating renal and hepatic function), complete blood count, ferritin, vitamins and folate levels [29].

Risk factor	Point scored
BMI > 50 kg/m^2	1
Male	1
Hypertension	1
Age > 45	1
Risk factors for PE (previous VTE, preoperative vena cava filter, OSA/OHS, right heart failure, pulmonary hypertension)	1

Table 3.
Obesity surgery mortality risk score (OS-MRS).

3. Intraoperative management

3.1 Patient preparation

Obese individuals are aware of societal perceptions regarding their size, and their self-image concerns are significant. Maintaining dignity is crucial for them. It's essential to have theater gowns in suitable sizes, provide appropriately sized underwear, and ensure rooms have accessible toilets and showers that can accommodate their size and weight [33].

Obesity increases the risk of deep vein thrombosis, with up to 10 times higher incidence post-surgery. Therefore, assessing the risk of deep vein thrombosis and implementing prophylaxis measures in accordance with national guidelines is necessary for all obese patients [34].

The current standard practice refrains from administering sedatives or hypnotics to these patients until they are on the operating room table, particularly in preparation for painful procedures like arterial line placement or airway management, including airway topicalization. Non-respiratory depressant premedication may be incorporated into multimodal analgesia for patients with morbid obesity. This approach holds the potential to alleviate preinduction anxiety, reduce anesthetic requirements, and mitigate immediate postoperative depressant effects of opioids in this high-risk population [35].

A backup plan for airway management, following Difficult Airway Society guidelines, must be communicated to the entire theater team. Front-of-neck airway access can be challenging, especially in high-risk cases. Identifying relevant landmarks, such as the cricothyroid membrane depth and vascular tissue, is crucial to improve the success rate of emergency procedures [35].

3.2 Transferring and positioning

It's crucial to ensure appropriate equipment availability for patient transfers, including transportation from home to the hospital, which may require suitable vehicles. Chairs, trolleys, beds, and operating tables must safely accommodate the patient's weight and movements. Prior to surgery, confirming that accommodations meet safety standards is essential for maintaining dignity. Gel pads should be used to prevent pressure points, and vigilance during anesthesia is vital to avoid crush injuries and rhabdomyolysis. Transitioning from the operating table to the ward bed can be facilitated with slide sheets or hover mattresses, which can also aid postoperative care [33].

3.3 Monitoring

Additionally, alongside standard ASA-required monitors such as ECG, non-invasive blood pressure, pulse oximetry, end-tidal CO2, and temperature, arterial line insertion may be necessary for continuous blood pressure monitoring in cardiac patients. To avoid interference with surgical procedures, temperature monitoring via an esophageal stethoscope with thermistor placement in the tympanic membrane or axilla is preferred over esophageal placement. Urinary drainage catheters are typically omitted. Peripheral nerve stimulators gauge muscle relaxant effects, while processed EEG like BIS® monitors anesthesia depth, particularly beneficial in laparoscopic bariatric surgeries due to unreliable vital sign proxies and frequent sympathomimetic support. Intraoperative spirometry and flow-volume loops provide valuable insights into surgical and patient status changes. The use of automatic peripheral nerve stimulators simplifies data recording on electronic medical records [36].

3.4 Airway management

Obesity is associated with known aspiration risk factors like hiatus hernia and diabetes mellitus with autonomic neuropathy, causing delayed gastric emptying. However, obesity alone does not increase reflux and aspiration risk. When there are no aspiration risk factors present, like an unfasted patient or intra-abdominal pathology, routine rapid sequence intubation (RSI) is not typically necessary [35].

A backup plan for airway management, following Difficult Airway Society guidelines, must be communicated to the entire theater team. Front-of-neck airway access can be challenging, especially in high-risk cases. Identifying relevant landmarks, such as the cricothyroid membrane depth and vascular tissue, is crucial to improve the success rate of emergency procedures [35].

3.5 Anesthetic medications

The ideal goal for an anaesthesiologist is to ensure a 100% success rate in achieving surgical anesthesia, coupled with complete reversibility of the condition and the absence of complications or side effects. To achieve this, the anaesthesiologist must meticulously adjust the drug doses based on individual patient characteristics, thereby providing comprehensive protection against surgical injury while minimizing the risk of adverse effects. Furthermore, modern balanced general anesthesia entails the intricate application of a combination of pharmacological agents, wherein multiple drugs are administered simultaneously to address the three primary components of anesthesia: hypnosis, muscle relaxation, and suppression of the sympathetic response triggered by surgical stress [37].

The physiological alterations induced by obesity can significantly influence the distribution, binding, and elimination of anesthetic drugs. Relying solely on actual body weight for drug dosing can lead to considerable risks of severe adverse events [38].

Obesity results in increased fat and lean masses compared to non-obese individuals of the same age, height, and sex. The rise in lean body mass constitutes 20–40%

of the total excess weight; however, the fat mass per kilogram of Total Body Weight (TBW) increases more significantly than lean mass, leading to a relative decrease in the percentage of lean mass and water in obese individuals compared to their non-obese counterparts of similar age, sex, and height. These alterations in tissue distribution induced by obesity can significantly impact the apparent volume of distribution of anesthetic drugs. Additionally, obesity triggers other changes that affect the pharmacokinetic profile of anesthetic drugs, such as an absolute increase in total blood volume and cardiac output (CO), as well as modifications in plasma protein binding. It's also worth noting that alterations in respiratory and cardiovascular functions resulting from obesity may influence the absorption and elimination of inhalation anesthetics, which play a crucial role in modern balanced anesthesia [39].

Changes in hemodynamic status and regional blood flow due to obesity can have additional implications for the pharmacokinetics of anesthetic drugs. While fat tissue typically receives approximately 5% of cardiac output (CO), viscera and lean tissues receive 73 and 22% of CO, respectively. Nevertheless, reports suggest that blood flow per gram of fat is diminished in obese individuals compared to non-obese counterparts, implying a potentially lower proportion of blood flow to fat compared to lean mass in obesity. Furthermore, the decrease in cardiac performance induced by obesity could exacerbate the reduction in tissue perfusion [37].

The impact of obesity on drug binding to plasma proteins remains uncertain. Reports suggest that elevated levels of triglycerides, lipoproteins, cholesterol, and free-fatty acids could hinder the protein binding of certain drugs, thereby elevating their free plasma concentrations. Conversely, the rise in concentrations of acute phase proteins, such as a1-acid glycoprotein, seen in obese individuals, may enhance the binding of other drugs, thereby lowering their free plasma concentrations [40]. Alterations in liver and kidney functions induced by obesity can influence the pharmacokinetics of anesthetic drugs. In obese patients, hepatic clearance may be impacted by fatty degeneration of the liver, which is a common occurrence, although typically hepatic clearance remains normal or may even increase. Concurrently, renal clearance tends to rise due to factors like increased kidney weight and glomerular filtration rate. However, prolonged exposure to obesity-related changes can lead to more profound kidney damage and the development of chronic renal disease over time. In obese patients with renal impairment, standard methods for estimating creatinine clearance may prove inaccurate, necessitating adjustments in dosing for drugs eliminated through renal pathways based on directly measured creatinine clearance [39].

The National Audit Project (NAP) 5 study uncovered a higher rate of awareness shortly after anesthesia induction in obese patients, which is attributed to the rapid redistribution of intravenous (IV) anesthetic agents. To minimize this risk, anaesthesiologists should ensure sufficient dosing of Intravenous anesthetic agents, promptly administer maintenance anesthetic agents, and consider additional IV boluses before airway manipulation or prolonged airway maneuvers [35, 41].

In situations where Total Intravenous Anesthesia (TIVA) is employed, the existing models are all based on assumptions derived from the normal-weight population, albeit they estimate effect-site and plasma concentrations differently. None of the common TIVA models—Marsh, Schnider, or Minto—have been validated for extreme weight ranges; all necessitate adjustment and precise titration [42].

The concentration of volatile agents at the effect site is contingent upon pulmonary uptake, the fraction of inspired anesthetic agent, and cardiac output. In obese individuals, functional residual capacity (FRC) decreases while cardiac output and the size of the poorly vascularized peripheral compartment increase. Consequently, the heightened pulmonary uptake (due to reduced FRC) is counterbalanced by extended equilibration (due to increased cardiac output). Furthermore, the impact of an enlarged peripheral compartment is lessened by its comparatively deficient vascularity. During prolonged procedures, lipid-soluble agents might accumulate, resulting in prolonged offset times. However, in practical usage and for shorter procedures, there's minimal disparity between obese and non-obese patients [43].

Various drugs require dose adjustments based on different body weight parameters, particularly when administering to obese individuals. Thiopental, for instance, requires adjustment during induction based on Lean Body Weight (LBW) and maintenance based on Total Body Weight (TBW). Simulations suggest a 60% reduction in peak plasma concentration in obese subjects compared to lean ones after a 250 mg dose, necessitating adjustment to achieve equivalent concentrations. Propofol also necessitates LBW-based induction and TBW-based maintenance for obese subjects, with similar induction requirements but increased volume of distribution and clearance at steady state with rising TBW. Fentanyl's clearance correlates with LBW, while Remifentanil requires LBW-based infusion to achieve plasma concentrations comparable to those in normal-weight subjects. Succinyl Choline, administered based on TBW, yields improved intubating conditions, and Vecuronium's TBW-based doses result in longer action durations in obese individuals. Similarly, Rocuronium and Cis/Atracurium administered based on Ideal Body Weight (IBW) lead to extended effects in obese individuals compared to doses based on TBW. These adjustments ensure optimal drug effects and patient safety across diverse body types [44].

Etomidate is suggested for individuals facing hemodynamic instability due to its minimal suppression of the cardiovascular system. However, its use raises concerns regarding potential adrenal insufficiency, which could lead to organ failure. Like propofol and thiopental sodium, when utilized for induction, necessary dosage adjustments should be based on non-fat body weight, considering both pharmacokinetic and pharmacodynamic characteristics [45].

When dosing ketamine, it is advisable to consistently utilize either ideal or adjusted body weight for weight-based dosing in obese patients, especially in those with more severe forms of obesity (e.g., BMI $\geq 40\ kg/m^2$).

The nutritional status influences the distribution and bonding of local anesthetics. Elevated levels of alpha-1 acid glycoprotein might diminish the unbound portion of local anesthetics, thereby raising the dosage needed for nerve blocks in obese individuals. Additionally, the impact of obesity on the epidural space can make central neuraxial blocks unpredictable. Generally, dosing based on lean body weight (LBW) is advised, although recommendations may differ [46].

Noradrenaline (norepinephrine) and adrenaline (epinephrine), crucial emergency medications, are administered based on ideal body weight. Conversely, the minimum dose of atropine is calculated according to lean body weight to mitigate the risk of paradoxical bradycardia, as lower doses may induce this adverse effect [33].

3.6 Postoperative care and recovery

Recovery should involve maintaining a 30–45 degrees head-up position, with early initiation of CPAP potentially aiding in restoring normal respiratory function. Opioids should be avoided, and early mobilization with regular monitoring by an experienced consultant is recommended. Intravenous opioid use should trigger continuous SpO2 monitoring and consideration for higher care levels. Patients with significant comorbidities should be evaluated for critical care admission [35].

DOI: http://dx.doi.org/10.5772/intechopen.1005827

4. Conclusion

The anesthetic management of obese patients requires careful consideration and tailored approaches to ensure optimal outcomes. Factors such as airway management, drug dosing, monitoring techniques, and positioning must be carefully addressed to mitigate risks associated with obesity-related complications. Utilizing a multidisciplinary approach involving anaesthesiologists, surgeons, and other healthcare professionals is essential for comprehensive preoperative assessment, intraoperative management, and postoperative care. By implementing evidence-based practices and individualized strategies, healthcare providers can enhance safety and efficacy in anesthetizing obese patients, ultimately improving patient outcomes and satisfaction.

Conflict of interest

The authors declare no conflict of interest.

Author details

Belal Khalil[1*], Koninica Sanyal[1], Mohamed Eshmandi[1], Ahmed Elfaioumy[2], Mohamed Mohamed[3], Amr Ashour[4], Amr Rashwan[5] and Mohamed Hussein[5]

1 Southend University Hospital, UK

2 Nottingham University Hospitals, UK

3 Tameside Hospital, UK

4 Milton Keynes University Hospital, UK

5 Calderdale and Huddersfield NHS Foundation Trust, UK

*Address all correspondence to: belal.khalil@nhs.net

References

[1] Obesity and Overweight. World Health Organization. Available from: https://www.who.int/news-room/fact-sheets/detail/obesity-and-overweight; [Accessed: March 04, 2024]

[2] Conway B, Rene A. Obesity as a disease: No lightweight matter. Obesity Reviews. 2004;**5**(3):145-151

[3] Zabena C, González-Sánchez JL, Martínez-Larrad MT, et al. The FTO obesity gene. Genotyping and gene expression analysis in morbidly obese patients. Obesity Surgery. 2009;**19**: 87-95

[4] Hensrud DD, Klein S. Extreme obesity: A new medical crisis in the United States. Mayo Clinic Proceedings. USA: Elsevier; 2006;**81**(10):S5-S10

[5] Schwartz MW, Seeley RJ, Zeltser LM, Drewnowski A, Ravussin E, Redman LM, et al. Obesity pathogenesis: An endocrine society scientific statement. Endocrine Reviews. 2017;**38**(4):267-296

[6] Nuttall FQ. Body mass index: Obesity, BMI, and health: A critical review. Nutrition Today. 2015;**50**(3):117

[7] Lister NB, Baur LA, Felix JF, et al. Child and adolescent obesity. Nature Reviews. Disease Primers. 2023;**9**:24

[8] Mafort TT, Rufino R, Costa CH, Lopes AJ. Obesity: Systemic and pulmonary complications, biochemical abnormalities, and impairment of lung function. Multidisciplinary Respiratory Medicine. 2016;11:1-1

[9] Palma G, Sorice GP, Genchi VA, Giordano F, Caccioppoli C, D'Oria R, et al. Adipose tissue inflammation and pulmonary dysfunction in obesity. International Journal of Molecular Sciences. 2022;**23**(13):7349

[10] Dixon AE, Peters U. The effect of obesity on lung function. Expert Review of Respiratory Medicine. 2018;**12**(9):755-767

[11] Salome CM, King GG, Berend N. Physiology of obesity and effects on lung function. Journal of Applied Physiology. 2010;**108**(1):206-211

[12] Salome CM, Munoz PA, Berend N, Thorpe CW, Schachter LM, King GG. Effect of obesity on breathlessness and airway responsiveness to methacholine in non-asthmatic subjects. International Journal of Obesity. 2008;**32**(3):502-509

[13] Arismendi E, Rivas E, Vidal J, Barreiro E, Torralba Y, Burgos F, et al. Airway hyperresponsiveness to mannitol in obesity before and after bariatric surgery. Obesity Surgery. 2015;**25**:1666-1671

[14] Jones RL, Nzekwu MM. The effects of body mass index on lung volumes. Chest. 2006;**130**(3):827-833

[15] Collins LC, Hoberty PD, Walker JF, Fletcher EC, Peiris AN. The effect of body fat distribution on pulmonary function tests. Chest. 1995;**107**(5):1298-1302

[16] Littleton SW. Impact of obesity on respiratory function. Respirology. 2012;**17**(1):43-49

[17] Steier J, Lunt A, Hart N, Polkey MI, Moxham J. Observational study of the effect of obesity on lung volumes. Thorax. 2014;**69**(8):752-759

[18] Shah NM, Kaltsakas G. Respiratory complications of obesity: From

early changes to respiratory failure. Breathe. 2023;**19**(1). Available from: https://breathe.ersjournals.com/content/19/1/220263

[19] Pankow W, Podszus T, Gutheil T, Penzel T, Peter JH, Von Wichert P. Expiratory flow limitation and intrinsic positive end-expiratory pressure in obesity. Journal of Applied Physiology. 1998;**85**(4):1236-1243

[20] Brazzale DJ, Pretto JJ, Schachter LM. Optimizing respiratory function assessments to elucidate the impact of obesity on respiratory health. Respirology. 2015;**20**(5):715-721

[21] DeLorey DS, Wyrick BL, Babb TG. Mild-to-moderate obesity: Implications for respiratory mechanics at rest and during exercise in young men. International Journal of Obesity. 2005;**29**(9):1039-1047

[22] Lorenzo S, Babb TG. Quantification of cardiorespiratory fitness in healthy nonobese and obese men and women. European Journal of Applied Physiology. 2008;**103**:707-717

[23] Ofir D, Laveneziana P, Webb KA, O'Donnell DE. Ventilatory and perceptual responses to cycle exercise in obese women. Journal of Applied Physiology. 2007;**102**:2217-2226

[24] American Academy of Sleep Medicine. Sleep-related breathing disorders in adults: Recommendations for syndrome definition and measurement techniques in clinical research. The Report of an American academy of Sleep Medicine Task Force. Sleep. 1999;**22**:667-689

[25] Epstein LJ, Dorlac GR. Cost-effectiveness analysis of nocturnal oximetry as a method of screening for sleep apnea-hypopnea syndrome. Chest. 1998;**113**(1):97-103

[26] Rudra A, Chatterjee S, Das T, Sengupta S, Maitra G, Kumar P. Obstructive sleep apnoea and anaesthesia. Indian Journal of Critical Care Medicine: Peer-reviewed, Official Publication of Indian Society of Critical Care Medicine. 2008;**12**(3):116

[27] Benalcazar DA, Cascella M. Obesity surgery preoperative assessment and preparation. In: StatPearls. Treasure Island (FL): StatPearls Publishing; 2024. Available from: https://www.ncbi.nlm.nih.gov/books/NBK546667/

[28] Bae E. Preoperative risk evaluation and perioperative management of patients with obstructive sleep apnea: A narrative review. Journal of Dental Anesthesia and Pain Medicine. 2023;**23**(4):179-192

[29] Adams JP, Murphy PG. Obesity in anaesthesia and intensive care. BJA: British Journal of Anaesthesia. 2000;**1**(1):91-108. 85

[30] Mozos I. Arrhythmia risk and obesity. Journal of Molecular and Genetic Medicine: An International Journal of Biomedical Research. 2014:s1. Available from: https://www.researchgate.net/publication/260287137_Arrhythmia_Risk_and_Obesity

[31] Poirier Paul A, Martin A, Fleisher Lee A, et al. Cardiovascular evaluation and management of severely obese patients undergoing surgery. Circulation. 2009;7(1):86-95

[32] Glance LG, Wissler R, Mukamel DB, et al. Perioperative outcomes among patients with the modifed metabolic syndrome who are undergoing noncardiac surgery. Anesthesiology. 2010;**113**(4):859-872

[33] Wynn-Hebden A, Bouch DC. Anaesthesia for the obese patient. BJA Education. 2020;**20**(11):388

[34] Nightingale CE, Margarson MP, Shearer E, et al. Guidelines for peri-operative management of the obese surgical patient. Anaesthesia. 2015;**70**(1):859-876

[35] Samuels JD, Yao F-SF. Morbid obesity, obstructive sleep apnea, and bariatric anesthesia. In: Yao and Artusio's Anesthesiology: Problem-Oriented Patient Management. 9th ed. Wolters Kluwer. pp. 2717-2802

[36] UpToDate. Available from: https://www.uptodate.com/contents/anesthesia-for-the-obese-patient [Accessed: March 18, 2024]

[37] Casati A, Putzu M. Anesthesia in the obese patient: Pharmacokinetic considerations. Journal of Clinical Anesthesia. 2005;**17**(2):134-145

[38] Jabbour H, Jabbour K, Abi Lutfallah A, Abou Zeid H, et al. Magnesium and ketamine reduce early morphine consumption after open bariatric surgery: A prospective randomized double-blind study. Obesity Surgery. 2020;**30**:1452-1458

[39] Barras M, Legg A. Drug dosing in obese adults. Australian Prescriber. 2017;**40**(5):189

[40] Hanley MJ, Abernethy DR, Greenblatt DJ. Effect of obesity on the pharmacokinetics of drugs in humans. Clinical Pharmacokinetics. 2010;**49**:71-87

[41] Pandit JJ, Andrade J, Bogod DG, et al. 5th National Audit Project (NAP5) on accidental awareness during general anaesthesia: Summary of main findings and risk factors. British Journal of Anaesthesia. 1 Oct 2014;**113**(4):549-459

[42] Hebbes CP, Thompson JP. Pharmacokinetics of anaesthetic drugs at extremes of body weight. BJA Education. 2018;**18**(12):364

[43] Arain SR, Barth CD, Shankar H, Ebert TJ. Choice of volatile anesthetic for the morbidly obese patient: Sevoflurane or desflurane. Journal of Clinical Anesthesia. 2005;**17**:413e9

[44] Ingrande J, Lemmens HJ. Dose adjustment of anaesthetics in the morbidly obese. British Journal of Anaesthesia. 2010;**105**(Suppl. 1):i16-i23

[45] Seyni-Boureima R, Zhang Z, Antoine MM, Antoine-Frank CD. A review on the anesthetic management of obese patients undergoing surgery. BMC Anesthesiology. 2022;**22**(1):98

[46] Nightingale CE, Margarson MP, Shearer E, et al. Peri-operativemanagement of the obese surgical patient 2015. Anaesthesia. 2015;**70**:859e76

Chapter 4

Optimizing Anesthesia: Challenges and Solutions in Bariatric Procedures

Halil Buluç

"Symptoms are not just the result of disease; they are also the result of a conflict within the person's inner world"

Carl Gustav Jung

Abstract

One of the most pressing issues arising from modern urban life is the excessive caloric intake leading to obesity. Metabolic surgical interventions offer a rapid solution to this global crisis. Although our experience with sleeve gastrectomy and other surgical procedures grows daily, consensus has yet to be achieved on key aspects such as ventilation strategies and the use of recruitment maneuvers. Techniques like abdominal plane blocks and opioid-free anesthesia and analgesia are increasingly employed, yet each approach carries its own advantages and limitations. Given the multifaceted nature of obesity, encompassing unique pathophysiology, pharmacodynamics, and perioperative considerations, it is clear that a comprehensive, multidisciplinary approach is essential for effective management.

Keywords: bariatric surgery, anesthetic management, ventilation strategies, pain management, difficult airway management

1. Introduction

Obesity is a global catastrophe requiring a multidisciplinary approach, now often regarded as an endemic disorder and one of the leading preventable causes of death [1]. Rather than addressing the underlying causes, humanity often opts for shortcuts to manage its problems. In the case of obesity, this approach has led to the increasing use of bariatric surgery as a primary intervention. Patients who undergo these types of surgeries frequently demonstrate significant improvement in comorbid conditions such as diabetes, dyslipidemia, hypertension, and obstructive sleep apnea [2].

As obesity continues to rise globally, the demand for bariatric surgery increases daily. Compared to our past experiences, surgery times have significantly decreased. As part of an international center, time management is a crucial aspect for our team. It has become essential to perform both endoscopy and surgery on the same day [3]. Predictive tools such as the apnea-hypopnea index and adipose tissue measurements are crucial in our assessments. However, unfortunately, none of these approaches provide one hundred percent accuracy [4]. Recent data indicate that opioid-free anesthesia demonstrate superiority over classical approaches [5]. The appropriate use of nonsteroidal anti-inflammatory drugs (NSAIDs) and abdominal blocks, such as the transversus abdominis plane (TAP) block and erector spinae plane (ESP) block, can reduce pain scores, decrease opioid requirements, and enhance ambulation following bariatric surgery [6–8].

2. Understanding obesity as a complex disease

The word "obesitas" itself is derived from the Latin verb "obedere," meaning "to eat up" or to devour. The World Health Organization defines obesity as a condition characterized by an excessive accumulation of body fat, which detrimentally impacts health and overall well-being [9]. As healthcare professionals, we categorize obesity into distinct classes to facilitate more precise management and treatment strategies. This classification enables us to tailor interventions according to the severity of the condition, improving the likelihood of successful outcomes and optimizing patient care (**Table 1**).

Body mass index (BMI) has several limitations. It may not accurately reflect body composition across different ethnic groups or among individuals with a high degree of muscular development. Additionally, BMI does not provide insight into the distribution of body fat or differentiate between fat and lean mass. Despite these shortcomings, BMI remains a prevalent tool for assessing obesity due to its simplicity and ease of calculation, relying solely on weight and height measurements. This widespread use is largely attributable to the minimal equipment and expertise required for its calculation, which makes it a convenient, albeit imperfect, measure of body fatness. The limitations of body mass index (BMI) could contribute to variability in obesity research outcomes. Alternative measures, such as the hip-to-abdominal girth ratio and skinfold thickness, may offer more precise insights into potentially hazardous patterns of fat distribution. Central obesity, characterized by an "apple-shaped" body type predominantly observed in males, is associated with higher health risks compared to peripheral obesity, which is often described as "pear-shaped" and more commonly seen in females. These alternative metrics can better reflect the distribution of adipose tissue and its implications for metabolic health.

Due to the limitations of BMI in predicting optimal ventilation strategies and pharmacological dosing, new alternative concepts have been needed. One method

Category	BMI (kg/m^2)
Underweight	<18.5
Normal	18.5–24.9
Overweight (pre-obese)	25–29.9
Obese Class I	30–34.9
Obese Class II (severe to morbid)	35–39.9
Obese Class III (morbid to super)	40+
Super obesity	45–50+

Table 1.
Obesity classification.

for estimating a healthy weight is the ideal body weight (IBW), which correlates with reduced mortality rates based on height and gender. The IBW can be calculated using Broca's index, a widely recognized formula [10].

Ideal body weight (kg) can be determined by subtracting a constant value X from the individual's height in centimeters. The value of X is typically 100 for adult man and 105 for adult women.

Another approach is predicted body weight (PBW), a concept akin to ideal body weight but more commonly cited in medical literature. Predicted body weight can be estimated using specific formulas based on the patient's height. For males, PBW (kg) is calculated by adding 50 to 0.91 times the difference between the individual's height in centimeters and 152.4. For females, the calculation starts with 45.5, and similarly, 0.91 times the difference between height in centimeters and 152.4 is added.

The third concept is lean body weight (LBW). LBW represents the total body weight minus the adipose tissue and includes body cell mass, extracellular water, and non-fat connective tissue. LBW typically approximates 80% of TBW in males and 75% in females.

In morbidly obese patients, an estimation of LBW can be obtained by increasing the ideal body weight by 20–30%, which provides a more accurate measure of lean tissue mass in this population [11]. Lean body weight can be a valuable parameter for calculating ventilation volumes and drug dosing.

Obesity can negatively impact multiple organ systems, leading to a range of adverse health outcomes. Excess adipose tissue contributes to systemic inflammation and alters metabolic processes, which can adversely affect cardiovascular, respiratory, endocrine, and musculoskeletal systems.

3. Respiratory system and pathophysiology

Fat accumulation in the thorax and abdomen reduces both chest wall and lung compliance, leading to shallow, rapid breathing and increased work of breathing, especially when lying down. This reduction in lung compliance is partly due to increased pulmonary blood volume, which accompanies the overall increase in blood volume. In individuals with obesity, the efficiency of respiratory muscles is reduced, leading to a decrease in functional residual capacity (FRC), vital capacity, and total lung capacity. The reduction in FRC is primarily caused by a diminished expiratory reserve volume (ERV), which in turn disrupts the balance between FRC and closing capacity, the stage when small airways start to close. Obese patients most commonly experience reductions in functional residual capacity and expiratory reserve volume as key pulmonary function abnormalities (**Figure 1**) [12].

Residual volume and closing capacity remain unchanged in obesity. However, the reduction in functional residual capacity (FRC), primarily due to a decrease in expiratory reserve volume (ERV), can cause lung volumes to fall below closing capacity during normal breathing. This situation can cause small airways to close, leading to ventilation-perfusion mismatch, right-to-left shunting, and low oxygen levels in the arteries (arterial hypoxemia). The effects are worsened by anesthesia and the supine position, causing FRC to drop by as much as 50% in anesthetized obese patients, compared to a 20% decrease in those who are not obese. While forced expiratory volume in 1 second (FEV1) and forced vital capacity (FVC) generally remain within normal ranges, ERV is the most sensitive measure of obesity's impact on lung function.

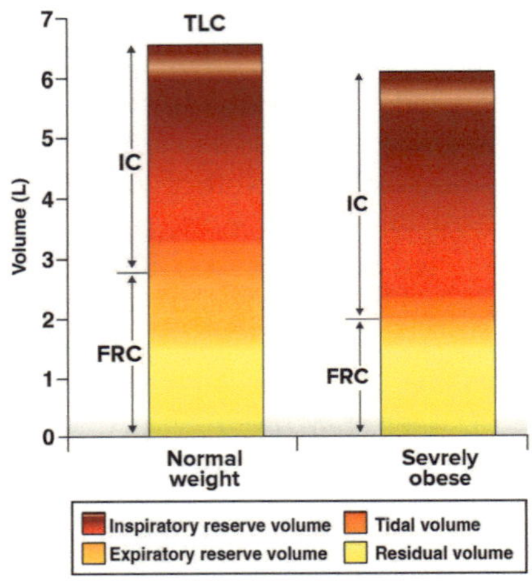

Figure 1.
Spirometric alterations in obesity highlight a significant decrease in functional residual capacity (FRC). Key parameters include total lung capacity (TLC) and inspiratory capacity (IC), with a notable reduction in FRC being a primary concern.

Obesity results in higher oxygen consumption and carbon dioxide production, even during rest. This is attributed to the metabolic demands of excess fat and the extra strain placed on the body's supporting tissues. To accommodate these increased metabolic needs, the body boosts both cardiac output and alveolar ventilation. Despite the basal metabolic rate staying within normal limits when adjusted for body surface area, normocapnia is usually preserved through an increase in minute ventilation. This process requires more oxygen, as most obese individuals retain their normal responses to hypoxemia and hypercapnia. In morbidly obese patients, arterial oxygen levels are lower than expected for non-obese individuals of similar age, both in sitting and supine positions. Chronic hypoxemia in these patients can lead to complications such as polycythemia, pulmonary hypertension, and cor pulmonale.

4. Obstructive sleep apnea -central sleep apnea -obesity hypoventilation syndrome

Patients with obesity frequently experience obstructive sleep apnea, which is marked by intermittent, partial, or complete blockage of the upper airway during sleep. In individuals with obesity, this condition is often caused by airway obstruction due to an accumulation of excess soft tissue. Nonetheless, central sleep apnea, which is driven by disruptions in the brain's signals to control breathing, can also occur.

OSA can cause several physiological issues, including low oxygen levels, high carbon dioxide levels, high blood pressure in the lungs, increased systemic blood pressure, and higher red blood cell count due to repeated low oxygen. These abnormalities elevate the risk of heart disease and stroke. Additionally, hypoxic pulmonary vasoconstriction can lead to right ventricular failure. Respiratory acidosis typically occurs only during sleep. The "gold standard" for diagnosing OSA is overnight polysomnography (OPS). However, due to its inconvenience, time requirements, and cost, many obese patients with suspected OSA may not receive a formal diagnosis [12]. During the preoperative visit, look for signs that suggest OSA, such as observed apnea episodes during sleep, a BMI of 35 or higher, a neck circumference of 16 inches (40 cm) or more, high insulin levels, and elevated hemoglobin A1c. While snoring, frequent nighttime awakenings, daytime drowsiness, trouble concentrating, memory issues, and morning headaches are common, they are not definitive indicators of OSA [13].

It is advisable to conduct a comprehensive preoperative evaluation for OSA well in advance of elective surgery. This allows time to develop a perioperative management plan. For severe OSA cases, starting continuous positive airway pressure (CPAP) before surgery should be considered [14]. Patients with confirmed or suspected OSA are at high risk for difficult airways and postoperative lung issues. They should be managed with this in mind [15].

Obesity hypoventilation syndrome (OHS), also known as Pickwickian syndrome, can develop from long-term OSA and affect 5–10% of severely obese patients. OHS combines obesity with chronic hypoventilation, leading to pulmonary hypertension and cor pulmonale. The diagnosis of obesity hypoventilation syndrome is supported by the combination of obesity (BMI >30 kg/m^2) and elevated arterial carbon dioxide levels ($PaCO_2$ >45 mm Hg), provided that there are no other known causes of hypoventilation. Prolonged OSA can alter breathing control, leading to CNS-mediated apneic events and increased dependence on hypoxic drive for ventilation. The primary issue in OHS is alveolar hypoventilation, not related to intrinsic lung disease. Other features of OHS include daytime sleepiness, high carbon dioxide levels, low oxygen levels, and increased red blood cell count. Right ventricular failure often develops, and these patients are also more sensitive to the respiratory depressant effects of general anesthetics [16].

5. Airway management

The airway of obese patients should be approached with caution, as traditional teachings and national audits suggest a higher likelihood of airway management challenges. However, several studies indicate that, in the hands of experienced practitioners, specific aspects of airway management particularly tracheal intubation may not be significantly more difficult than in non-obese patients. Difficulty with laryngoscopy and intubation in obese patients typically arises from anatomical factors such as a short, thick neck, a large tongue, and excessive pharyngeal soft tissue. Success in airway management often depends on a straightforward approach, with careful attention to patient positioning before inducing general anesthesia. Proper positioning is crucial for creating the best conditions to successfully place the endotracheal tube under direct vision.

In our clinical practice, two approaches are crucial. The first is preoxygenation or nitrogen washout. Traditional methods recommend administering 100% oxygen for two min, but recent research suggests that using 80% oxygen for two min before anesthesia induction results in better outcomes and fewer postoperative complications. A video laryngoscope, with which the practitioner has prior experience, should be readily available and prepared for use during intubation.

Factors linked to difficult intubation include being over 46 years old, male gender, a Mallampati score of 3 or 4, a thyromental distance of less than 6 cm, and intact dentition. Male patients with severe obesity, particularly those with a BMI over 50, OSA, or a neck circumference greater than 42 cm, face an increased risk of challenging mask ventilation and intubation [17].

In patients with suspected or known difficult intubation, the use of a simple nasal cannula or high-flow nasal cannula should be considered as an adjunct during mask ventilation. This approach has been shown to extend apnea time by up to 40% and help maintain oxygenation, thereby reducing the risk of desaturation during anesthesia induction [18].

When difficult intubation is anticipated, performing the procedure with the patient awake, using topical or regional anesthesia along with a fiberoptic device, is advisable to maintain spontaneous breathing. It is important to minimize the use of sedative-hypnotic medications during awake intubation. Using dexmedetomidine for sedation during awake intubation offers sufficient anxiolysis and pain relief without causing respiratory depression [19]. Preventing hypoxia and aspiration during endotracheal intubation is critical. Having an experienced colleague present or nearby during induction can assist with mask ventilation or intubation attempts. It is also essential to have a surgeon available who can perform a surgical airway if needed. Positioning the obese patient in a "ramped" position, where the upper body is elevated, enhances the laryngoscopic view compared to the standard "sniffing" position [20]. If oxygen levels cannot be quickly stabilized following extubation, continuous positive airway pressure (CPAP) therapy is advised. CPAP should be continued until the patient's breathing rate and effort return to normal, with no occurrences of hypopnea or apnea for at least one hour [21].

Tools to predict difficult intubation in obese patients include ultrasound, which quantifies the thickness of soft tissue between the skin and the trachea's anterior surface at the level of the vocal cords. Researchers besides evaluated respiratory tract characteristics via measuring distance from the thyroid notch to the mentum, maximum mouth gap, neck rotational and flexional capacity, Mallampati grading system, circumferential measurement of the neck, and the existence of obstructive sleep apnea. Among these factors, an increased thickness of soft tissue in the pretracheal region, as calculating using ultrasound, and larger cervical circumference has been identified as factors suggesting difficulty in difficult intubation when laryngoscopy was carried out with the patient in the position with head extended and neck flexed [22].

6. Ventilation strategies

Obesity complicates the selection of ventilator settings because weight gain does not correspond directly to a proportional increase in lung size. Although similar ventilatory parameters used for non-obese patients can be applied, it may be challenging to keep plateau pressures below 30 cm H_2O in obese patients. Higher inflation pressures may be more acceptable and tolerated in this population [23].

Various strategies can contribute to protective ventilation. Recommended measures to prevent ventilator-induced lung injury include using low tidal volumes (VT) and maintaining low levels of positive end-expiratory pressure (PEEP) without employing recruitment maneuvers [24]. When estimating tidal volume, using predicted body weight which accounts for the patient's height and sex may be preferred over actual body weight. A low physiological VT is considered lung-protective in patients with acute respiratory distress syndrome (ARDS) [25].

Contemporary data indicate that using 6 to 8 mL/kg of tidal volume of predicted body weight can help diminish the likelihood of respiratory issues. This approach is recommended to be used for patients in general, including those with normal lung function, irrespective of overweight status [26]. Obese individuals are at higher risk for developing atelectasis, particularly in the dependent regions of the lungs. Combining recruitment maneuvers (RMs) with positive end-expiratory pressure (PEEP) can be an effective strategy to enhance gas exchange and improve lung mechanics [27].

In our clinical practice, we have observed that each obese patient requires individualized management. This variability may explain the lack of consensus on optimal ventilation strategies, PEEP values, and recruitment maneuvers for obese patients. During anesthesia, three key parameters can guide our management: delta PEEP, peak plateau pressures, and end-tidal CO_2 values. Values slightly above normal ranges may be acceptable. Occasionally, end-tidal CO_2 values may exceed expected levels. This highlights the need for further understanding of how obesity affects human physiology.

There is considerable uncertainty about the optimal PEEP level for obese patients with healthy lungs, and the effectiveness of PEEP and recruitment maneuvers in preventing postoperative pulmonary complications is still not well defined [28]. PEEP requirements can vary significantly among patients. Administering low tidal volumes during anesthesia and adjusting PEEP settings individually can help reduce postoperative atelectasis while enhancing intraoperative gas exchange and driving pressures. This suggests that tailoring PEEP levels to specific physiological goals may be beneficial for lung protection [29].

High driving pressure (the difference between plateau pressure and PEEP) may be linked to a greater risk of severe adverse outcomes in patients with acute respiratory distress syndrome (ARDS) [30]. Obese patients may need higher cut-off values for protective driving pressure compared to non-obese patients. This is due to their lower lung capacity and the physiological changes that occur during surgery [31].

Pressure-controlled ventilation (PCV) can enhance ventilation uniformity across different lung regions, reducing the risk of alveolar overdistension and improving oxygenation [32]. Conversely, volume-controlled ventilation (VCV) offers more precise control over tidal volume during procedures that intermittently impact chest wall compliance. This method may be associated with a lower incidence of postoperative pulmonary complications [33]. A recent systematic review assessed various ventilatory strategies for obese patients undergoing bariatric surgery. The review compared pressure-controlled ventilation (PCV) versus volume-controlled ventilation (VCV), different recruitment maneuvers, varying levels of PEEP, and ratios of 1:1 versus 2:2. It included 14 studies with a total of 574 participants. The review revealed significant variability in the interventions used, highlighting the ongoing lack of consensus on the optimal ventilation approach for obese patients undergoing surgery [34].

7. Cardiovascular pathophysiology

In obese individuals, blood volume is augmented nevertheless based on the ratio of volume to weight, and the condition is lower compared to non-obese individuals (50 mL/kg vs. 70 mL/kg). The majority of this additional volume is stored in adipose tissue. Blood flow to the kidneys and digestive organs is elevated. Cardiac output rises with increased body weight, adding 20 to 30 mL/kg of excess fat due to ventricular dilation and higher stroke volume. This increased stress on the left ventricle results in hypertrophy, reduced compliance, impaired filling (diastolic dysfunction), elevated left ventricular diastolic pressure, and pulmonary edema [35].

Echocardiographic studies reveal three predominant pathological patterns in obesity: concentric remodeling (thickening of the left ventricular wall without hypertrophy), concentric hypertrophy (hypertrophy with increased wall thickness relative to the chamber), and eccentric dilated hypertrophy (thickened left ventricular wall with reduced wall-to-cavity ratio due to dilation). These patterns indicate early reduced ventricular wall compliance and diastolic dysfunction. As cardiac dilation progresses, there is a gradual decrease in systolic contractility. Obesity indeed has detrimental effects on the cardiopulmonary system (**Figure 2**).

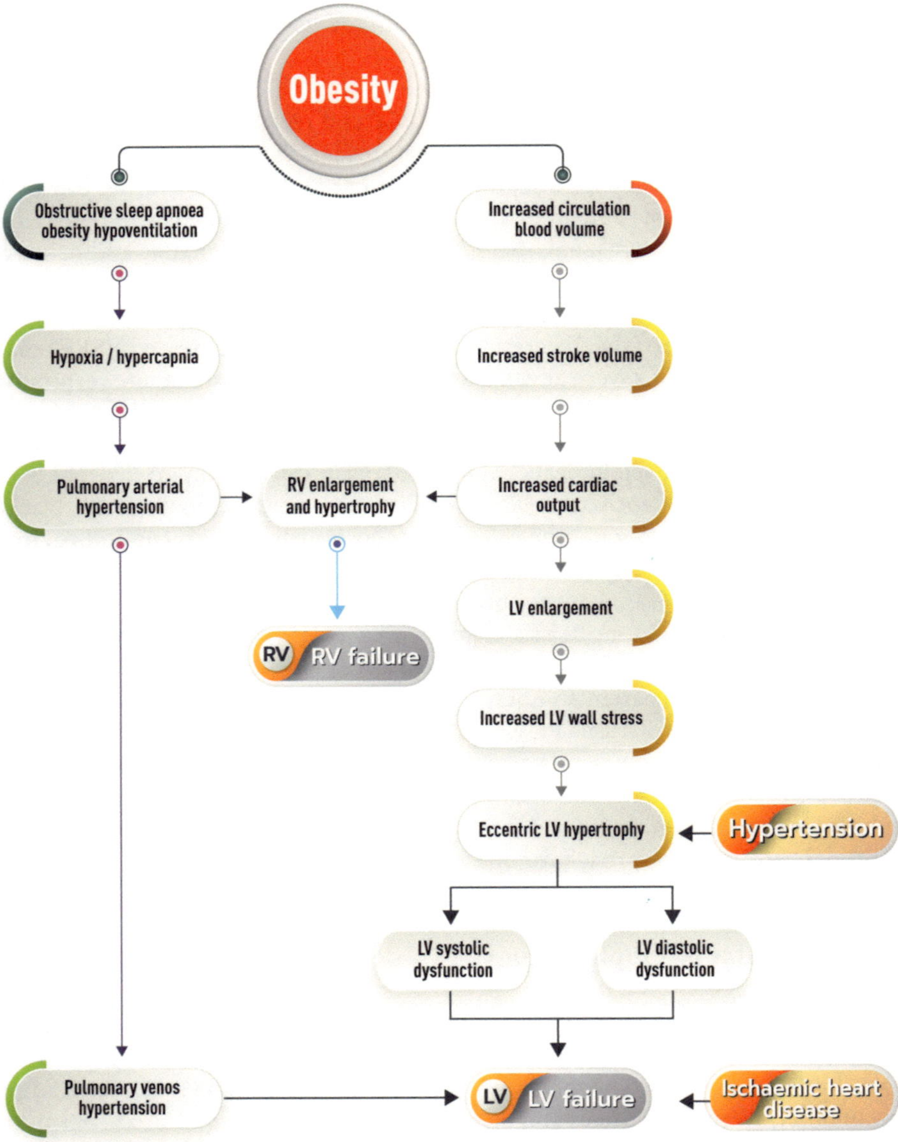

Figure 2.
Impact of obesity-induced cardiomyopathy.

However, it is noteworthy that lower cardiac mortality rates have been observed in individuals with mild obesity, a phenomenon known as the "obesity paradox." This paradox refers to the counterintuitive observation that mild obesity might be associated with better cardiac outcomes compared to normal weight or more severe obesity.

Obesity paradox: Arterial disease is linked to both primary obesity and its associated comorbid conditions, such as hyperlipidemia and diabetes mellitus. Some studies suggest that coronary artery disease risk increases by 50% between normal weight and overweight individuals, with the risk rising to a hazard ratio greater than 2.5 in severely morbidly obese individuals. Despite this, lower cardiac mortality rates have been reported in those with mild obesity. This discrepancy may stem from the limitations of body mass index as a measure of central obesity, which is a more accurate indicator of vascular risk. For instance, peripheral vascular disease does not correlate with BMI when adjusted for comorbid conditions. In contrast, measures of obesity such as waist circumference, waist-to-hip ratio, or waist-to-thigh ratio are associated with higher vascular risk. This paradoxical observation, known as the "obesity paradox," refers to the phenomenon where obesity is linked to lower mortality rates in various conditions, including critical illness, congestive heart failure, and eccentric versus concentric cardiac hypertrophy.

Blood flow to fat tissue is about 2 to 3 mL per 100 grams. Excess fat increases cardiac output to meet higher oxygen demand, maintaining a normal or slightly elevated arteriovenous oxygen difference in the systemic circulation. Ventricular dysfunction during surgery can develop due to the immediate delivery of IV fluids rapid intravenous fluid administration (pointing to left ventricular diastolic impairment), the undesirable inotropic effects of anesthetic medications, or increased pulmonary vascular resistance from low oxygen levels or elevated carbon dioxide. Abnormal heart rhythms may be triggered by fatty deposits in the cardiac conduction pathways, oxygen deficiency and high carbon dioxide concentrations, electrolyte imbalances, atherosclerotic coronary disease, higher concentrations of circulating catecholamines, obstructive sleep apnea, and hypertrophy of the myocardium. Common ECG results in individuals with severe obesity frequently exhibit diminished QRS voltage, evidence of left-ventricular thickening, enlargement of the left atrium, and depressed T-wave morphology in inferior and lateral leads [36].

Among morbidly obese individuals, cardiac output increases more rapidly in response to exercise and is often accompanied by elevated pressure in the left ventricle at the end of diastole and wedge pressure in the pulmonary capillary bed. Corresponding variations can take place in the perioperative timeframe that necessitates a low threshold for thorough cardiac evaluation. A significant portion of obese patient experience mild-to-moderate elevated blood pressure, accompanied by systolic pressure rising by 3 to 4 mm Hg and diastolic pressure by 2 mm Hg for every 10 kg of weight gained. Even normotensive obese individuals typically have reduced systemic vascular resistance, which increases when hypertension develops. Their expanded blood volume leads to higher cardiac output and a lower calculated systemic vascular resistance for a given arterial blood pressure.

Right ventricular dysfunction is notably associated with sleep-disordered breathing. The interplay of chronic pulmonary hypertension, often resulting from nocturnal hypoxemia, combined with the effects of chronic volume overload due to obesity, contributes to progressive changes in the left ventricle. These factors lead to right-sided ventricular dilation, along with both systolic and diastolic dysfunctions, ultimately resulting in right heart failure.

7.1 Anesthetic agents: Key pharmacologic principles and dosing strategies

Obese patients may exhibit changes in both pharmacokinetics and pharmacodynamics, which have significant clinical implications. Understanding fundamental concepts such as drug solubility, compartment volumes, distribution, and metabolism can be beneficial. However, these interactions are complex, and consulting published data are crucial. This complexity contributes to ongoing debate, and special caution is advised when using target-controlled infusion algorithms designed for individuals of normal weight (**Table 2**).

In general pharmacokinetic principles, drug dosing typically depends on the volume of distribution (VD) for determining the loading dose and the clearance rate for setting the maintenance dose, though there are exceptions to this rule [37]. For drugs primarily distributed to lean tissues, the loading dose should be based on lean body weight. If the drug is distributed equally between adipose and lean tissues, the loading dose should be calculated using total body weight. For maintenance dosing, if the drug's clearance is similar in obese and non-obese individuals, LBW is used. However, if the drug's clearance increases with obesity, the maintenance dose should be based on TBW. In obese patients, there are often exceptions to standard dosing calculations. Even with precise dosing based on lean body weight or total body weight, it may be necessary to administer additional doses. This patient population requires careful monitoring and adjustment to ensure effective and safe drug administration.

Anesthetic agents such as opioids, propofol, and benzodiazepines are known to have amplified effects in patients with obstructive sleep apnea. These drugs can reduce the tone of the pharyngeal muscles, which is crucial for maintaining airway patency [38]. Volatile anesthetics can reduce the ventilatory response to carbon dioxide, particularly in children with tonsillar hypertrophy and obstructive sleep apnea. In spontaneously breathing, tracheally intubated children with a history of OSA, even a small dose of intravenous fentanyl (0.5 μg/kg) can significantly impair ventilation and may induce apnea. An opioid-sparing anesthetic approach, including the use of local anesthesia, is supported by high levels of evidence and carries a strong recommendation grade. Doses of commonly used anesthetic drugs can be based on either total body weight or ideal body weight, depending on the drug's lipid solubility. Historically, ideal body weight was equated with non-fat weight, suggesting it may substitute for lean body weight or lean body mass (LBM), typically approximated as 120% of IBW. LBM is particularly useful for dosing hydrophilic medications. In obese patients, the volume of distribution for lipophilic drugs,

Kinetic property	Impact of escalating obesity
Blood volume and cardiac output	İncrease
Adipose and lean body mass	İncrease
Hepatic blood flow and glucuronidation rate	increase
GFR and renal excretion	increase
Cytochrome P450 isoenzymes	Variable
Renal tubular reabsorption	Decrease

Table 2.
Factors influencing drug pharmacokinetics and pharmacodynamics in obesity.

such as benzodiazepines and barbiturates, is notably altered, affecting their dosing requirements. Two exceptions to this rule are procainamide and remifentanil. Despite being highly lipophilic, their volume of distribution does not correlate with the drug's lipid solubility [39].

For vecuronium or rocuronium, the initial dose should be calculated using ideal body weight (IBW), with subsequent doses adjusted based on peripheral nerve stimulator monitoring. Achieving complete neuromuscular blockade in morbidly obese patients is crucial not only for the convenience of the surgeon but also to ensure effective mechanical ventilation. The specific neuromuscular blocker used is less important than ensuring adequate depth of paralysis.

Deep neuromuscular blockade (NMB) necessitates timely and thorough reversal at the conclusion of surgery. Although the impact of residual NMB has not been extensively studied in bariatric surgery, the physiological effects linked to residual NMB are likely to be particularly significant in this patient population [40]. Patients should undergo complete reversal of neuromuscular blockade and be closely monitored using objective methods for assessing residual blockade both during surgery and after reversal at the end of the procedure [41]. Achieving a nerve-stimulated TOF ratio of ≥ 0.9 is crucial for ensuring recovery, as it helps prevent recurarization and the need for reintubation due to persistent neuromuscular blockade [42]. Sugammadex provides significantly faster reversal of neuromuscular blockade compared to neostigmine, reversing moderate block 6.5 times faster and deep blockade 16.8 times more rapidly. Additionally, its use is associated with fewer adverse events than traditional reversal agents [43]. The dosing of Sugammadex should be tailored to the degree of neuromuscular blockade and the patient's body weight to ensure swift and complete reversal. Administering a dose of 2 mg/kg IBW ± 40% appears to strike an optimal balance between rapid recovery and a favorable side effect profile [44].

The confirmed incidence of hypersensitivity reactions to Sugammadex is approximately 5%, with anaphylaxis occurring in 0.3% of cases, predominantly at the higher dose of 16 mg/kg. However, in practice, hypersensitivity reactions are reported at a significantly lower rate. For bariatric surgery patients, a dose of 2 mg/kg IBW ± 40% is generally considered the most appropriate and safe, minimizing the risk of adverse reactions while ensuring effective neuromuscular blockade reversal [45].

Even with the aid of TOF monitoring and the use of Sugammadex, physicians must remain vigilant for the possibility of recurarization. Recurarization refers to the redistribution of rocuronium or other muscle relaxants, which can be life-threatening. Patients who have undergone such surgeries require meticulous postoperative care to monitor for any signs of residual neuromuscular blockade and ensure their safety.

7.2 Standardized anesthetic protocol and opioid-free anesthesia

The use of short-acting anesthetic agents and minimizing opioid administration during surgery are critical components for optimizing postoperative recovery. Anesthesia induction should be ideally calculated based on lean body weight to mitigate the risk of hypotension [46]. Anesthesia necessitates a comprehensive array of pharmacologic agents to formulate an effective anesthetic regimen that ensures adequate sedation, analgesia, amnesia, muscle relaxation, and suppression of reflexes. Opioid administration, whether as a bolus or continuous infusion, is commonly employed in both major and ambulatory surgical procedures. However, the consumption of opioids is connected to a range of negative effects, including reduced breathing rate, breathing suppression, increased sensitivity to pain caused by opioids, queasiness and emesis, inability to pass urine, bowel immobility, and potential mental and sleep disturbances. The adverse effect profile of opioids can lead to delayed recovery and prolonged discharge times from the post-anesthesia care unit. Additionally, these effects may contribute to increased rates of unplanned hospital readmissions [47]. Given the array of adverse effects associated with opioids, there is a growing need for alternative strategies such as opioid-free anesthesia. This approach aims to mitigate the complications and enhance patient recovery by avoiding the use of opioids altogether.

Propofol is the most commonly utilized agent for induction and has not been demonstrated to elevate the risk of rhabdomyolysis associated with propofol infusion syndrome in individuals with extreme obesity receiving typical bariatric surgical procedures [48]. When volatile anesthetics are employed for maintenance, desflurane may provide more rapid emergence compared to sevoflurane or isoflurane in patients with a body mass index exceeding 30 kg/m^2 [49]. On the other hand, in contrast to sevoflurane, which has bronchodilator effects, desflurane can increase airway resistance, as well as cause hypertension and tachycardia. Therefore, the choice of inhalational agent should be guided by the patient's comorbidities and other relevant factors.

In an opioid-free anesthesia regimen, patients received a dexmedetomidine infusion at a rate of 0.5 mcg/kg/h and started 10 minutes prior to induction, and an intravenous bolus of ketamine at 0.35 mg/kg was administered before the skin incision. The combination of lidocaine, dexmedetomidine, ketamine, and magnesium, when used in opioid-free anesthesia, may offer enhanced anti-inflammatory effects compared to traditional opioid-based approaches, potentially making it a preferable alternative [50].

The bispectral index (BIS) is one of several methods employed to monitor the depth of anesthesia, aiming to minimize intraoperative awareness and optimize the dosage of anesthetic agents. For the assessment of intraoperative awareness, both BIS and end-tidal anesthetic gas (ETAG) monitoring are utilized. Studies have demonstrated that these methods are similarly effective in reducing the incidence of intraoperative awareness when compared to reliance solely on clinical signs [51].

Additionally, the judicious use of nonsteroidal anti-inflammatory drugs (NSAIDs) can reduce opioid consumption. However, a limitation of most NSAIDs is their "low-ceiling" analgesic effect. In contrast, paracetamol does not carry the same risk of bleeding, gastric, or renal side effects that can constrain the use of NSAIDs [52]. Infiltration of bupivacaine 0.5% before incision has been shown to significantly reduce postoperative opioid consumption and alleviate pain following surgery [53].

7.3 Postoperative pain management and abdominal plane blocks

Effective pain management is crucial in the postoperative care of obese patients. The primary objectives are to provide sufficient analgesia while promoting early mobilization and maintaining optimal respiratory function. Although mobilization can be challenging in this population, it is essential for preventing complications such as pressure ulcers, pulmonary embolism, deep vein thrombosis, and pneumonia.

Pain management strategies should encompass the following options: the use of multimodal analgesics, regional anesthesia or analgesia techniques, encouraging early patient mobilization, providing supplemental oxygen, and elevating the head of the bed. Alongside the implementation of a safe analgesic approach, thorough postoperative monitoring is essential to ensure patient safety.

For individuals suffering from obstructive sleep apnea, consideration should be given to regional anesthetic approaches to lessen or eradicate the necessity for systemic opioid use, which can pose additional risks in this population. When neuraxial anesthesia is used, it is important to carefully assess the positive aspects and potential drawbacks of administering an opioid or an opioid-local anesthetic combination, as opposed to a local anesthetic alone. If patient-managed systemic opioid therapies are necessary, constant baseline infusions should generally be avoided or applied solely with careful consideration. To further minimize opioid use, nonsteroidal anti-inflammatory drugs (NSAIDs) and other alternative pain management strategies should be employed. Additionally, patients at increased perioperative risk due to OSA should receive continuous supplemental oxygen until they are able to maintain their baseline oxygen saturation while breathing room air. After discharge from the recovery room, these patients should be closely monitored with continuous pulse oximetry to detect any respiratory compromise.

Bariatric surgery typically causes moderate-to-severe pain, and in patients with obesity, the use of opioids can lead to breathing difficulties, so their use should be minimized. This study aimed to compare the effectiveness of the newer ultrasound-guided erector spinae plane block (ESPB) technique and the transversus abdominis plane (TAP) block technique against standard care in reducing intraoperative opioid use and managing postoperative pain. Both of these techniques are commonly used for postoperative pain relief in various types of surgeries. The TAP block, in particular, is also frequently employed for pain management after a cesarean section performed under general anesthesia (**Figure 3**) [54].

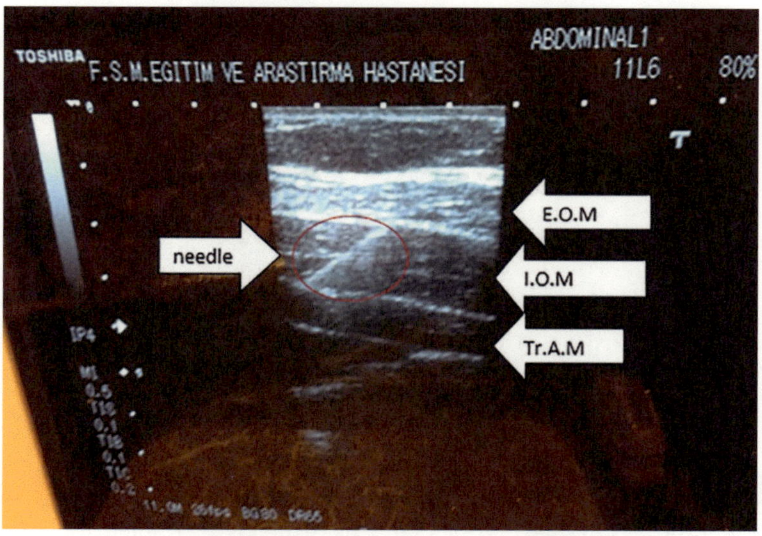

Figure 3.
Ultrasound visualization of initial TAP block injection: Needle placement and muscle layer identification.

8. Conclusion

In conclusion, bariatric surgery and the management of obesity represent a multifaceted medical journey, demanding a nuanced understanding of every aspect involved. This chapter has endeavored to shed light on these complexities, particularly in the realm of anesthetic management where significant uncertainties persist. Despite the advancements made, there remain unexplored territories and numerous gray areas that call for deeper investigation. The field is ripe for further research, and as we continue to unravel these complexities, our knowledge and practices will evolve, ultimately leading to improved outcomes for bariatric patients.

Acknowledgements

The author acknowledges the usage of ChatGPT for language editing and grammar correction of this manuscript. My sincere appreciation goes to my academic mentor, Associate Professor Dr. Barış Güven, whose guidance and expertise were instrumental in shaping the research direction of this book.

Author details

Halil Buluç
Acıbadem University, Türkiye

*Address all correspondence to: buluchalil@gmail.com

References

[1] Ng M, Fleming T, Robinson M, et al. Global, regional, and national prevalence of overweight and obesity in children and adults during 1980-2013: A systematic analysis for the global burden of disease study 2013. Lancet. 2014;**384**:766-781

[2] Buchwald H, Avidor Y, Braunwald E, Jensen MD, Pories W, Fahrbach K, et al. Bariatric surgery: A systematic review and meta-analysis. Journal of the American Medical Association. 2004;**292**:1724-1737

[3] American Society for Metabolic and Bariatric Surgery. Bariatric Surgery in Class I Obesity [Internet]. Available from: http://asmbs.org/resources/bariatric-surgery-in-class-i-obesity. [Accessed: March 21, 2020]

[4] Neto AS, Hemmes SN, Barbas CS, et al. Association between driving pressure and development of postoperative pulmonary complications in patients undergoing mechanical ventilation for general anesthesia: A meta-analysis of individual patient data. The Lancet Respiratory Medicine. 2016;**4**(4):272-280

[5] Mulier J. Opioid-free general anesthesia: A paradigm shift? Revista Española de Anestesiología y Reanimación. 2017;**64**(8):427-430

[6] Govindarajan R, Ghosh B, Sathyamoorthy MK, et al. Efficacy of ketorolac in lieu of narcotics in the operative management of laparoscopic surgery for morbid obesity. Surgery for Obesity and Related Diseases. 2005;**1**(6):530-535

[7] Foldi M, Soos A, Hegyi P, et al. Transversus abdominis plane block appears to be effective and safe as a part of multimodal analgesia in bariatric surgery: A meta-analysis and systematic review of randomized controlled trials. Obesity Surgery. 2021;**31**(2):531-543

[8] Chin KJ, Malhas L, Perlas A. The erector spinae plane block provides visceral abdominal analgesia in bariatric surgery: A report of three cases. Regional Anesthesia and Pain Medicine. 2017;**42**(3):372-376

[9] World Health Organization. Obesity: Preventing and managing the global epidemic. Report of a WHO consultation. World Health Organization Technical Report Series. 2000;**894**:1-253

[10] Acute Respiratory Distress Syndrome Network. Ventilation with lower tidal volumes as compared with traditional tidal volumes for acute lung injury and the acute respiratory distress syndrome. The New England Journal of Medicine. 2000;**342**:1301-1308

[11] Leykin Y, Miotto L, Pellis T. Pharmacokinetic considerations in the obese. Best Practice and Research. Clinical Anaesthesiology. 2011;**25**:27-36

[12] Kaw R, Michota F, Jaffer A, et al. Unrecognized sleep apnea in the surgical patient: Implications for the perioperative setting. Chest. 2006;**129**:198-205

[13] Dixon JB, Schachter LM, O'Brien PE. Predicting sleep apnea and excessive daytime sleepiness in the severely obese: Indicators for polysomnography. Chest. 2003;**123**:1134-1141

[14] Gross JB, Bachenberg KL, Benumof JL, et al. Practice guidelines for the perioperative management of patients with obstructive sleep apnea. Anesthesiology. 2006;**104**:1081-1093

[15] Memtsoudis S, Liu SS, Ma Y, et al. Perioperative pulmonary outcomes in patients with sleep apnea after noncardiac surgery. Anesthesia and Analgesia. 2011;**112**:113-121

[16] Olson AL, Zwillich C. The obesity hypoventilation syndrome. The American Journal of Medicine. 2005;**118**:948-956

[17] Moon TS, Fox PE, Somasundaram A, et al. The influence of morbid obesity on difficult intubation and difficult mask ventilation. Journal of Anesthesia. 2019;**33**(1):96-102

[18] Wong DT, Dallaire A, Singh KP, et al. High-flow nasal oxygen improves safe apnea time in morbidly obese patients undergoing general anesthesia: A randomized controlled trial. Anesthesia and Analgesia. 2019;**129**(4):1130-1136

[19] Abdelmalak B, Makary L, Hoban J, et al. Dexmedetomidine as sole sedative for awake intubation in management of the critical airway. Journal of Clinical Anesthesia. 2007;**19**:370-373

[20] Collins JS, Lemmens HJ, Brodsky JB, et al. Laryngoscopy and morbid obesity: A comparison of the "sniff" and "ramped" positions. Obesity Surgery. 2004;**14**:1171-1175

[21] Nightingale CE, Margarson MP, Shearer E, et al. Perioperative management of the obese surgical patient: Guidelines from the Association of Anaesthetists of Great Britain and Ireland. Anaesthesia. 2015;**70**(7):859-876

[22] Ezri T et al. Anesthesia for obese patients. Anaesthesia. 2003;**58**:1111-1115

[23] Lewandowski K, Lewandowski M. Intensive care in the obese. Best Practice and Research. Clinical Anaesthesiology. 2011;**25**:95-108

[24] Bluth T, Serpa Neto A, Schultz MJ, Pelosi P, Gama de Abreu M. Effect of intraoperative high positive end-expiratory pressure (PEEP) with recruitment maneuvers vs low PEEP on postoperative pulmonary complications in obese patients: A randomized clinical trial. Journal of the American Medical Association. 2019;**321**(23):2292-2305

[25] Rackley CR, MacIntyre NR. Low tidal volumes for everyone? Chest. 2019;**156**(4):783-791

[26] Futier E, Constantin JM, Paugam-Burtz C, et al. A trial of intraoperative low-tidal-volume ventilation in abdominal surgery. The New England Journal of Medicine. 2013;**369**(5):428-437

[27] Aldenkortt M, Lysakowski C, Elia N, Brochard L, Tramer MR. Ventilation strategies in obese patients undergoing surgery: A quantitative systematic review and meta-analysis. British Journal of Anaesthesia. 2012;**109**(4):493-502

[28] Ball L, Hemmes SNT, Serpa Neto A, et al. Intraoperative ventilation settings and their associations with postoperative pulmonary complications in obese patients. British Journal of Anaesthesia. 2018;**121**(4):899-908

[29] Pereira SM, Tucci MR, Morais CCA, et al. Individual positive end-expiratory pressure settings optimize intraoperative mechanical ventilation and reduce postoperative atelectasis. Anesthesiology. 2018;**129**(6):1070-1081

[30] Amato MB, Meade MO, Slutsky AS, et al. Driving pressure and survival in the acute respiratory distress syndrome. The New England Journal of Medicine. 2015;**372**(8):747-755

[31] Ball L, Pelosi P. How I ventilate an obese patient. Critical Care. 2019;**23**(1):176

[32] Cadi P, Guenoun T, Journois D, Chevallier JM, Diehl JL, Safran D. Pressure-controlled ventilation improves oxygenation during laparoscopic obesity surgery compared with volume-controlled ventilation. British Journal of Anaesthesia. 2008;**100**(5):709-716

[33] Bagchi A, Rudolph MI, Ng PY, et al. The association of postoperative pulmonary complications in 109,360 patients with pressure-controlled or volume-controlled ventilation. Anaesthesia. 2017;**72**(11):1334-1343

[34] Costa Souza GM, Santos GM, Zimpel SA, Melnik T. Intraoperative ventilation strategies for obese patients undergoing bariatric surgery: Systematic review and meta-analysis. BMC Anesthesiology. 2020;**20**:36

[35] Finer N. Medical consequences of obesity. Medicine. 2011;**39**:18-23

[36] Fraley MA, Birchem JA, Senkottaiyan N, et al. Obesity and the electrocardiogram. Obesity Reviews. 2005;**6**:275-281

[37] Casati A, Putzu M. Anesthesia in the obese patient: Pharmacokinetic considerations. Journal of Clinical Anesthesia. 2005;**17**:134-145

[38] Dhonneur G et al. Anesthesia and Analgesia. 1999;**89**:762-767

[39] Ogunnaike BO et al. Anesthesia and Analgesia. 2002;**95**:1793-1798

[40] Schreiber JU. Management of neuromuscular blockade in ambulatory patients. Current Opinion in Anaesthesiology. 2014;**27**(6):583-588

[41] Kopman AF, Naguib M. Laparoscopic surgery and muscle relaxants: Is deep block helpful? Anesthesia and Analgesia. 2015;**120**(1):51-58

[42] Sauer M, Stahn A, Soltesz S, Noeldge-Schomburg G, Mencke T. The influence of residual neuromuscular block on the incidence of critical respiratory events. European Journal of Anaesthesiology. 2011;**28**(12):842-848

[43] Hristovska AM, Duch P, Allingstrup M, Afshari A. Comparative efficacy and safety of sugammadex and neostigmine in reversing neuromuscular blockade in adults. Anaesthesia. 2018;**73**(5):631-641

[44] Badaoui R, Cabaret A, Alami Y, et al. Reversal of neuromuscular blockade by sugammadex in laparoscopic bariatric surgery: In support of dose reduction. Anaesthesia Critical Care and Pain Medicine. 2016;**35**(1):25-29

[45] Min KC, Bondiskey P, Schulz V, et al. Hypersensitivity incidence after sugammadex administration in healthy subjects: A randomized controlled trial. British Journal of Anaesthesia. 2018;**121**(4):749-757

[46] Ingrande J, Brodsky JB, Lemmens HJ. Lean body weight scalar for the anesthetic induction dose of propofol in morbidly obese subjects. Anesthesia and Analgesia. 2011;**113**(1):57-62

[47] Dinges HC, Otto S, Stay DK, Bäumlein S, Waldmann S, Kranke P, et al. Side-effect rates of opioids in equianalgesic doses via intravenous patient-controlled analgesia: A systematic review and network meta-analysis. Anesthesia and Analgesia. 2019;**129**:1153-1162

[48] Lehavi A, Sandler O, Mahajna A, Weissman A, Katz YS. Comparison of rhabdomyolysis markers in patients undergoing bariatric surgery with propofol and inhalation-based anesthesia. Obesity Surgery. 2015;**25**(10):1923-1927

[49] Singh PM, Borle A, McGavin J, Trikha A, Sinha A. Comparison of the recovery profile between desflurane and sevoflurane in patients undergoing bariatric surgery: A meta-analysis of randomized controlled trials. Obesity Surgery. 2017;**27**(11):3031-3039

[50] Mulier JPDB. A prospective randomized controlled trial comparing a multitarget opioid-free anesthesia (OFA) and a 3-Liter volume calculated airseal carbon dioxide insufflator with a balanced anesthesia using sufentanil-sevoflurane and a standard 15 mmHg carbon dioxide pressure pneumoperitoneum insufflator. Journal of Clinical Anesthesia and Pain Management. 2018;**2**(2):6

[51] Avidan MS, Jacobsohn E, Glick D, et al. Prevention of intraoperative awareness in a high-risk surgical population. The New England Journal of Medicine. 2011;**365**(7):591-600

[52] Beloeil H, Albaladejo P, Sion A, et al. Multicentre, prospective, double-blind, randomised controlled clinical trial comparing different non-opioid analgesic combinations with morphine for postoperative analgesia: The OCTOPUS study. British Journal of Anaesthesia. 2019;**122**(6):106

[53] Boerboom SL, de Haes A, Vd Wetering L, et al. Preperitoneal bupivacaine infiltration reduces postoperative opioid consumption, acute pain, and chronic postsurgical pain after bariatric surgery: A randomized controlled trial. Obesity Surgery. 2018;**28**(10):3102-3110

[54] Buluc H, Yildirim A, Turan G, Karadogan F, Sargin MA, Akgun N. The efficacy of transversus abdominis plane block for post-operative analgesia after cesarean section performed under general anesthesia. Northern Clinics of Istanbul. 2019;**6**(4):368-373

Section 3

Surgical and Endoscopic Bariatric Procedures

Chapter 5

Sleeve Gastrectomy: Surgical and Endoscopic Approaches

Sedat Carkit and Mustafa Karaagac

Abstract

Sleeve gastrectomy (SG) is the most frequently performed bariatric procedure worldwide, accounting for more than 55% of all bariatric procedures. Due to its prevalence and its numerous costly complications, such as diabetes and heart disease, as well as disability and loss of productivity, obesity is more expensive than any other health issue. Diet, exercise, and behavior modification are the foundational elements of any meaningful initiative for significant and lasting weight loss. Unfortunately, for the morbidly obese, these measures alone almost invariably fail to achieve acceptable long-term weight loss. This article will be comprehensive and detail all approaches used in the implementation of sleeve gastrectomy, providing readers with all the necessary tools to perform an excellent SG.

Keywords: sleeve gastrectomy, obesity, bariatric surgery, weight loss surgery, metabolic surgery

1. Introduction

Sleeve gastrectomy is not an independent procedure but has emerged as a staged surgery in bariatric surgeries. Historically, it began with gastroplasty, which was performed in anti-reflux surgeries [1]. The first known procedure was carried out in March 1988 by Dr. Doug Hess in Bowling Green, Ohio, as part of a more extensive duodenal switch operation [2]. But as time has gone on, sleeve gastrectomy has emerged as a stand-alone therapeutic option thanks to its high rate of weight loss and favorable safety profile [3]. In high-risk patients with a body mass index (BMI) > 50 kg/m^2, Almogy et al. suggested longitudinal gastrectomy (LG) as a safe substitute for duodenal switch, which was thought to be the most successful weight loss procedure at the time [4]. The procedure's popularity has increased because of its high success rate in weight loss and relative simplicity when compared to other bariatric operations. The eighth report from the International Federation for the Surgery of Obesity and Metabolic Disorders (IFSO) in 2023 states that, with 60.4% of all metabolic procedures performed worldwide, sleeve gastrectomy (SG) is presently the most often performed bariatric procedure [5].

2. Epidemiology

Obesity has been recognized as a chronic disease requiring a multifactorial, multidisciplinary approach by the American Medical Association in 2013. This definition includes several subcategories: deviations from routine physiology, persistence for over a year, the necessity for continuous medical treatment, and impairment in daily living activities. The prevalence of obesity continues to rise at an alarming rate [6, 7]. This increase in obesity prevalence also raises the burden of chronic diseases and comorbidities associated with obesity. Therefore, managing obesity has become a public health priority. Obesity was always thought to be a problem that primarily affected high-income nations, but in recent years, it has become a major public health concern in low- and middle-income nations, encompassing both urban areas and underserved regions. The etiology of obesity is complex and only partially understood. Genetic, epigenetic, environmental, and psychological factors all play varying roles, but conceptually, obesity is an energy imbalance disorder characterized by an increase in stored fat that endangers an individual's organ function, disease susceptibility, and overall health. Obesity has been shown to predispose individuals to numerous diseases, including cardiovascular disease, diabetes mellitus, sleep apnea, and osteoarthritis.

3. Financial impact

There are studies indicating that obesity significantly increases annual medical expenses [8]. This increase correlates with the severity of obesity. Specifically, the costs associated with morbid obesity, including hypertension, diabetes mellitus, joint diseases, and related surgeries, are substantial.

4. Psychological impact

The stigma attached to obesity might worsen the problem by encouraging bad eating patterns and a decrease in physical activity [9]. Additionally, it has been noted that obese people frequently cancel or significantly delay their doctor appointments. This avoidance feeds the cycle of health problems associated with obesity and makes it more difficult for them to receive the essential healthcare.

5. Indications and contraindications

Morbid obesity is defined as a body mass index (BMI) of 40 kg/m^2 or higher, which indicates an individual's body weight in relation to their height in square meters. Overweight is defined as a BMI greater than 25 kg/m^2; class I obesity ranges from 30 to 34.9 kg/m^2; class II obesity from 35 to 39.9 kg/m^2; class III obesity $\geq$40 kg/m^2; and super morbid obesity is defined as a BMI greater than 50 kg/m^2 [10]. Patients with severe obesity who are unable to lose enough weight with diet, exercise, or other non-surgical means may benefit from bariatric surgery. The 1991 National Institutes of Health bariatric surgery recommendations were revised in 2022 by the American Society for Metabolic and Bariatric Surgery (ASMBS) and the International Federation for the

Surgery of Obesity and Metabolic Disorders (IFSO) [11]. The initially defined eligibility criteria stipulated that a BMI of ≥40 kg/m^2 without accompanying diseases or a BMI of 35–40 kg/m^2 with some associated disorders (hypertension, dyslipidemia, diabetes, and severe sleep apnea) qualifies for the procedure. Additionally, the American Academy of Pediatrics and the ASMBS recommend the consideration of metabolic and bariatric surgery (MBS) in children and adolescents whose BMI exceeds 120% of the 95th percentile or surpasses 140% of the 95th percentile and have serious comorbidities [12]. In this patient group, sleeve gastrectomy is the most commonly performed surgical intervention due to comparative weight loss outcomes and desired safety profiles [12]. For morbidly obese patients with gastrointestinal stromal tumors (GISTs), gastric neuroendocrine tumors, or illnesses requiring endoscopic evaluation of the stomach, sleeve gastrectomy (SG) is a great choice for weight management [13]. Recent years have seen growing awareness of the relationship between obesity and transplantation. Numerous studies have demonstrated that obesity causes glomerular hyperfiltration in patients with chronic kidney disease (CKD), leading to structural abnormalities in glomeruli similar to those seen in cases with reduced renal mass [14]. From a bariatric perspective, approximately 21% of patients with CKD are obese [15]. An estimated 750 MBS procedures are performed annually in CKD patients, and 400 to 450 in patients with end-stage renal disease (ESRD) [16]. These figures indicate that only a small portion of these patients are directed toward or undergo these surgeries. However, MBS is used to make CKD and ESRD patients suitable candidates for transplantation. According to a 2013 statement from the American Association for the Study of Liver Diseases (AASLD), having a BMI of 40 or higher puts a person at high risk of complications after receiving a liver transplant [17]. Patients who are extremely obese and have liver disease can benefit from bariatric surgery as a bridge to liver transplantation (LT). For this patient population, SG is becoming the go-to choice both before and after transplantation [18].

There are very few absolute contraindications for laparoscopic sleeve gastrectomy, and they usually correspond with the lists of contraindications for other elective surgical operations. Patients who are considered to be at high risk for surgery should not be suggested to have surgery, including those who have uncorrectable coagulopathy or are contraindicated for general anesthesia.

Patients with metastatic or incurable cancers, as well as those with irreversible cardiopulmonary failure or other organ failures that reduce life expectancy, should not have a sleeve gastrectomy. Furthermore, patients who are pregnant or intend to get pregnant within a year after surgery should postpone the procedure.

A restricted ability to understand the surgical procedure or the lifelong behavioral modifications required for postoperative success and safety are examples of relative contraindications. Patients also need to be able, willing, and motivated to follow through on dietary supplements, follow-up care, and lifestyle modifications following surgery. Relative contraindications for surgery include untreated serious psychological illnesses and active substance misuse, particularly drug or alcohol dependency. Sleeve gastrectomy should be delayed in individuals with active peptic ulcer disease until evidence of successful treatment is obtained.

6. Surgical procedure

Preoperative antibiotics and venous thromboembolic prophylaxis are given, or at least before induction. The patient is placed in a split-leg or supine position.

To get into the reverse Trendelenburg posture, utilize a footboard. Port placement is comparable to gastric bypass; however, since stapling is done with one or two ports, fewer 12-mm ports are needed. In addition to the additional incision for the liver retractor, four or five ports are employed. Two ports measuring 15 and 12 mm are used, with the remaining ports measuring 5 mm. After then, the 15-mm port is utilized, for instance, to remove samples. The gastroesophageal junction and the proximal stomach are visible due to the retraction of the left liver lobe. The Trendelenburg position is reversed for the patient. After locating the pylorus, a location on the stomach's larger curvature that is 4 cm from the pylorus is chosen for the first dissection. The antral pump mechanism is maintained at this 4 cm separation. Alternatively, the dissection could begin at this place and work its way back to the mid-body on the greater curvature. It is easy to enter the smaller pouch at this point. The gastroepiploic arcade is separated along the full length of the greater curvature of the stomach, including short gastric arteries, and the entrance to the decreased pouch is produced using an ultrasonic scalpel or bipolar energy device. In order to minimize the quantity of fat linked to the gastrectomy specimen and facilitate its removal, dissection should occur extremely close to the larger curvature and cut the gastroepiploic veins that are attached to it (**Figure 1**). The fundus is fully mobilized upon division of the phrenoesophageal ligament, which also facilitates the diagnosis of hiatal hernias. The distal esophagus is pulled into the abdominal cavity and released from mediastinal attachments if a hiatal hernia is discovered. With permanent sutures, the crura are approximated posteriorly (**Figure 2**). The mobility of the stomach body is finished with the dissection of adhesions to the posterior stomach that are connected to the pancreas and retroperitoneum (**Figure 3**). The anesthetist inserts a bougie and

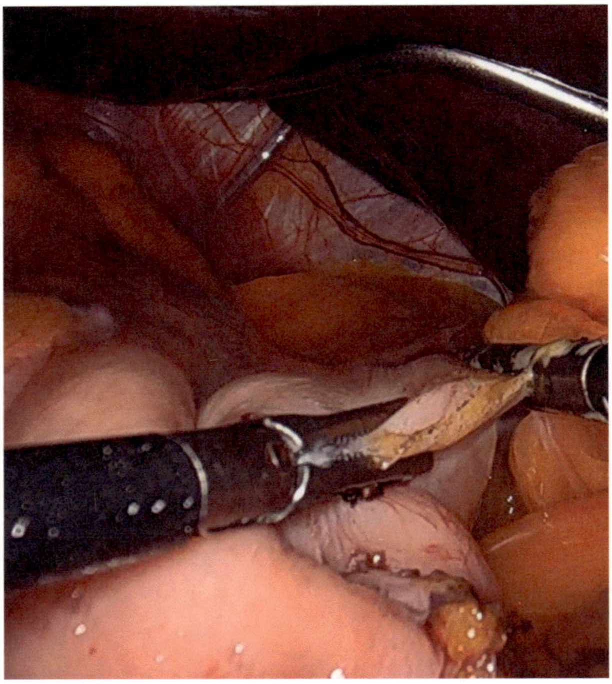

Figure 1.
Release of the greater curvature of the stomach from the omentum.

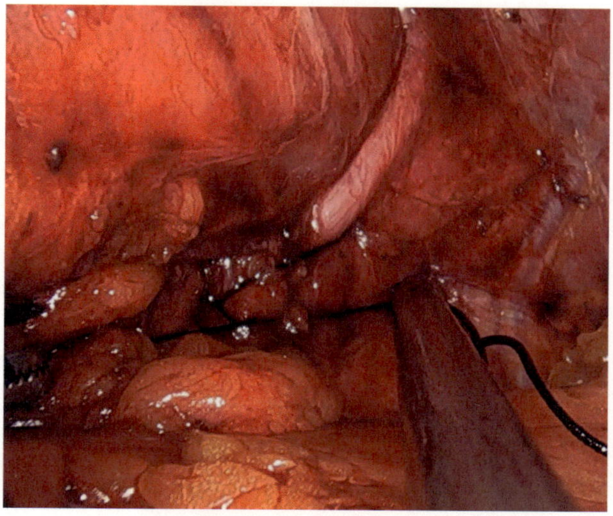

Figure 2.
Discovered hiatal hernia repair by permanent sutures.

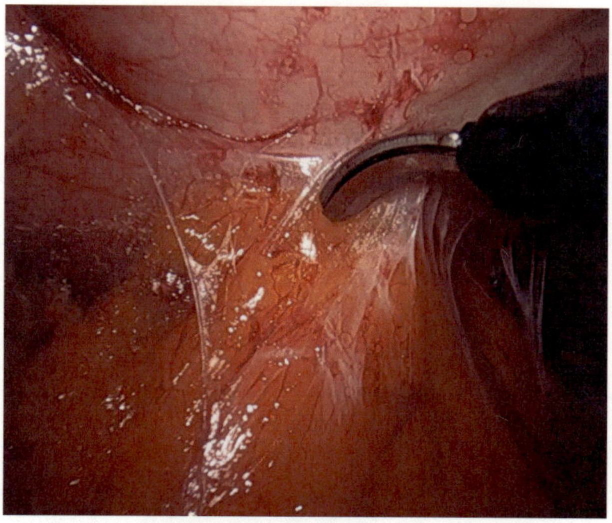

Figure 3.
Dissection of adhesions to the posterior stomach with connection to the pancreas and retroperitoneum.

removes any orogastric tubes that have been previously inserted before stapling. With the surgeon's assistance and guidance, the bougie is placed along the lesser curvature and directed toward the pylorus (**Figure 4**).

The bougie dilator comes in sizes ranging from 32 to 50 French, however 36 French is the most popular size. An Ewald gastric lavage tube, measuring 34 French sizes, is a large size that works well for methylene blue leakage testing. It is crucial to keep the bougie and stapler separated by 1–2 mm when using a bougie with a smaller diameter. With the use of a grasper, the surgeon evaluates this. The right upper quadrant port is used to insert the first linear stapler loading, and the sleeve resection is started at 4–5 cm in front of the pylorus. For the first firing, 60 mm stapler cartridges with a closed height of 2.3 or 2 mm are utilized; as the fundus's tissue thickness lowers, blue

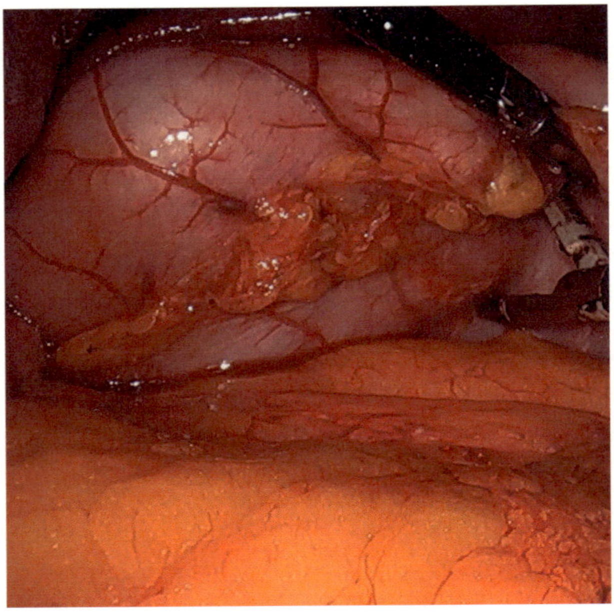

Figure 4.
The bougie is placed along the lesser curvature and directed toward the pylorus.

(1.5 mm) cartridges are employed. Hemostasis is aided by adjusting the stapler height to match tissue thickness. Because stenosis is typical at this level, care is exercised when stapling in close proximity to the incisura angularis. The anterior and posterior walls are taken in equal amounts to prevent the stapler line from bending or spiraling (**Figure 5**). This is facilitated by stretching the greater curvature when placing the stapler. Usually, the stapler needs to be fired six or seven times. It is debatable if the stapler line should be reinforced. Roughly 80% of surgeons utilize reinforcing

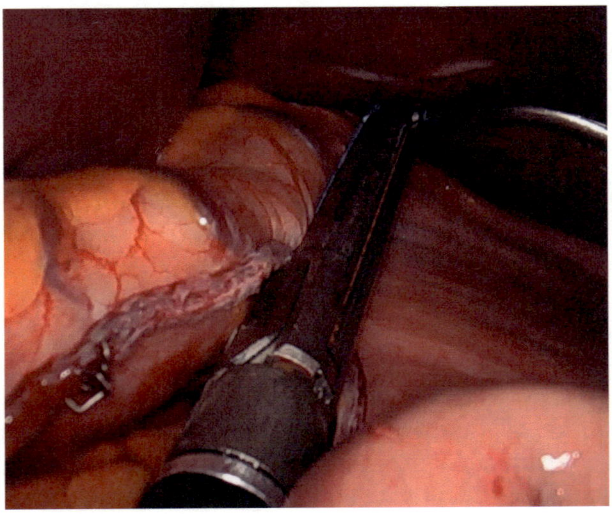

Figure 5.
The stapling procedure was performed with the removal of equal amounts of tissue from both the anterior and posterior walls.

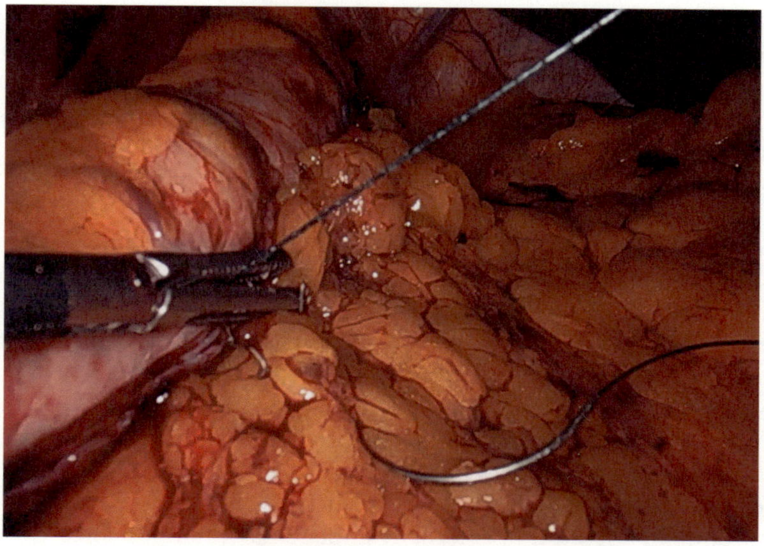

Figure 6.
Suturing staple line.

material of some kind; 60% use absorbable materials, while the remaining physicians suture the stapler line (**Figure 6**). The use of reinforcing material was linked to a lower incidence of stapler line bleeding, according to a 2016 meta-analysis, although there was no discernible drop in leakage rates [19]. Suturing the stapler line has not shown a clear advantage. The integrity of the stapler line can be tested by injecting 50–100 mL of methylene blue into saline solution or intraoperative endoscopy, which facilitates the detection of stenosis or intraluminal bleeding. Routine intraoperative leakage tests lack supporting data for their ability to detect leaks, although they are common. Some surgeons perform omentoplasty to restore the natural direction of the sleeve, reduce twisting, and further support the stapler line by suturing the gastric omentum to the stapler line or reinforcement material. However, data supporting this practice are lacking. Drains aren't utilized frequently. One of the port sites is used to remove the specimen. It is usually not necessary to widen the site when using a 15 mm port. Every port site with a diameter of 12 mm or more is closed. Using a transabdominal suture technique, we typically place two sutures in the 15 mm port site and one suture in the 12 mm site. It is not necessary to close the 12 mm sites while using non-cutting trocars.

7. Endoscopic procedure

Endoscopy has become an essential part of managing complications after sleeve gastrectomy, and a variety of endoscopic weight loss procedures are being used or developed. The American Society for Gastrointestinal Endoscopy's Standards of Practice Committee and representatives from the Society of Gastrointestinal and Endoscopic Surgeons and ASMBS published guidelines regarding this matter in 2015. They concluded that the use of endoscopy should be decided in close consultation between the patient and the surgeon. The ASMBS recommends considering endoscopy in the evaluation of patients with a history of gastroesophageal reflux disease

(GERD). The largest unknown is the number of asymptomatic patients who have significant endoscopic findings. In a large review of 28 studies involving 6616 patients, it was found that the majority of preoperative endoscopic findings (92.4%) did not alter the treatment course, but 7.6% had findings that delayed or changed the surgery [20]. This supports performing routine preoperative endoscopy to avoid unexpected situations during surgery. Therefore, before bariatric surgery, symptomatic patients must undergo endoscopy, and preoperative endoscopy should be considered for asymptomatic patients.

Many surgeons perform intraoperative leakage tests in the operating room to prevent complications after the procedure. The leakage test method can vary from using methylene blue via an orogastric tube to insufflation with air through a tube or endoscope. When using the insufflation test, the stapler line and any proximal anastomosis are submerged under sterile saline, and air is insufflated into the gastric pouch. The presence of air bubbles is then assessed to determine if the stapler lines are air-tight under hyper-distension. The advantage of an endoscope is that it can be both diagnostic and therapeutic during surgery. If a leak is detected, it can be managed with endoscopic clips or sutured externally under endoscopic guidance. Furthermore, any bleeding along the stapler line can be managed immediately when clinically apparent rather than deferring to a potential return to the operating room later. Finally, endoscopy allows the surgeon to assess the postoperative anatomy thoroughly and ensure that it appears as intended.

After the anatomy of a patient is altered for a weight loss procedure, endoscopy is invaluable for assessing patients who return with abdominal complaints, regain weight, or develop complications related to their procedures. Understanding the surgical anatomy after a bariatric procedure can be challenging, especially if the surgery was performed many years ago. The most commonly known procedures include gastric bypass, vertical Laparoscopic Sleeve Gastrectomy (LSG), gastric banding, and vertical banded gastroplasty. Leaks are one of the most feared complications following bariatric surgery. They carry a high mortality rate and are among the complications that surgeons most want to avoid. One of the most frequently used interventions for a leak is the use of a fully covered stent. The endoscopically placed stent traverses the perforation to decrease further contamination. This may allow the patient to continue oral intake during the postoperative period. A study describing stenting reported a 90% success rate with a healing time of 6 weeks. Stent migration occurred in 8/20 patients, indicating an important concern related to these stents and appearing as the Achilles' heel of this management approach [21]. Several preventive methods have been described to prevent migration, including suturing or clipping the stent in place. Clips often fail because they detach quickly, and stents are usually left in place for four to 6 weeks. Suturing can be placed endoscopically, but these devices can be cumbersome in such small areas. A sutured stent can be bridged to the nose. Fluoroscopy is necessary to ensure proper stent placement. Leaks following LSG can be particularly challenging, as existing stents in the United States are not long enough to traverse the entire sleeve. Many individuals use two overlapping stents to alleviate this issue. Another approach to leak management is the use of endoscopic clips over fluoroscopic guidance. This technology typically works better for small, chronic leaks or fistulas measuring less than 1 cm, provided the opening is not too small and the edges are fresh. Endoscopic vacuum-assisted closure is now being used for sealing large leaks. This technique involves placing a vacuum sponge at the end of an orogastric tube into the cavity outside the leak to promote closure over time. This is effective for encapsulated leaks. This technique requires intensive management, as it necessitates changing the device every few days like conventional vacuum devices. Overall, patients may require 8 to 12 procedures over weeks. The benefit of this technique is that it can significantly shorten recovery times compared to traditional methods. If the opening is small but the external cavity is larger, a double pigtail stent can be used for internal drainage. This allows the internal drainage of the extraluminal cavity, which is especially useful in situations where placing an external drain is difficult. In cases where the opening is small, endoscopic septotomy has also been performed to ensure better drainage of the extraluminal cavity.

8. Postoperative care

The defined postoperative care protocol emphasizes a comprehensive approach to the patient's recovery that focuses on pain management, nutritional support, and the prevention of complications.

8.1 Pain management

A multimodal pain control strategy is implemented to ensure the effective alleviation of pain. This includes the administration of regular and breakthrough analgesics, as well as antiemetic therapy as needed. The goal is to ensure a pain score of less than 4 on an 11-point scale within 30 minutes post-surgery and to keep patients pain-free at rest. Regular assessment of pain and prompt adjustments to the analgesic regimen are particularly important for patients with a higher risk of complications due to cardiopulmonary issues.

8.2 Nutritional support

Nutritional care begins on postoperative day zero with a liquid diet of clear fluids necessary for hydration without overstressing the digestive system. On the first postoperative day, the diet is advanced to full liquids as tolerated. To enhance recovery and wound healing, routine meals along with three daily protein supplement servings are provided. A dietitian consults with patients on the first postoperative day to ensure understanding and compliance with nutritional plans.

8.3 Deep vein thrombosis

To reduce the risk of deep vein thrombosis (DVT), chemoprophylaxis is initiated in most patients on postoperative day zero. However, in patients with coagulopathy or those who have undergone complex surgeries, prophylaxis may be delayed until the first postoperative day. Decisions regarding extended thromboprophylaxis after discharge are based on the patient's risk assessment tool [22].

8.4 Discharge criteria

Patients are generally discharged on the first or second postoperative day based on their ability to tolerate oral intake, effective symptom management, and stable lab results along with vital signs. This comprehensive assessment ensures that patients are ready to continue their recovery process at home.

This structured approach to postoperative care aims to optimize recovery outcomes, enhance patient comfort, and reduce the risk of complications.

9. Outcomes

LSG (Laparoscopic Sleeve Gastrectomy) is associated with permanent weight loss and resolution of accompanying medical issues. While weight loss is somewhat lower than that following gastric bypass, it is greater than that achieved with gastric banding [23]. The literature reports that excess weight loss within 1 year following LSG varies between 51 and 71% [24, 25]. It has been demonstrated that LSG improves accompanying medical issues comparably to gastric bypass. Hutter et al. [23] found no significant difference in the resolution of medical issues following LSG compared to LRYGB, with the notable exception of GERD (Gastroesophageal Reflux Disease), which poses a significant risk in LSG procedures. According to one study, patients with preoperative GERD do worse after LSG than individuals without a history of GERD, especially in terms of morbidity and reoperation rates [26]. Two major consensus conferences have been conducted among experts regarding sleeve gastrectomy, and their findings were published in the literature. The first consensus conference [24] confirmed that this procedure provides a weight loss of 59% excess weight in 1 year, decreasing to 50% in 6 years. The mortality rate is 0.33%, and serious complications are rare, with leakage (1.1%), bleeding (1.8%), and stenosis (0.9%) reported. Experts at the second consensus conference stated that while preoperative GERD may not always imply total contraindication, it should be carefully evaluated. Randomized, prospective studies have demonstrated that LSG can effectively address medical problems and help people lose weight. The STAMPEDE trial showed a 24% resolution rate of type 2 diabetes with LSG at 5 years, compared to a 5% resolution in the medical therapy group [27]. It was established by the Swiss Randomized Trial [25] that LSG and LRYGB both offer similar weight loss benefits. Prospective studies continue to show the benefit of LRYGB for type 2 diabetes, despite a recent assessment of the data suggesting that LSG may offer similar rates of remission [27].

10. Complications

A relatively low rate of morbidity and mortality is linked to LSG. A recent study using a large database found that the risk of significant morbidity was 3.8% and the rate of 30-day mortality was 0.1%. Reoperation rates are 1.6% on record [28].

After LSG, stapler line leakage and stapler line bleeding are the most frequent consequences. The standard report for stapler line bleeding is approximately 1%; the rate drops to 0.75 percent when tissue support material is used. Similar reports place stapler line leak rates at around 1%; however, the incidence of leaks could rise from 0.65% to 0.96% if support material is used [29].

Another frequently reported complication following LSG is stapler line stenosis, which typically has an incidence of between 1% and 2% and may require reoperation if dilation does not sufficiently relieve obstructive symptoms.

Adapting to the anatomy of LSG may be challenging for some patients. Even if it is confirmed that there is no obstructive anatomy after surgery, a small percentage of patients (4–6%) experience persistent nausea up to 3 months after the procedure.

The incidence of late complications following LSG is relatively low, particularly compared to LRYGB, which can lead to issues such as bowel obstruction and marginal ulcers in the long term. New-onset GERD may develop post-LSG, with an estimated incidence of 8% [30].

Data regarding weight regain following LSG has only recently begun to emerge, with results approaching 10 years post-application indicating the incidence may not be significantly higher than that of LRYGB.

11. Revision surgery after sleeve gastrectomy

Weight gain, insufficient weight loss, and gastroesophageal reflux illness are the most frequent reasons to convert SG to Roux-en-Y gastric bypass (RYGB) [31]. Clapp et al. did a meta-analysis assessing the long-term (7 years or more) outcomes of SG and found no heterogeneity in the recurrence rate of 27.8% (<50% EWL) (95% CI: 22.8–32.7%). Weight gain and GERD were reported to have caused revision rates of 13.1% (95% CI: 5.6–20.6%) and 2.9% (95% CI: 1.0–4.9%), respectively [32]. To gain a better understanding of the safety profile of SG-RYGB, Dang and colleagues compared this revision metabolic treatment with primary RYGB (P-RYGB) using the Metabolic and Bariatric Surgery Accreditation and Quality Improvement Program (MBSAQIP) database.

They found that the probability of major problems was higher for SG-RYGB than for P-RYGB (%7.2 versus %5, respectively, $p < 0.001$). Additionally, there was a statistically significant increase in the incidence of readmission (7.3% compared to 4.8%, $p < 0.001$), reoperation (3% versus 1.9%, $p < 0.001$), deep surgical site infection (1% versus 0.5%, $p < 0.001$), sepsis (0.3% versus 0.1%, $p < 0.001$), and postoperative hemorrhage (2% versus 1.6%, $p < 0.001$). The 30-day death rate, however, did not differ statistically significantly (1% versus 1%, $p = 0.385$) [31]. A thorough systematic review and meta-analysis was carried out by Dantas and associates with the aim of assessing one-anastomosis gastric bypass (OAGB) as a feasible and safe alternative after sleeve gastrectomy (SG) that failed because of weight increase or insufficient weight loss.

It was observed that the duration from SG entrance to OAGB conversion ranged from 38.5 to 68.4 months. The results of the investigation demonstrated that, on average, OAGB produces superior results for total weight loss (TWL) than does Roux-en-Y gastric bypass (RYGB) ($p < 0.01$) [32]. Despite the fact that there was no statistically significant difference in the overall incidence of complications between the two surgical techniques, the researchers warn against bias because of study heterogeneity. Furthermore, the study indicated that further research should be done in this area as there is currently insufficient long-term nutritional data required to support the safety profile of OAGB [33].

In a modified Delphi consensus on reoperation after sleeve gastrectomy, published recently by Kermansaravi et al., 91.3% of participants agreed that all revision procedures after SG should undergo evaluation by a multidisciplinary team (MDT). Moreover, 95.6% advised endoscopy (EGD) prior to starting any conversion or revision. Moreover, 97.8% of respondents said RYGB was a suitable choice. On the other hand, the majority (93.3%, 93.3%, and 95.5%, respectively) did not view biliopancreatic diversion/duodenal switch (BPD/DS), single-anastomosis duodenal ileal bypass (SADI-S), and single-anastomosis sleeve ileal bypass (SASI) as viable alternatives for revision following sleeve gastrectomy [34].

12. Conclusions

It is evident that the rise in obesity rates is not just affecting adults; younger groups are also starting to express concern about it. This pattern is especially concerning since it creates the foundation for several health issues in the future. The expanding obesity pandemic emphasizes how urgently a comprehensive plan of action is required to address this escalating health issue.

All things considered, sleeve gastrectomy is a dependable and successful surgical option, especially for young patients and those with complicated medical requirements associated with immune system compromised states or transplants. In comparison to previous bariatric operations, this method not only offers a lower risk profile but also enables significant weight loss. Future developments in sleeve gastrectomy procedures might make use of advances in technologies and surgical methods to boost accuracy and design individualized patient care plans based on comprehensive preoperative screening to maximize results.

Conflict of interest

The authors declare no conflict of interest.

Financial support and sponsorship

The authors report no funding sources for this article.

Author details

Sedat Carkit* and Mustafa Karaagac
Erciyes University Faculty of Medicine, Kayseri, Turkey

*Address all correspondence to: opdrsedatcarkit@gmail.com

References

[1] DeMeester T, Fuchs KH, Ball CS, Albertucci M, Smyrk T, Marcus JN. Experimental and clinical results with proximal end-to-end duodenojejunostomy for pathologic duodenogastric reflux. Annals of Surgery. 1987;**206**(4):414

[2] Hess DS, Hess DW. Biliopancreatic diversion with a duodenal switch. Obesity Surgery. 1998;**8**(3):267-282

[3] Stefura T, Kacprzyk A, Droś J, Chłopaś K, Wysocki M, Rzepa A, et al. The hundred most frequently cited studies on sleeve gastrectomy. Wideochir Inne Tech Maloinwazyjne. 2020;**15**(2):249-267

[4] Almogy G, Crookes PF, Anthone GJ. Longitudinal gastrectomy as a treatment for the high-risk super-obese patient. Obesity Surgery. 2004;**14**(4):492-497

[5] Tish S, Corcelles R. The art of sleeve gastrectomy. Journal of Clinical Medicine. 2024;**13**(7):1954

[6] Hales CM, Fryar CD, Carroll MD, Freedman DS, Ogden CL. Trends in obesity and severe obesity prevalence in US youth and adults by sex and age, 2007-2008 to 2015-2016. Journal of the American Medical Association. 2018;**319**(16):1723-1725

[7] Yoon K-H, Lee J-H, Kim J-W, Cho JH, Choi Y-H, Ko S-H, et al. Epidemic obesity and type 2 diabetes in Asia. The Lancet. 2006;**368**(9548):1681-1688

[8] Cawley J, Biener A, Meyerhoefer C, Ding Y, Zvenyach T, Smolarz BG, et al. Direct medical costs of obesity in the United States and the most populous states. Journal of Managed Care & Specialty Pharmacy. 2021;**27**(3):354-366

[9] Forse RA, Betancourt-Garcia MM, Kissee MC. Epidemiology and discrimination in obesity. In: The ASMBS Textbook of Bariatric Surgery. Cham, Switzerland: Springer; 2020. pp. 3-14

[10] Mokdad AH, Bowman BA, Ford ES, Vinicor F, Marks JS, Koplan JP. The continuing epidemics of obesity and diabetes in the United States. Journal of the American Medical Association. 2001;**286**(10):1195-1200

[11] Eisenberg D, Shikora SA, Aarts E, Aminian A, Angrisani L, Cohen RV, et al. 2022 American Society of Metabolic and Bariatric Surgery (ASMBS) and International Federation for the Surgery of Obesity and Metabolic Disorders (IFSO) Indications for Metabolic and Bariatric Surgery. Cham, Switzerland: Springer; 2023

[12] Pratt JS, Browne A, Browne NT, Bruzoni M, Cohen M, Desai A, et al. ASMBS pediatric metabolic and bariatric surgery guidelines, 2018. Surgery for Obesity and Related Diseases. 2018;**14**(7):882-901

[13] Hashimoto K, Sakaguchi Y, Nambara S, Kudou K, Kusumoto E, Yoshinaga K, et al. Laparoscopic sleeve gastrectomy performed in a morbidly obese patient with gastrointestinal stromal tumor: A case report and literature review. Surgical Case Reports. 2020;**6**:1-5

[14] Tsuboi N, Utsunomiya Y, Kanzaki G, Koike K, Ikegami M, Kawamura T, et al. Low glomerular density with glomerulomegaly in obesity-related glomerulopathy. Clinical Journal of the American Society of Nephrology. 2012;7(5):735-741

[15] Silveira FC, Martin WP, Maranga G, le Roux CW, Ren-Fielding CJ. The impact of CKD on perioperative risk and mortality after bariatric surgery. Kidney360. 2021;**2**(2):236-244

[16] Cohen JB, Tewksbury CM, Torres Landa S, Williams NN, Dumon KR. National postoperative bariatric surgery outcomes in patients with chronic kidney disease and end-stage kidney disease. Obesity Surgery. 2019;**29**:975-982

[17] Martin P, DiMartini A, Feng S, Brown R Jr, Fallon M. Evaluation for liver transplantation in adults: 2013 practice guideline by the American Association for the Study of Liver Diseases and the American Society of Transplantation. Hepatology. 2014;**59**(3):1144-1165

[18] Ahmed Z, Khan MA, Vazquez-Montesino LM, Ahmed A. Bariatric surgery, obesity and liver transplantation. Translational Gastroenterology and Hepatology. 2022;**7**:25

[19] Wang Z, Dai X, Xie H, Feng J, Li Z, Lu Q. The efficacy of staple line reinforcement during laparoscopic sleeve gastrectomy: A meta-analysis of randomized controlled trials. International Journal of Surgery. 2016;**25**:145-152

[20] Parikh M, Liu J, Vieira D, Tzimas D, Horwitz D, Antony A, et al. Preoperative endoscopy prior to bariatric surgery: A systematic review and meta-analysis of the literature. Obesity Surgery. 2016;**26**:2961-2966

[21] Aryaie AH, Singer JL, Fayezizadeh M, Lash J, Marks JM. Efficacy of endoscopic management of leak after foregut surgery with endoscopic covered self-expanding metal stents (SEMS). Surgical Endoscopy. 2017;**31**:612-617

[22] MacDougall K, Spyropoulos AC. New paradigms of extended thromboprophylaxis in medically ill patients. Journal of Clinical Medicine. 2020;**9**(4):1002

[23] Hutter MM, Schirmer BD, Jones DB, Ko CY, Cohen ME, Merkow RP, et al. First report from the American College of Surgeons bariatric surgery center network: Laparoscopic sleeve gastrectomy has morbidity and effectiveness positioned between the band and the bypass. Annals of Surgery. 2011;**254**(3):410-422

[24] Gagner M, Deitel M, Erickson AL, Crosby RD. Survey on laparoscopic sleeve gastrectomy (LSG) at the fourth international consensus summit on sleeve gastrectomy. Obesity Surgery. 2013;**23**:2013-2017

[25] Peterli R, Wölnerhanssen BK, Vetter D, Nett P, Gass M, Borbély Y, et al. Laparoscopic sleeve gastrectomy versus Roux-Y-gastric bypass for morbid obesity—3-year outcomes of the prospective randomized Swiss Multicenter Bypass or Sleeve Study (SM-BOSS). Annals of Surgery. 2017;**265**(3):466-473

[26] DuPree CE, Blair K, Steele SR, Martin MJ. Laparoscopic sleeve gastrectomy in patients with preexisting gastroesophageal reflux disease: A national analysis. JAMA Surgery. 2014;**149**(4):328-334

[27] Cho J-M, Kim HJ, Menzo EL, Park S, Szomstein S, Rosenthal RJ. Effect of sleeve gastrectomy on type 2 diabetes as an alternative treatment modality to Roux-en-Y gastric bypass: Systemic review and meta-analysis. Surgery for Obesity and Related Diseases. 2015;**11**(6):1273-1280

[28] Singhal R, Cardoso VR, Wiggins T, Super J, Ludwig C, Gkoutos GV, et al. 30-day morbidity and mortality of sleeve

gastrectomy, Roux-en-Y gastric bypass and one anastomosis gastric bypass: A propensity score-matched analysis of the GENEVA data. International Journal of Obesity. 2022;**46**(4):750-757

[29] Berger ER, Clements RH, Morton JM, Huffman KM, Wolfe BM, Nguyen NT, et al. The impact of different surgical techniques on outcomes in laparoscopic sleeve gastrectomies: The first report from the metabolic and bariatric surgery accreditation and quality improvement program (MBSAQIP). Annals of Surgery. 2016;**264**(3):464-473

[30] Woźniewska P, Diemieszczyk I, Hady HR. Complications associated with laparoscopic sleeve gastrectomy - a review. Przegląd Gastroenterologiczny. 2021;**16**(1):5-9

[31] Dang JT, Vaughan T, Mocanu V, Mubashir H, Barajas-Gamboa JS, Codina RC, et al. Conversion of sleeve gastrectomy to Roux-en-Y gastric bypass: Indications, prevalence, and safety. Obesity Surgery. 2023;**33**(5):1486-1493

[32] Clapp B, Wynn M, Martyn C, Foster C, O'Dell M, Tyroch A. Long term (7 or more years) outcomes of the sleeve gastrectomy: A meta-analysis. Surgery for Obesity and Related Diseases. 2018;**14**(6):741-747

[33] Dantas ACB, Branco LT, Tustumi F, de Oliveira DRCF, Pajecki D, Santo MA. One-anastomosis gastric bypass versus Roux-en-Y gastric bypass as revisional surgery after sleeve gastrectomy: A systematic review and meta-analysis. Obesity Surgery. 2022;**32**(12):4082-4088

[34] Kermansaravi M, Parmar C, Chiappetta S, Shikora S, Aminian A, Abbas SI, et al. Best practice approach for redo-surgeries after sleeve gastrectomy, an expert's modified Delphi consensus. Surgical Endoscopy. 2023;**37**(3):1617-1628

Chapter 6

Tips and Tricks in Sleeve Gastrectomy

Anıl Ergin and İksan Taşdelen

Abstract

Obesity has become a serious health problem worldwide. Surgery is seen as the most important weapon in the fight against obesity. Laparoscopic Sleeve Gastrectomy is the most widely practiced obesity surgery technique worldwide. Today, this surgery is safely applied to a large number of patients. With the development of technology and surgical experience, the mortality and morbidity of obesity surgeries have decreased considerably. However, these surgeries still require serious experience and knowledge. In this book chapter, we have compiled the technical tips of laparoscopic sleeve gastrectomy, key points that will increase the comfort of the surgeon and the patient, and tricks that will facilitate the operation and shorten the operation time.

Keywords: obesity, bariatric surgery, laparoscopic sleeve gastrectomy, technical tips, weight loss surgery

1. Introduction

Obesity is considered a serious health problem all over the world. Surgery is the most effective method in the treatment of obesity. Although many surgical methods have been tried in the treatment of obesity, some of them have been abandoned due to the difficulty of application and high complication rates. Today, Sleeve Gastrectomy (SG) is the most widely used surgical technique in the treatment of obesity worldwide. SG has become the most preferred surgery because it is relatively easier to perform than other techniques, has a low complication rate, and has similar benefit rates to other techniques. With the development of the technique, improvement in the quality of the materials used, and the demonstration of long-term results, SG has become a more reliable and predictable operation [1]. As the experience and knowledge about this operation, which is performed so frequently worldwide, increases, experienced surgeons recognize that there are many tricks that facilitate the operation, increase the comfort of both the surgeon and the patient, reduce postoperative complications, shorten the hospitalization period, and increase patient satisfaction. In this book chapter, we aim to share the algorithms and technical details that we have applied in our clinic with over 2000 cases of SG experience.

2. Patient selection and indications

Patients with a BMI between 30 and 34.9 kg/m^2 (Class 1 Obesity) with comorbid diseases and patients with BMI >35 kg/m^2 (Class 2 and Class 3 Obesity) are candidates for bariatric surgery regardless of the presence of comorbid diseases [1].

Of course, patient selection cannot be based solely on body mass index. The patient's psychological state, eating habits, socioeconomic level and treatment compliance, comorbidities, and many other parameters significantly affect the success of treatment and are very important in patient selection for bariatric surgery.

3. Preoperative evaluation and consultations

A multidisciplinary approach is one of the most fundamental steps in preparing patients for surgery. The patient's suitability for surgery should be determined by a multidisciplinary team. In our clinic, cardiology, pulmonologist, psychiatry, anesthesiology, and endocrinology consultations are routinely performed for all patients before LSG and surgery plans are made in line with the recommendations of all branches [2].

In addition to the expert evaluation of the relevant branches, all patients undergo preoperative upper gastrointestinal system endoscopy (UGISE) and preoperative upper GIS pathologies are also investigated.

All patients receive thromboembolism (TE) prophylaxis with anticoagulant at 8 hours postoperatively and preoperative compression stockings.

4. Peroperative approach

4.1 Position of the patient and surgeons

The secret of success in obesity surgeries is a uniform surgery and an established system. All surgeries are performed by specialized surgeons who have received special training in bariatric surgery and have adopted the same surgical technique. Patients are placed in the French position and surgeons and equipment are arranged as shown in **Figure 1** [3].

4.2 Trocar entry sites and placement of materials

For LSG, 5 trocars are routinely used in our clinic. One 12 mm, one 10 mm, two 5 mm, and one liver retractor are used. Liver retraction is routinely performed with Nathanson Retractor in every case. Trocar placement is very important for the surgeon's ergonomics during surgery. For this reason, entering the trocars too close to each other during trocar insertion will cause the instruments to interfere with each other during the operation and will hinder the surgeon. In addition, entering the trocars in a direction other than the surgical site will make it very difficult to use the instruments in obesity patients with high subcutaneous adipose tissue. Therefore, these points should be considered during trocar entry.

4.3 Entry of the first trocar

The entry site and shape of the first trocar is the most important step in the ergonomics of the entire operation. Due to obesity, the thickness of the subcutaneous fatty

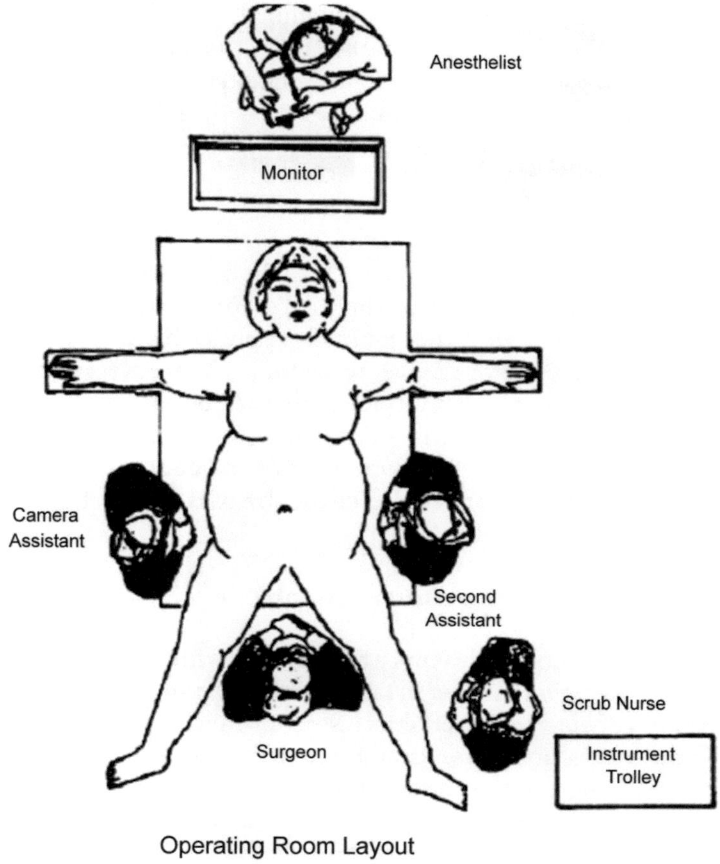

Figure 1.
Operating room layout [3].

tissue is very high, which causes the standard trocar size to be insufficient. Therefore, we routinely choose a 12 mm long trocar as the first trocar in our clinic. There are many techniques for introducing the first trocar; however, we routinely use the direct trocar method (Hasson technique). In the absence of a long trocar, pneumoperitoneum can be created with the help of a Verres needle before the first trocar is inserted and the subsequent insertion of the first trocar will reduce the risk of injury [4].

4.4 Pneumoperitoneum

Following the insertion of the first trocar, we wait until pneumoperitoneum is achieved. The pressure value we routinely use for LSG is 14 mmHg. Since the intra-abdominal pressure is higher in patients with obesity, performing the operation at the lowest pressure level that can be achieved will be advantageous for the patient in many ways. After reaching the desired pressure, the working trocars are entered [5].

4.5 Intra-abdominal exploration

Following the placement of the camera trocar, intra-abdominal structures must be evaluated with the help of a camera. Pathologies that may interfere with surgery may be encountered. For this reason, intra-abdominal exploration should be performed prior to intra-abdominal exploration in order to avoid wasting other trocars. Conditions such as intra-abdominal adhesions, solid organ tumors, and anatomical anomalies due to previous operations should be revealed, and the surgical plan should be revised if necessary.

4.6 Liver retraction

In patients with obesity, the size of the liver can be considerably larger than expected. Although there are clinics that apply a diet for a certain period of time before surgery to reduce this, we do not routinely apply such a diet. Regardless of the size of the liver, we use a retractor for liver retractor in all cases (**Figure 2**).

Although there are many types of retractors that can be used for liver retraction (Nathanson, Pretzelflex, and Crow's foot retractors), we routinely use the Nathanson Retractor (NR), which is fixed to the operating table and does not require assistance. After intra-abdominal exploration, we decide the size of the NR to be used according to the size of the liver [6].

4.7 Emptying the stomach with an orogastric tube

It is very important to routinely empty the stomach with an orogastric tube before starting the operation in order to facilitate the manipulation of the stomach, to increase the field of view in the left crus dissection, and to select the appropriate stapler during the transection phase. In addition to the use of the orogastric tube to determine the remaining gastric volume after gastric transection, its use in gastric aspiration following trocar insertion is also facilitated by the fact that it is wider and easier to apply than aspiration tubes.

4.8 Dissection of gastrocolic ligament

Dissecting the gastrocolic ligament is one of the first and important steps of the operation (**Figure 3**). Bleeding that may occur during this process contaminates the surgical field and can distort the surgeon's view by causing accurate plans to be lost. It is best to start the dissecting of the gastrocolic ligament at the level of the incisura

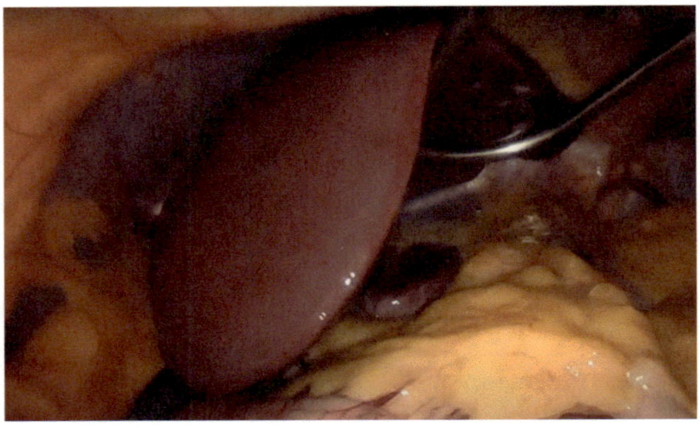

Figure 2.
Nathanson retractor placement.

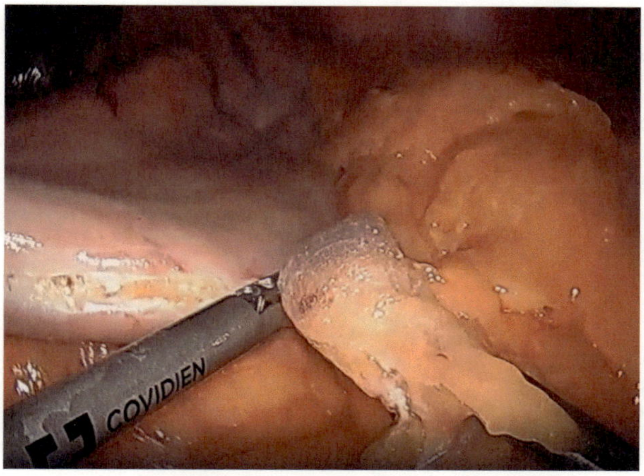

Figure 3.
Dissection of Gastrocolic ligament.

angularis or slightly superior to it. This is because that the easiest access to the lesser sac. Dissection should start as close to the stomach as possible and continue in that direction. The reason for this is to avoid damaging the gastroepiploic vessel, which is located very close to the stomach and whose tracing can easily enter the dissection area.

4.9 Inferior dissection border

In gastrocolic ligament dissection, the distal gastric transection limit should be decided and dissection should be performed up to that region of the stomach. Excessive dissection may cause disruption of blood supply in this region of the stomach. It is generally known that gastric transection can be started at a distance of approximately 2 cm to 6 cm from the pylorus. However, we should keep in mind that the closer we transect to the pylorus, the more postoperative nausea and vomiting will occur and the greater the possibility of pyloric deformation will be [7]. Therefore, starting gastric transection with a distance of 4 cm to the pylorus is the ideal approach.

4.10 His angle and crus dissection

This step is one of the most important steps of the surgery. It is one of the indispensable steps for the complete release of the great curvature of the stomach; that is, the gastric fundus should not be left wide. Failure of the releasing His angle and failure to expose the left crus and completely release the fundus may lead to failure of the surgical technique and an increase in the regain rate [8]. Therefore, in our clinic, we routinely perform left crus dissection in all patients and make sure that we completely free the gastric fundus before transection (**Figure 4**).

4.11 Routine crus dissection and investigation of hiatal hernia

After LSG, lower esophageal sphincter insufficiency is predisposed due to impaired His angle and increased gastric mobilization. In addition, bile reflux may

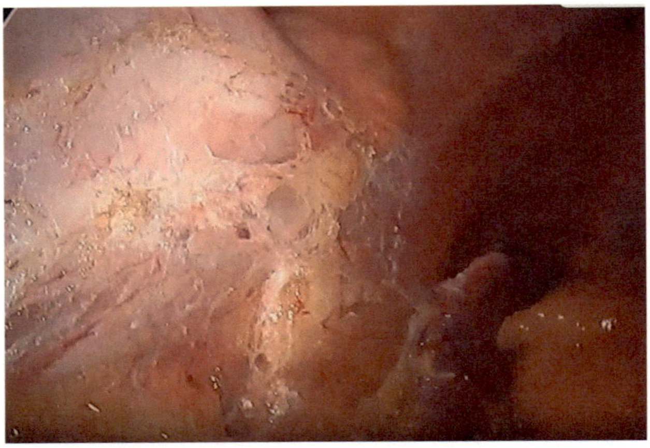

Figure 4.
Dissection of left crus.

also be seen due to increased intragastric pressure after LSG. These conditions may turn into a misery for patients. Therefore, it is very important to perform hiatus repair by crus dissection in patients with hiatal hernia and lower esophageal sphincter insufficiency in preoperative UGISE. In patients in whom UGISE was not performed preoperatively, intraoperative crus dissection should be performed to investigate the presence of hiatal hernia [9]. In our clinic, we routinely perform hiatal repair in all patients in whom hiatal hernia is detected during routine preoperative upper GI endoscopy (**Figure 5**).

4.12 Release of posterior gastric adhesions

Adhesions located in the posterior part of the stomach may occur for many unknown reasons. These adhesions encountered during surgery prevent full mobilization of the stomach and may cause shifts and rotations in the staple line. Therefore,

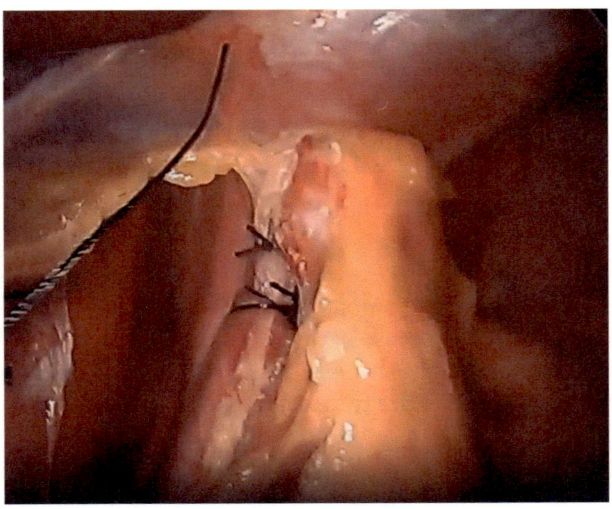

Figure 5.
Peroperative hiatal hernia repair.

these adhesions in the posterior part of the stomach should be opened by treating the small curvature vessels with care and the stomach should be fully mobilized. This will prevent rotations in the staple line and distortions in the formation of the B formation. Since bleeding can be seen during the separation of these adhesions, they should be separated with energy devices and the tissue should be treated very carefully. Blunt dissection should be avoided as much as possible [10].

4.13 Placement of the orogastric tube

It is preferred that the anesthesiologist in charge of obesity surgeries has special training and experience in this field. The anesthesiologist is expected to master the interventions performed by the anesthesiologist at some stages of the surgery. Before transection of the stomach, an orogastric tube extending to the pylorus is inserted into the stomach to ensure lumen patency. Since passing the orogastric tube through the pylorus may cause deformity and curvature in the stomach, it should be left at the transection start line. While the orogastric tube is brought to this area, the anesthesiologist and surgeon should work in coordination and the surgeon should guide the orogastric tube to the position where it should be with the dressing method.

The size of the orogastric tube depends entirely on the surgeon's choice. It is known that thin tubes can cause strictures and thick tubes can cause insufficient weight loss. Therefore, very narrow and very wide orogastric tubes should not be chosen. It would be appropriate to choose orogastric tubes with thicknesses between 32 and 40 French [11]. In our clinic, 36 French orogastric tubes are routinely used (**Figure 6**).

4.14 Stapler selection and transection of the stomach in accordance with gastric wall thickness

It is known that gastric wall thickness may vary depending on many factors (age, gender, body mass index, infectious pathologies of the stomach, etc.). It has been

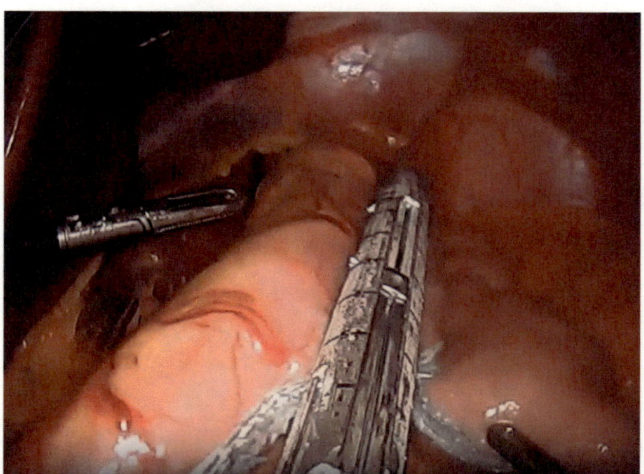

Figure 6.
Orogastric tube-guided transection of the stomach.

determined in many studies that the antrum is the thickest part of the stomach wall and the thickness decreases as you go to the fundus. Therefore, it is necessary to make sure that the stapler to be used in the antrum is compatible with thick tissue and the stapler to be used in the fundus is suitable for thinner tissues. Staple thickness is distinguished by colors and different companies have different color options. Regardless of the manufacturer's preference, staples with the ability to close thicker tissues in the antrum region where the gastric wall thickness is the highest and staples with the ability to close thinner tissues as they approach the fundus region should be preferred [12]. In our clinic, we complete the gastric transection by using the thickest cartridge for the first staple (**Figure 7**) and a medium-thick cartridge for the remaining gastric tissue.

When determining the superior border during transection of the stomach, a distance of 1 cm to the esophagus must be left (**Figure 8**). Structured tissue corresponding to this distance should be separated from the stomach and prevented from entering the staple line.

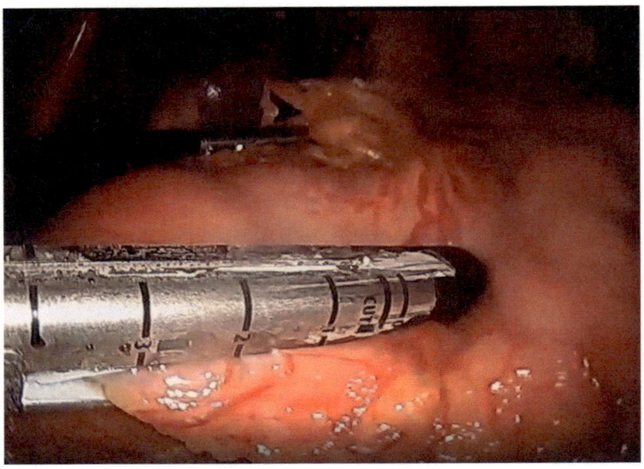

Figure 7.
Inserting the first cartridge.

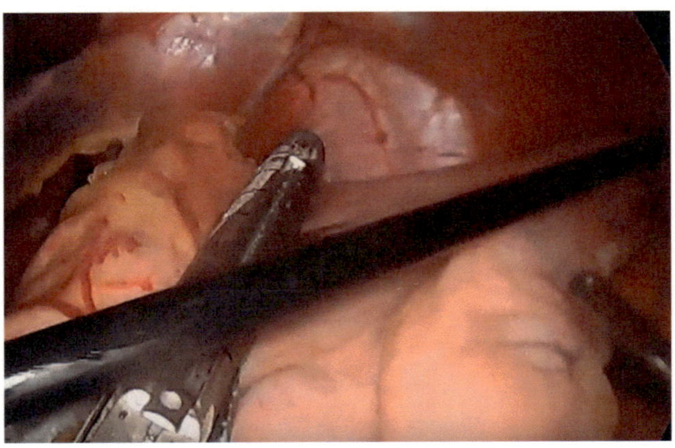

Figure 8.
Inserting the last cartridge.

4.15 Hemostasis in the stapler line

After complete transection of the stomach, bleeding seen on the stapler line should be stopped with the help of clips. Bleeding control should be done very carefully. Bleeding from the stapler line may occur due to postoperative hypertension or increased intra-abdominal pressure. Continued suturing of this line is another option to control bleeding in the stapler line [13, 14]. In our clinic, both clip application and continue suturing of the stapler line are routinely performed. Sheathed staples can also be used to control bleeding.

4.16 Removal of the specimen

Specimen removal is performed through 12 mm trocars. In the removal of the specimen, the gastric specimen is grasped from the antrum by sending a grasping device through the trocar and pulled out of the abdomen with the trocar (**Figure 9**). Since the antrum wall is thicker, the strength of this region is stronger. Therefore, the removal process should start from the antrum. During the removal of the specimen, great care should be taken not to open the stomach and not to spill secretions or tissue fragments into the abdomen. The stomach should be taken out of the abdomen in one piece and with the staple line intact [15].

4.17 Leakage test

Nowadays, many surgeons have abandoned the traditional methylene blue leak test after transection of the stomach. However, in our clinic, methylene blue leakage test is routinely performed by closing the stomach from the pylorus with an instrument following removal of the specimen. During this test, both the B formation of the stapler line can be easily evaluated and the bleeding that may occur due to increased pressure can be revealed [16].

4.18 Suturing of the stapler line

Suturing the stapler line to the gastrocolic ligament or omentum is practiced by many surgeons because it is effective in both controlling bleeding and preventing

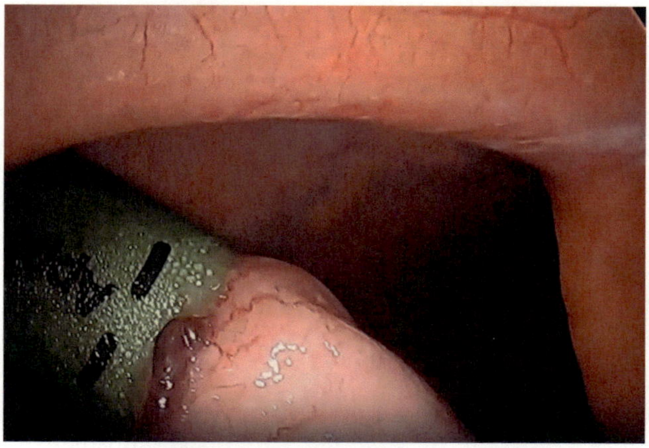

Figure 9.
Removal of the specimen.

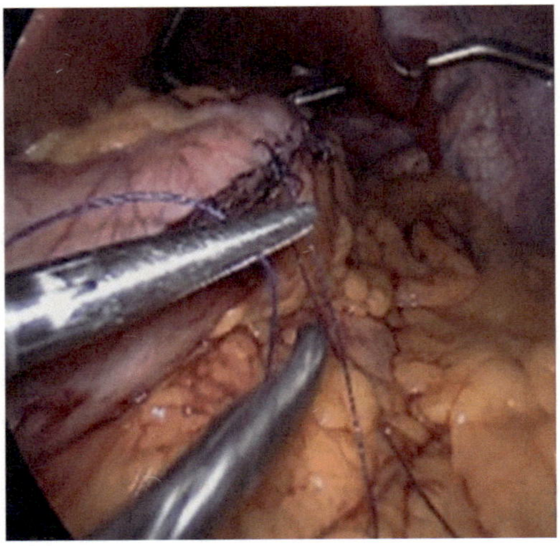

Figure 10.
Suturing the stapler line.

the possibility of twist in the postoperative period (**Figure 10**). Suturing the stapler line from the superior border to the inferior border contributes to the return of the stomach to its former anatomy and reduces the possibility of stapler line adhesion to the liver [17]. In our clinic, the entire stapler line is routinely sutured from superior to inferior to the gastrocolic ligament at the end of surgery.

4.19 Drain placement

Placement of a drain at the end of surgery is not routine. This depends entirely on the surgeon's preference. However, routine drain placement after every bariatric surgery is not a correct approach. Placing the drain only in cases where there is a possibility of bleeding or when the surgeon needs it for any reason will prevent unnecessary drain complications [18].

4.20 Closure of trocar sites

Patients with obesity are candidates for incisional hernia due to the higher intra-abdominal pressure compared to normal people. Therefore, it is very important to close trocar defects larger than 5 mm. Closure of trocar sites can be quite challenging due to the high amount of subcutaneous fatty tissue. There are many instruments that facilitate closure of fascia defects. Help can be obtained from these instruments [19]. In our clinic, fascia defects larger than 5 mm are routinely closed and Carter-Thomasson Suture Passer is used for this purpose (**Figure 11**).

5. Postoperative approach

Patients should be provided with adequate analgesia and antiemesis in the postoperative period. In addition, early mobilization and use of anticoagulants for TE prophylaxis are very important. In our clinic, patients are routinely mobilized at the 4th hour postoperatively and anticoagulation with low molecular weight heparin is provided at the 8th hour postoperatively.

DOI: http://dx.doi.org/10.5772/intechopen.1005856

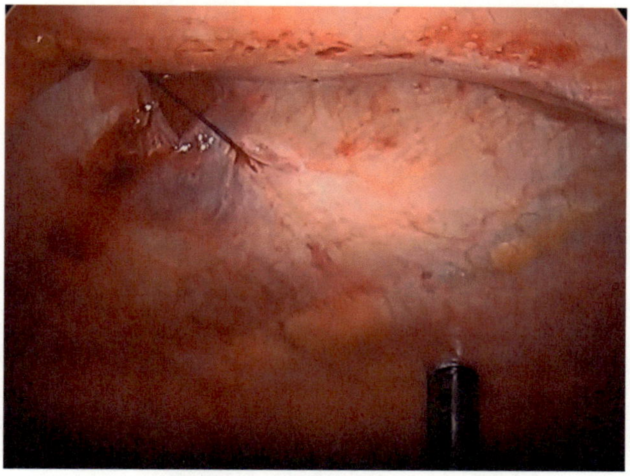

Figure 11.
Closure of trocar sites.

Following mobilization, patients are started on oral water. Water and clear fruit juices are given to all patients on the first postoperative day and grain-free soup and liquid foods can be given on the second postoperative day.

Although there are approaches such as X-ray-assisted passage radiographs, computed tomography, and methylene blue test to evaluate the stapler line after surgery, we do not apply any of these to our patients. In our clinic, we perform amylase measurement in the drain fluid, which is both radiation-free and easy to perform. If the salivary amylase level measured in the drain fluid is above 400 U/L and if the amylase level increases in the follow-up, we apply advanced imaging tests to the patients. There are also studies that we have proved the effectiveness of drain amylase measurement in determining leakage in our clinic, and we have brought it to the literature [20]. In addition, we perform additional tests in cases such as tachycardia, hypotension, fever, and severe abdominal pain that may suggest postoperative leakage. Apart from this, we do not perform postoperative leakage test in patients who do not have any postoperative problems and no drain is placed.

Patients are discharged on postoperative day 3, and anticoagulant use continues for 10 days.

Postoperative controls are performed on the 7th day, 1st month, 3rd month, 6th month, 9th month, 12th month, 18th month, and 24th month. Afterwards, annual follow-up is continued. Dietitian, endocrinology, and psychiatry controls are routinely performed for all patients in the postoperative period.

Author details

Anıl Ergin* and İksan Taşdelen
Istanbul Fatih Sultan Mehmet Research and Training Hospital, Istanbul, Turkey

*Address all correspondence to: dranilergin@gmail.com

References

[1] Eisenberg D, Shikora SA, Aarts E, Aminian A, Angrisani L, Cohen RV. 2022 American Society for Metabolic and Bariatric Surgery (ASMBS) and International federation for the surgery of obesity and metabolic disorders (IFSO): Indications for metabolic and bariatric surgery. Surgery for Obesity and Related Diseases. 2022;**18**(12):1345-1356. DOI: 10.1016/j.soard.2022.08.013. Epub 2022 Oct 21

[2] Carr P, Keighley T, Petocz P, Blumfield M, Rich GG, Cohen F, et al. Efficacy and safety of endoscopic sleeve gastroplasty and laparoscopic sleeve gastrectomy with 12+ months of adjuvant multidisciplinary support. BMC Primary Care. 5 Feb 2022;**23**(1):26. DOI: 10.1186/s12875-022-01629-7. PMID: 35123409; PMCID: PMC8817771

[3] Chowbey PK, Dhawan K, Khullar R, Sharma A, Soni V, Baijal M, et al. Laparoscopic sleeve gastrectomy: An Indian experience—Surgical technique and early results. Obesity Surgery. Oct 2010;**20**(10):1340-1347. DOI: 10.1007/s11695-009-9973-9. Epub 2009 Sep 29. PMID: 19787412

[4] Miti C, Busuulwa P, Scott R, Bloomfield-Gadelha H. Primary entry trocar design and entry-related complications at laparoscopy in obese patients: Meta-analysis. BJS Open. 5 May 2023;**7**(3):zrad047. DOI: 10.1093/bjsopen/zrad047. PMID: 37352873; PMCID: PMC10289830

[5] Brunaud L, Ayav A, et al. Effect of pneumoperitoneum on postoperative pain after laparoscopic gastric bypass: A randomized study. Obesity Surgery. 2011;**21**(7):980-985. DOI: 10.1007/s11695-011-0402-8

[6] Ayav A, Brunaud L, et al. Comparison of the Pretzelflex and Nathanson retractors in laparoscopic sleeve gastrectomy: Efficacy and safety. Obesity Surgery. 2021;**31**(4):1645-1653. DOI: 10.1007/s11695-020-05172-8

[7] Aktokmakyan TV, Gungor O, Sumer A. Technical details of laparoscopic sleeve gastrectomy. Mini-invasive Surgery. 2020;**4**:23. DOI: 10.20517/2574-1225.2019.72

[8] Parikh M, Kole KL, Ali MR. The significance of left crus dissection in laparoscopic sleeve gastrectomy. Journal of Clinical Medicine. 2024;**13**(7):1954. DOI: 10.3390/jcm13071954

[9] Northup CJ. Dissection of the crus in laparoscopic sleeve gastrectomy: A necessity or an option? Journal of Clinical Medicine. 2024;**13**(7):1954. DOI: 10.3390/jcm13071954

[10] Jawad AA et al. The role of posterior adhesion dissection in laparoscopic sleeve gastrectomy. International Journal of Surgery. 2020;**76**:112-118. DOI: 10.1016/j.ijsu.2020.02.034

[11] Helmy MMD, MRCS. Bougie size 32 versus 40 french in laparoscopic sleeve gastrectomy. The Egyptian Journal of Surgery. 2018;**37**(2):200-208. DOI: 10.4103/ejs.ejs_1_18

[12] Barski K, Binda A, Kudlicka E, Jaworski P, Tarnowski W. Gastric wall thickness and stapling in laparoscopic sleeve gastrectomy - A literature review. Wideochir Inne Tech Maloinwazyjne. 2018;**13**(1):122-127. DOI: 10.5114/wiitm.2018.73362. Epub 2018 Feb 7

[13] Naeem MS, Ul Ain R, Sadiq Z, Ejaz A, Rafi U, Awais M, et al.

Gastric staple line reinforcement with ligation clips for Hemostasis in laparoscopic sleeve gastrectomy. Cureus. 2023;**15**(4):e37271. DOI: 10.7759/cureus.37271

[14] Siddiq G, Dr AW, Khizar S, Haider MI, Razzaq A, Ahmad Z, et al. Laparoscopic sleeve gastrectomy: To suture or not to suture staple line? Cureus. 2018;**10**(7):e2992. DOI: 10.7759/cureus.2992

[15] Shoar S, Aboutaleb S, Karem M, Bashah MM, AlKuwari M, Sargsyan D, et al. Comparison of two specimen retrieval techniques in laparoscopic sleeve gastrectomy: What is the role of endobag? Surgical Endoscopy. 2017;**31**(12):4883-4887. DOI: 10.1007/s00464-017-5434-z. Epub 2017 Mar 24

[16] Mayir B. Is intraoperative leak test required in laparoscopic sleeve gastrectomy? Journal of the College of Physicians and Surgeons–Pakistan. 2021;**31**(3):318-321. DOI: 10.29271/jcpsp.2021.03.318

[17] Aiolfi A, Gagner M, Zappa MA, et al. Staple line reinforcement during laparoscopic sleeve gastrectomy: Systematic review and network meta-analysis of randomized controlled trials. Obesity Surgery. 2022;**32**:1466-1478. DOI: 10.1007/s11695-022-05950-z

[18] Albanopoulos K, Alevizos L, Linardoutsos D, Menenakos E, Stamou K, Vlachos K, et al. Routine abdominal drains after laparoscopic sleeve gastrectomy: A retrospective review of 353 patients. Obesity Surgery. 2011;**21**(6):687-691. DOI: 10.1007/s11695-010-0343-4

[19] Karampinis I, Lion E, Hetjens S, Vassilev G, Galata C, Reissfelder C, et al. Trocar site hernias after bariatric laparoscopic surgery (HERBALS): A prospective cohort study. Obesity Surgery. 2020;**30**(5):1820-1826. DOI: 10.1007/s11695-020-04400-y

[20] Karip B, Atabekoğlu S, Altun H, Yılmaz A. Drain amylase levels in the early diagnosis of gastric leak after laparoscopic sleeve gastrectomy. Turkish Journal of Surgery. 2020;**36**(4):245-252. DOI: 10.5152/turkjsurg.2020.4802

Chapter 7

Standardization of the Fully Stapled Roux-En-Y Gastric Bypass

Isabelle Debergh

Abstract

The laparoscopic Roux-en-Y gastric bypass (RYGB) is a commonly performed bariatric procedure known for many years as an effective treatment for morbid obesity, and associated comorbidities, such as diabetes mellitus type 2 (DM2), arterial hypertension, and obstructive sleep apnea syndrome (OSAS). In the technical evolution of bariatric surgery, this procedure became more and more professionalized and standardized. The fully stapled RYGB has emerged as a gold standard technique, with excellent consistency, safety, and efficiency. Also, preoperative and postoperative care evolved toward standardized obesity care pathways to enhance a swift recovery. This chapter will highlight the surgical technique and detailed principles of the standardized fully stapled RYGB and obesity care pathway in our center to optimize patient outcomes.

Keywords: obesity, gastric bypass, bariatric surgery, standardization, roux-en-Y gastric bypass, fully stapled gastric bypass, RYGB

1. Introduction

The concept of RYGB was introduced in the 1960s by Dr. Edward Mason [1], initially an open procedure, incorporating both hand-sewn and stapled techniques.

Over time, advancements in surgical technology and an increased understanding of bariatric surgery led to the adoption of laparoscopy and fully stapled anastomoses, which provided more uniform results and reduced operative and admission time.

In 2009, Dr. Bruno Dillemans described the standardization of the fully stapled Roux-en-Y gastric bypass (RYGB) with the circular technique in a large volume center [2]. In 2606 patients, minimal morbidity and mortality were reported, proving that this procedure ensured patient safety. As streamlined training became possible with the introduction of clear, standardized procedures, the education and training of surgical teams was facilitated and reproducibility was confirmed a few years later [3].

Continuous improvements were added to this technique, leading to reduced risks of complications by adhering to consistent surgical practices [4, 5]. Moreover, the beneficial effect of this standardized procedure concerning feasibility and safety in complex revisional procedures was investigated and proven on large groups of patients that underwent conversion from vertical banded gastroplasty (VBG) to RYGB [6–8], or laparoscopic adjustable gastric band (LAGB) to RYGB [9, 10].

New small improvements were made to this classic and solid technique, which we describe in this chapter.

A precise and replicable surgical method and a standardized obesity care pathway will lead to improved outcomes, enhanced weight loss, and comorbidity resolution in the long term. Data on the weight loss of all RYGB patients in our center between 2019 and 2024 are depicted in **Figure 1**. Further long-term analysis will be made in the future.

We must embrace exciting surgical innovations such as novel types of surgery or robotic procedures and also test them against proven ones. This professionalization of obesity care is now more than ever necessary to counter criticism from other healthcare workers in the near future and the pharmaceutical industry.

2. Preoperative standardization

Patient selection and preparation is of the utmost importance for good short, intermediate, and long-term results. In our center, obese patients undergo a complete dietetic, endocrinological, and psychological evaluation. The nutritional and psychological evaluation will ensure that patients are mentally and physically prepared for bariatric surgery and subsequent lifestyle changes. Laboratory tests may rule out hormonal dysfunctions, nutritional deficiencies, and other relevant conditions affecting pre- and postoperative health. Gastroscopy, and sometimes upper gastrointestinal series, can identify anatomical anomalies that can affect surgery. Depending on the severity of obesity, comorbidities, and motivation, the patient is allocated to conservative treatment with/without medication (incretin mimetics) or a surgical pathway. The demographic data of the RYGB patients in our obesity center are depicted in **Figure 2**.

Preoperatively, patients can gain access to a digital tool with information, postoperative questionnaires, and measurements for enhancing compliance in the long run. All patients will follow a preop diet for 2 weeks, to reduce liver volume and steatosis.

In our obesity clinic, several surgeons perform the fully stapled RYGB: more than half of the cases are performed with the circular gastroenteric anastomosis, as described by Dillemans [2, 4–10] and the remaining part with the linear technique. This chapter will describe in detail the circular gastrojejunostomy technique.

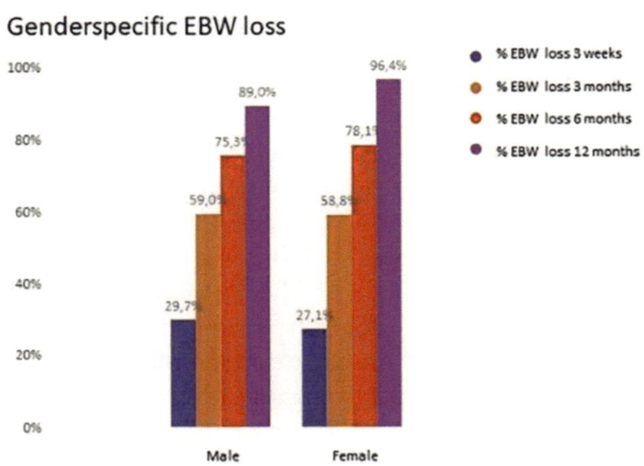

Figure 1.
Excessive body weight loss (EBW) in all RYGB patients between 2019 and 2024 in our obesity center.

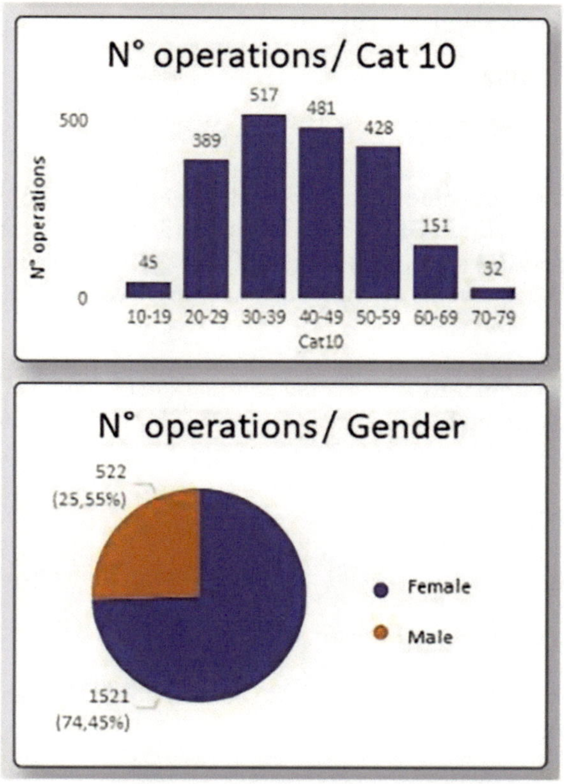

Figure 2.
Age and gender distributions of all RYGB patients between 2019 and 2024 in our obesity center.

3. Operative technique

3.1 Material list

- Knife with N 11 blade
- Veress needle (Covidien, USA or Ethicon, USA)
- Trocars: 1 × 5 mm, 4 × 12 mm
- Insufflation tubing
- Suction device
- Orogastric tube: 34 French Calibration Tube (Bariatric Solutions, Switzerland)
- 30° laparoscope
- Light cable
- Ultrasonic dissecting device Harmonic™ AceR laparoscopic shears (Ethicon, USA) or Sonicision™ (Covidien, USA)

- Three laparoscopic clamps (Conmed, USA)
- One Babcock (Conmed, USA)
- Laparoscopic needle holder (Ethicon, USA)
- Echelon flex™ 60 mm blue (3.5 mm): 3 cartridges; white (2.5 mm): 3 cartridges (Ethicon, USA); or Endo GIA™ 60 mm purple (3–4 mm): 3 cartridges; 60 mm tan: 3 cartridges (Covidien, USA); or IntoCare™ Disposable Powered Endoscopic Linear Cutting Stapler IEC 60 mm blue (3.5 mm): 3 cartridges; white (2.5 mm): 3 cartridges (IntoCare, China)
- DST SERIES™ circular EEA ™ stapler 25 mm blue (3.5 mm) (Covidien, USA); or Endoscopic Curved Intraluminal Stapler™ ILS 25 mm (Ethicon, USA); or IntoCare™ Disposable Powered Circular Stapler ICS 25 mm (IntoCare, China)
- Two towel clamps
- One polydioxa-none suture (PDS) 3/0 cut at 22 cm (Ethicon, USA)
- Two PDS 4/0 cut at 15 cm (Ethicon, USA)
- Multifire Endo Hernia™ (Covidien, USA) or Filbock™ Non-absorbable 15 cm (Duomed, Belgium)
- Endo Close™ (Covidien, USA)
- One Polysorb 1 suture (Covidien, USA)

3.2 Patient positioning and trocar placement

The patient is not wearing antithrombotic stockings. Underpants are allowed, must be comfortable, but do not need to be removed. Hair is already removed between the nipples and the umbilicus. The patient receives an intravenous dose of prophylactic antibiotic (cefazoline or clindamycin in case of penicillin allergy) and put under general anesthesia, and a 34-French orogastric tube is placed by the anesthesiologist. The patient is placed in a 30° reverse Trendelenburg beach-chair position with split legs. This position is not difficult for the obese body and allows optimal workspace and access to the upper part of the abdomen. The legs and wrists are fixed in a safe and pressure-free position. After disinfection and draping of the patient, the surgeon will take place between the patient's legs. The video processor, the light source, and the insufflator are placed on the right side of the patient, next to the head. The first assistant will hold the camera and stands at the surgeon's left. The dedicated obesity nurse stands at the surgeon's right-hand side. Sometimes a second assistant is available, but this is not obligatory (right side). After installation of insufflation, suction, camera, and an ultrasonic device, the region of all incisions is infiltrated with a long-acting local anesthetic. Then, a horizontal 1.5-cm incision is made 8–10 cm below the xiphoid. The Veress needle is inserted, intra-abdominal pressure is set at 15 mmHg, and the abdomen is insufflated with carbon dioxide (CO_2). A 12-mm scope trocar is placed at first, the 30° angled scope is introduced, the abdomen is inspected, and four additional working trocars are placed under direct vision: a 5-mm port high in the epigastric area in the midline, a 12-mm port in the right upper quadrant, and two 12-mm ports in the left upper quadrant (**Figure 3**). Once the insertion of trocars is completed, the procedure begins with the creation of the gastric pouch.

3.3 Construction of the gastric pouch

We ask the anesthesiologist to control systolic blood pressure <100 mmHg during the construction of the gastric pouch and gastroenterostomy. The 34-French gastric tube is positioned in the esophagus.

In general, the size of the pouch is standardized, typically around 15–30 mL, to ensure consistent restriction and weight loss outcomes.

The first assistant (left-side surgeon) keeps the liver aside using the right trocar. The Babcock forceps are introduced via the left lateral trocar (nurse/second assistant) and hold traction on the lesser curvature of the stomach at the level of the antrum. The crow's foot of the nerve of Latarjet is identified and spared. The bursa omentalis is accessed 4–5 cm below the gastroesophageal junction by creating a small window in the lesser omentum (**Figure 4**) using a grasper (cranial trocar) and the ultrasonic device (left medial trocar). The first assistant will introduce a linear stapler (right trocar) through this window. The stomach is horizontally cut over approximately 60 mm (**Figure 5**), without completely transecting the stomach. Mostly, a blue/purple cartridge is used, but cartridges with higher stapler height are necessary when tissue is thicker, for example, in redo cases.

Subsequently, the Babcock forceps is repositioned at the lateral part of the newly formed stapler line and holds upward and caudal traction on the stomach to reveal the posterior gastric wall. The first assistant retracts the liver. Now, posterior gastric adhesions are divided with the ultrasonic device, and the grasper (cranial trocar) is placed

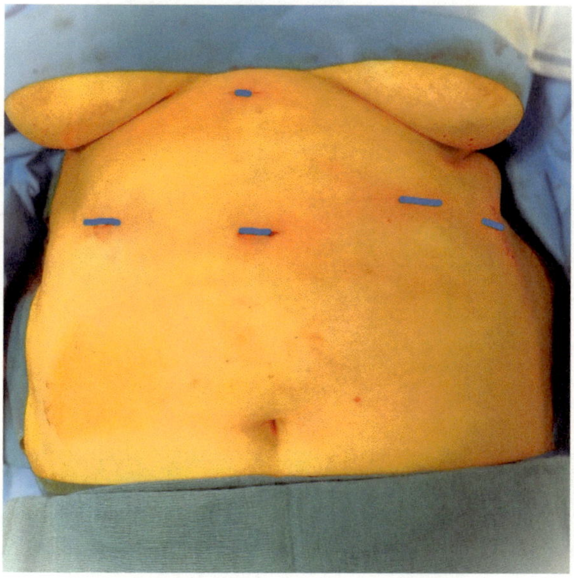

Figure 3.
Position of trocars. Cranial trocar (5 mm) predominantly used by the surgeon. Right trocar (12 mm) mainly used by the first assistant. Middle trocar (12 mm) for the camera. Left medial trocar (12 mm) only used by the surgeon. Left lateral trocar (12 mm) used by the second assistant or dedicated obesity nurse and dilated for the introduction of the circular stapler device.

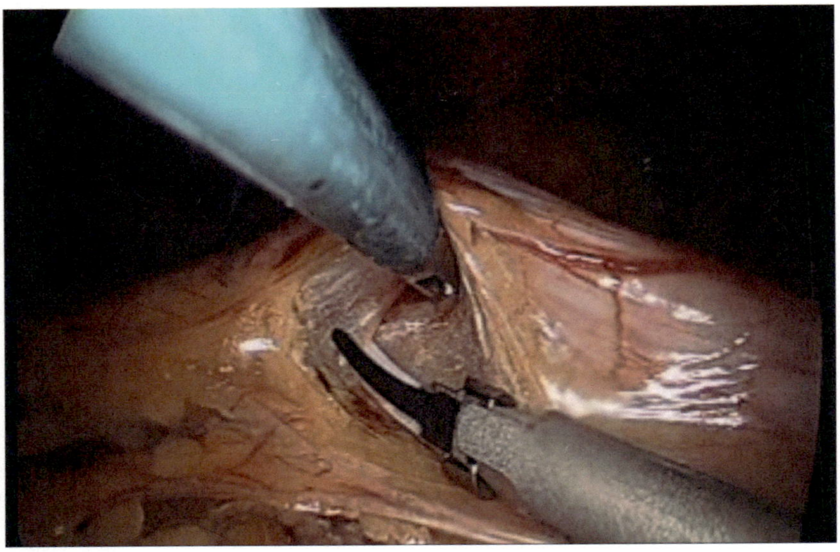

Figure 4.
Entering the bursa omentalis through ultrasonic dissection of the lesser omentum.

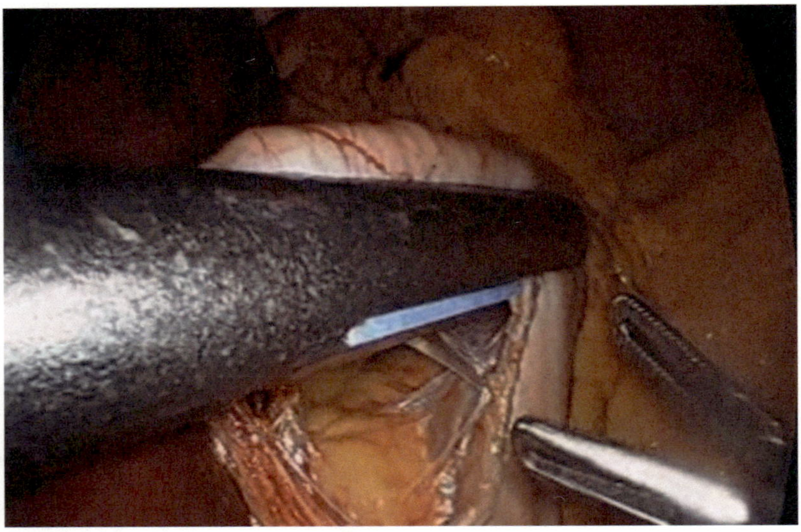

Figure 5.
First horizontal stapler transects the stomach.

under the stomach, against the left crus toward the angle of His (**Figure 6**). The posterior dissected tunnel is completed by dividing the last tissue fibers at the angle of His with blunt dissection or the ultrasonic device. A second linear 60-mm stapler is introduced through the left medial trocar and positioned toward the angle of His starting from the most lateral point of the horizontal transection. If visualization is too difficult, the Babcock forceps can be placed in this tunnel to aid positioning of the stapler device, preventing to leave a posterior sac. The anesthesiologist will guide and check the gastric tube, and the stapler is closed and fired (**Figure 7**). At last, the pouch is finalized by vertically firing the last 60-mm cartridges in the direction of and through the created

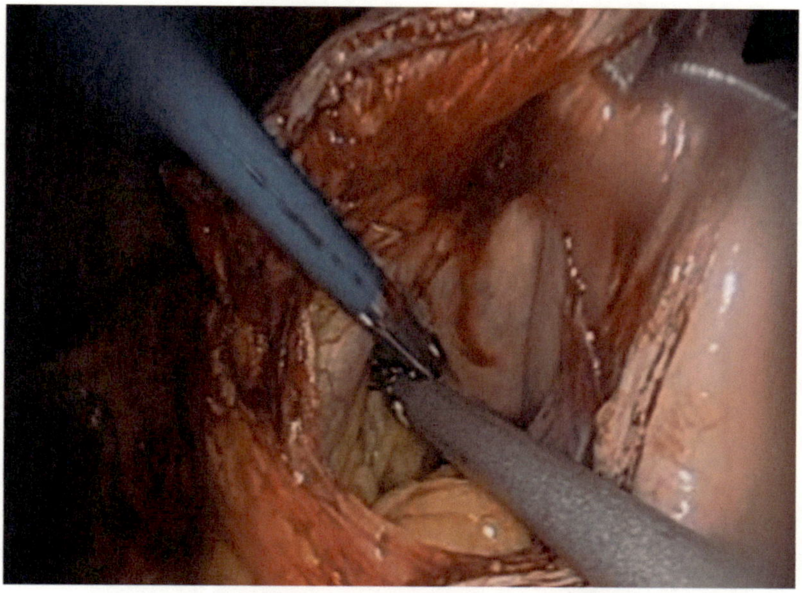

Figure 6.
Dissection of the posterior stomach tunnel toward the angle of His.

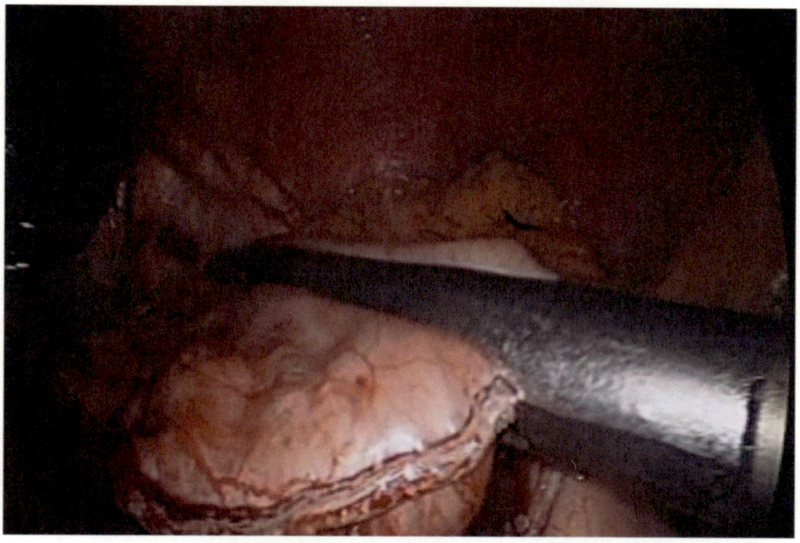

Figure 7.
First vertical stapler, guided by the orogastric tube.

window, along the gastric tube, and well aligned to the previous vertical stapler line (**Figure 8**). Now, the orogastric tube is pulled back into the esophagus.

3.4 Creation of the gastrojejunostomy

Two tissue bites of the lower left corner of the pouch are excised using the ultrasonic device (**Figure 9**). The opening is stretched with two graspers, and a 3/0 PDS 22 cm purse-string suture is sewn (**Figure 10**).

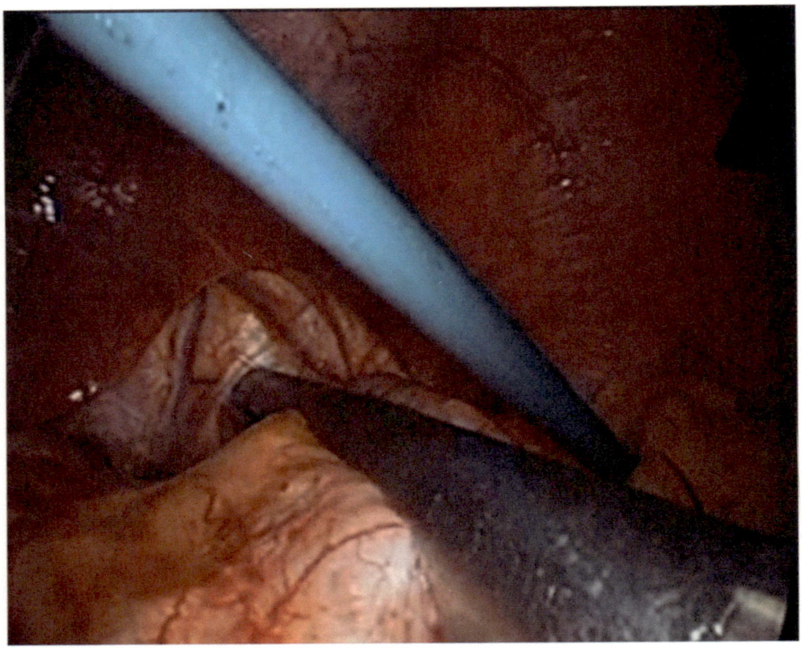

Figure 8.
Placement of the second vertical stapler toward the angle of His.

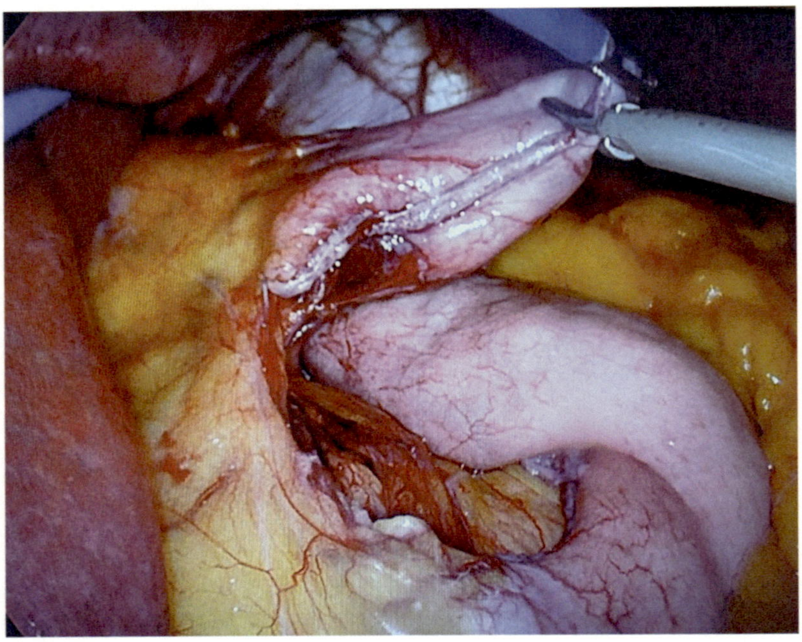

Figure 9.
Opening the gastric pouch with an ultrasonic device.

The second assistant or the dedicated obesity nurse (right-side surgeon) is performing some important steps now. The left lateral trocar port is enlarged up to 2.5 cm, and the interior opening in the abdominal wall is bluntly dilated with a pair of

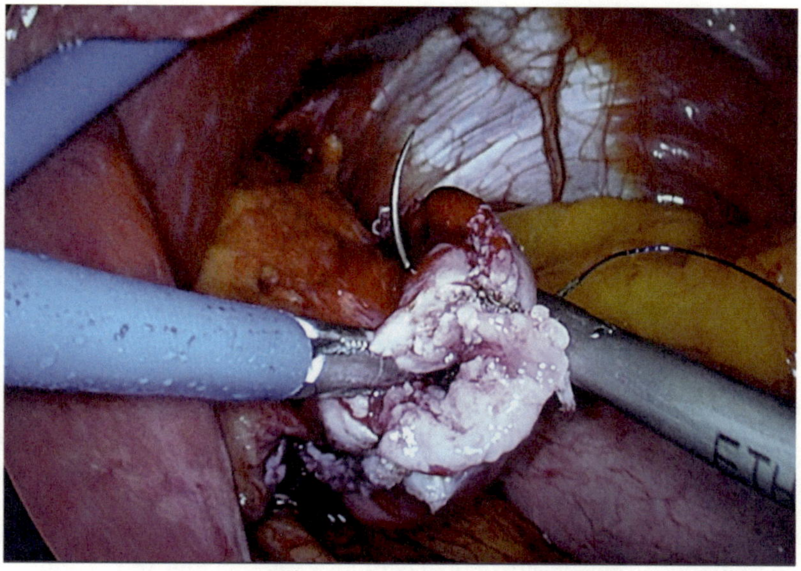

Figure 10.
Sewing of the purse-string suture.

scissors. Two fingers can be introduced in this port site, allowing the circular 25-mm stapler to enter the body. To prevent losing pneumoperitoneum, the skin is closed tight around the stapler device using one towel clamp. The anvil is introduced into the gastric pouch opening (**Figure 11**). The body of the stapler device is temporarily removed from the abdomen, allowing maximal workspace for the team. The last step is completed by tying the purse-string tightly around the anvil. We inspect the future

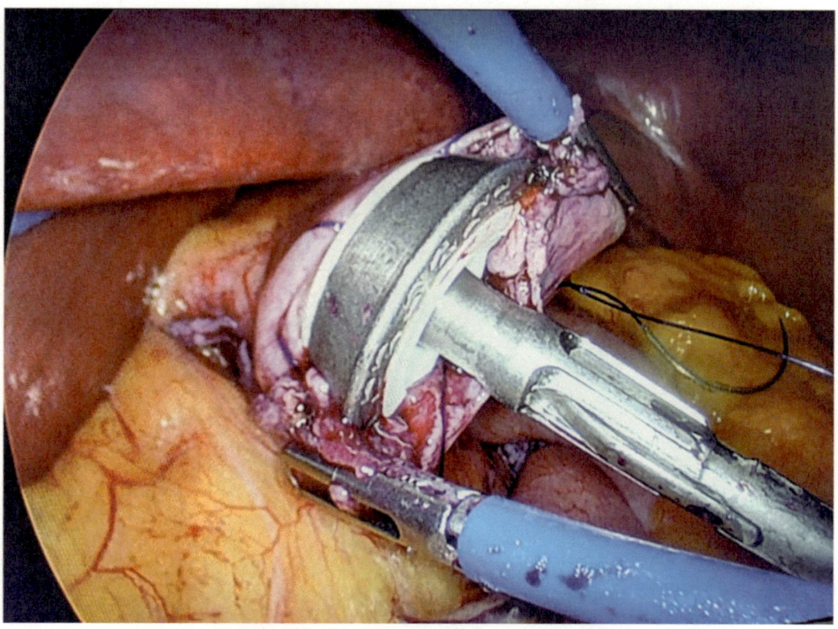

Figure 11.
Introduction of the anvil in the purse-string at the gastric pouch.

anastomosis and remove potential disturbing excess mucosa or fat, and veins or arteries to prevent bleeding.

During the next phase, the greater omentum is lifted and the transverse colon is visualized. Now and then, the greater omentum is heavy and causes traction on the future anastomotic region, obliging us to split the omentum. The first assistant holds the transverse mesocolon with a grasper via the right trocar. Now, the ligament of Treitz is located, as well as the inferior mesenteric vein, and the root of the transverse mesocolon as anatomical landmarks to ensure the start of the jejunum. The jejunum is stretched up by the surgeon from this point in an anticlockwise and antecolic antegastric direction to the gastric pouch. The length of the biliary limb varies mostly between 60 and 80 cm and is rarely longer than 100 cm, depending on the degree of tension on the gastrojejunostomy.

The first assistant holds and stretches the jejunum with a grasper at the antimesenteric side toward the liver, at 2 cm distally (aboral) of the designated anastomotic point. An enterotomy is created by the surgeon 6–8 cm proximal to the future gastroenterostomy, and this opening is stretched by two graspers. The second assistant or the obesity nurse introduces the circular stapler through the left lateral port site into the jejunal loop toward the designated anastomotic region (**Figure 12**) and perforates carefully the spike of the stapler device at the antimesenteric side of the bowel. Next, the spike of the stapler is connected to the anvil (**Figure 13**), and the anastomosis is completed by closing and firing the stapler (**Figure 14**). Afterward, the stapler device is removed from the abdomen, the left lateral trocar is replaced with two towel claps preventing a leaking pneumoperitoneum, and the tissue donuts are verified on completeness. The future biliopancreatic limb is disconnected from the alimentary limb, by making a mesenteric window with the ultrasonic device (surgeon) 1 cm proximal to the gastrojejunostomy and transecting the tissue using a linear stapler with a 60-mm white/tan cartridge, thus, avoiding a long blind loop ("candy cane") of the

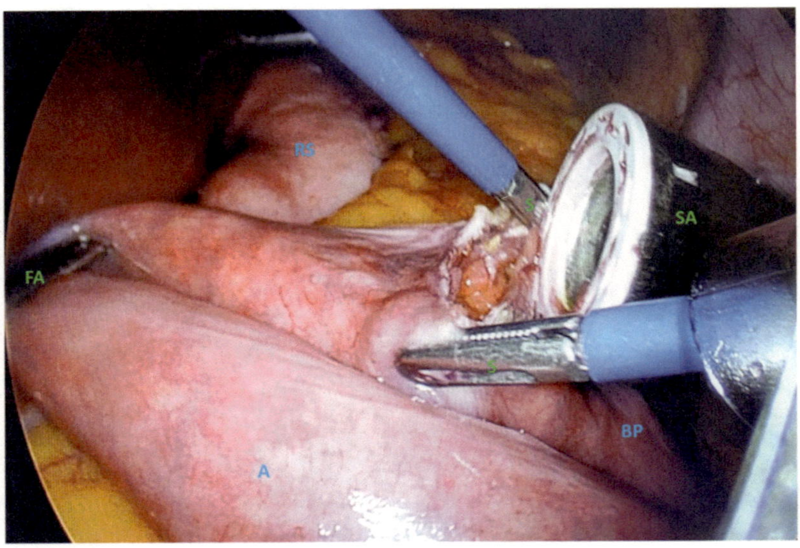

Figure 12.
Introduction of the circular stapler device in the enterotomy. RS: Remnant Stomach; BP: BilioPancreatic limb; A: Alimentary limb. S: Surgeon; FA: First Assistant; SA: Second Assistant or dedicated obesity nurse.

DOI: http://dx.doi.org/10.5772/intechopen.1005852

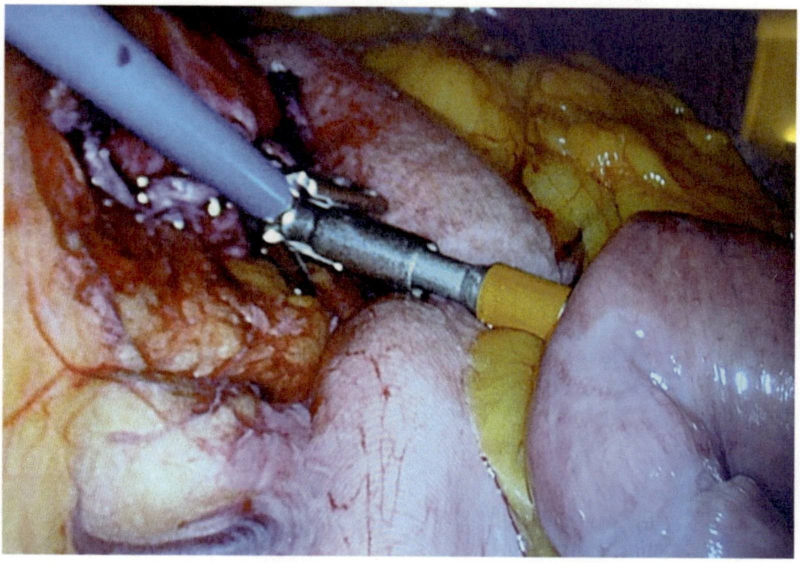

Figure 13.
Connection of the anvil to the spike of the circular stapler.

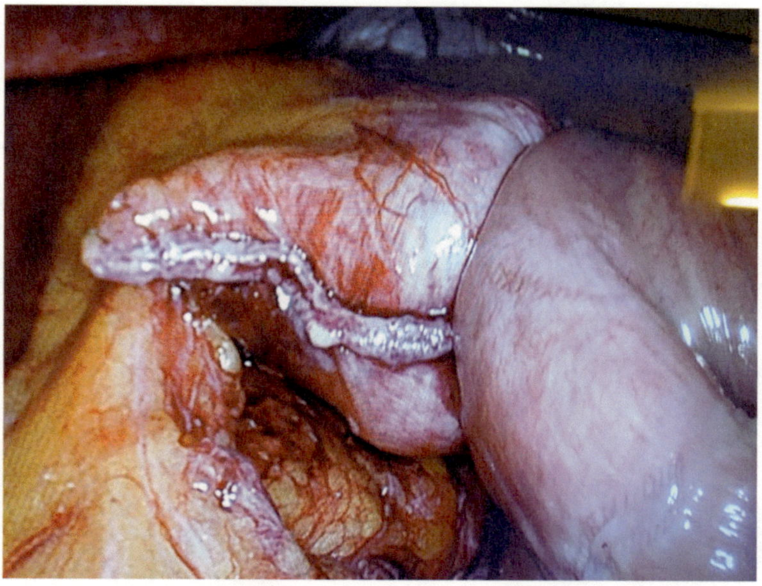

Figure 14.
Circular stapler device is fired.

jejunum (**Figure 15**). Finally, the gastrojejunostomy is inspected, and an extra "good night" PDS stitch is placed in case of hematoma, serosal weakness, or high traction.

Ensuring tension-free and well-perfused anastomosis is crucial. The main advantages of the circular technique are that it is a reliable and reproducible technique, with a standardized diameter of 25 mm, offering a homogenous blood perfusion, and a balanced distribution of traction.

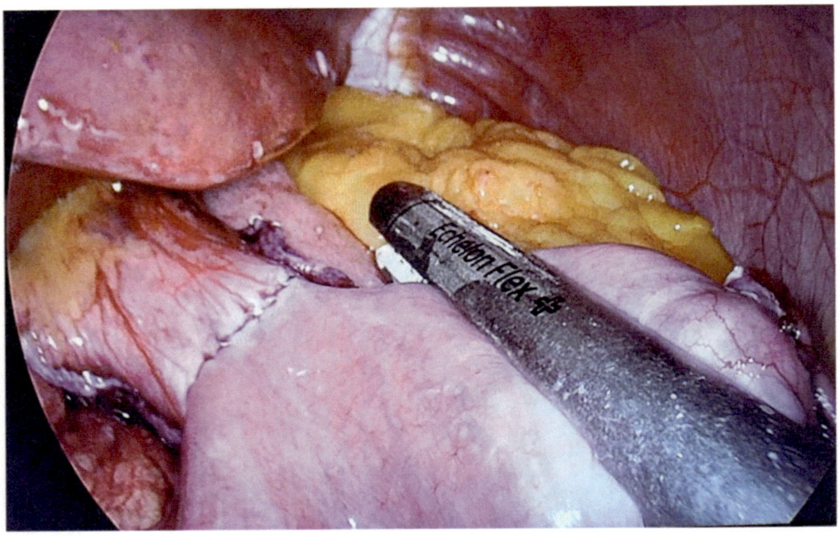

Figure 15.
Disconnecting the alimentary limb from the future biliopancreatic limb with a linear stapler.

3.5 Construction of the Roux-en-Y jejunojejunostomy

The alimentary limb is measured in a distal direction by the surgeon until 100 to 130 cm, and a small antimesenteric opening is created in the jejunum using the ultrasonic device (**Figure 16**). This opening is stretched with a grasper. The nurse or

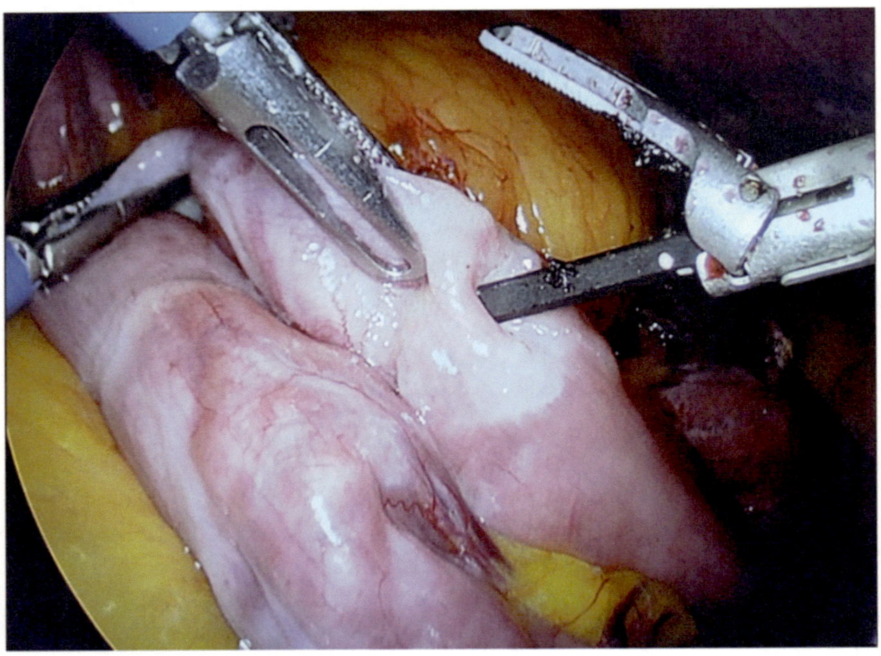

Figure 16.
Making an antimesenteric opening in the alimentary limb, at the site of the future jejunojejunostomy.

the second assistant holds this bowel with a grasper (left lateral trocar) placed 1 cm distal of this opening, stretching the bowel toward the left lower quadrant.

Secondly, a similar opening is made in the biliopancreatic limb, 5–8 cm proximal to the enterotomy, and stretched with a grasper. The first assistant (left hand) uses the most cranial trocar and holds the jejunum 1 cm distal from the small opening, toward the left upper quadrant. The surgeon takes the camera. A linear 60-mm stapler with a white/tan cartridge is introduced by the first assistant (right hand) via the right trocar in the biliopancreatic limb with help from the surgeon. The other part of the linear stapler is then placed in the opening of the alimentary limb by aiming toward the left lower quadrant. At this part, the grasper of the left lateral trocar must let go. After positioning both sides of the stapler in the small bowel, the stapler and the future jejunojejunostomy have to be stretched toward the left upper quadrant (**Figure 17**). An inspection is necessary to verify whether both sides of the stapler device are well in place, leaving no unused stapler line, and placing the stapler in a perfect antimesenteric position preventing bleeding before the device is finally fired. The side-to-side jejunostomy is now completed, and the stapler removed.

The first assistant takes the camera with the right hand and is still holding the jejunum with the left hand (cranial trocar). The resulting enterotomy needs to be closed in the next step. The surgeon uses the right and left medial trocar to put a PDS traction stitch at the alimentary side of the enterotomy (**Figure 18**). Then, the excess biliopancreatic mesentery is removed toward the aimed jejuno-jejunostomy (Barcelona-type principle) with the ultrasonic device (**Figure 19**). Make sure to not cause thermal injuries on the jejunum, or to devascularize the anastomosis. The defect is closed by a linear stapler through the right trocar

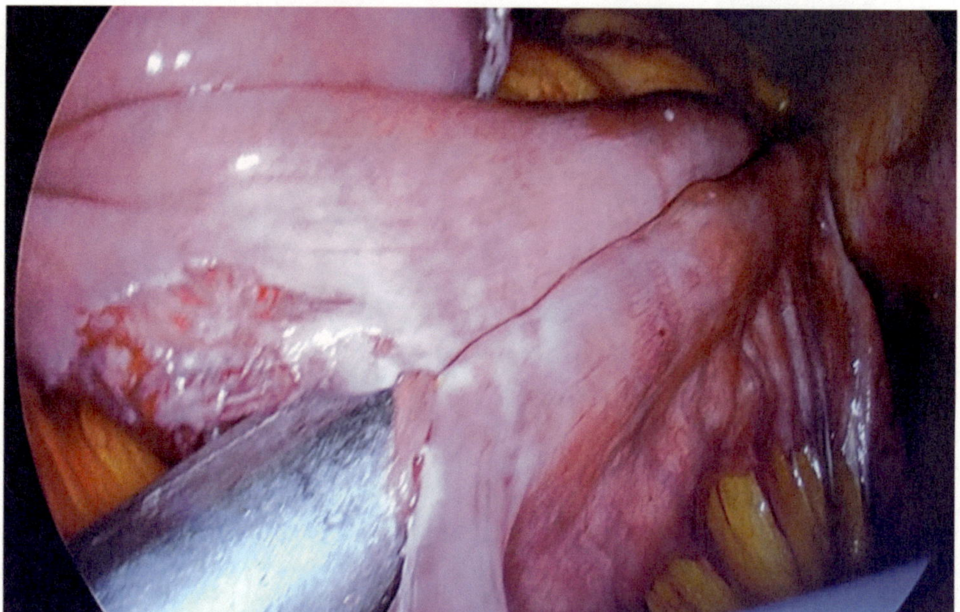

Figure 17.
The first assistant ensures a perfect antimesenteric positioning of the linear stapler device, before firing the jejunojejunostomy.

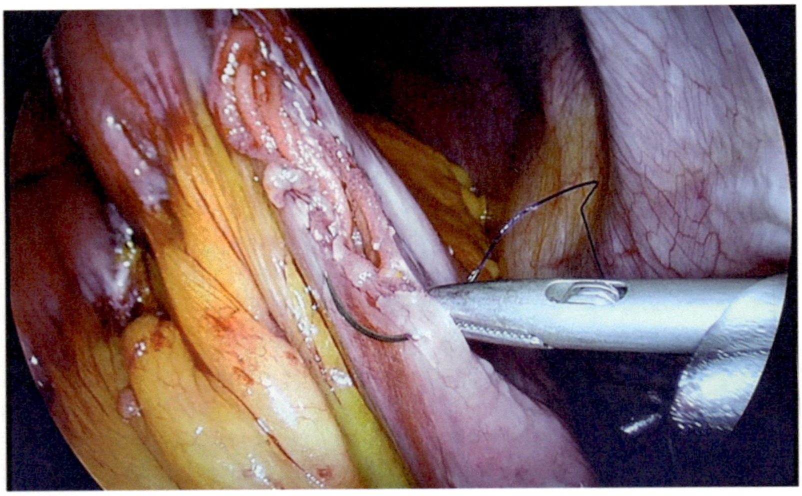

Figure 18.
Temporary traction suture at the alimentary side of the enterotomy.

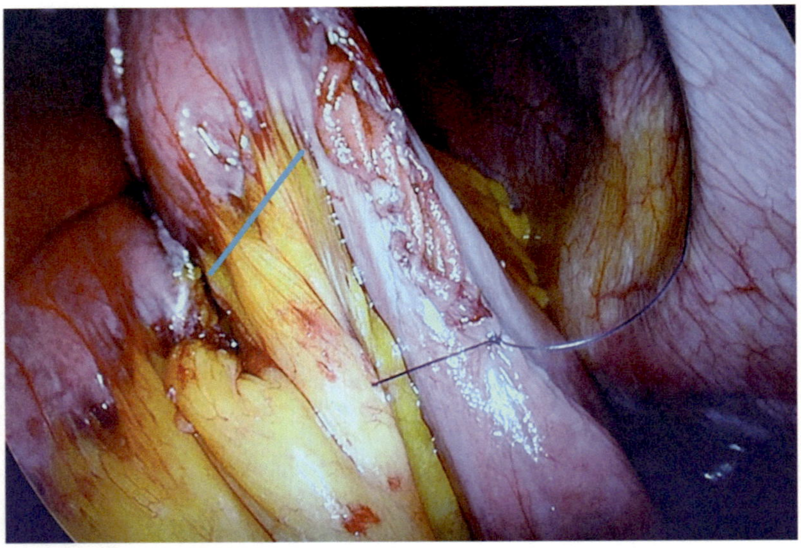

Figure 19.
The blue line depicts the dissection line of the abundant mesentery at the excess loop of the jejunojejunostomy.

(first assistant) (**Figure 20**). Before firing, the diameter of the alimentary limb entrance toward the enteroenterostomy is verified and the surgeon might carefully pull out some extra millimeters of bowel tissue to prevent a narrow entrance. The first assistant is still holding the jejunal loop that will soon be removed and pulls this excess loop well into the stapler. After firing, this resected piece of bowel is removed via the left lateral trocar.

At this moment, the anesthesiologist is asked to start raising the systolic blood pressure gently above 130 mmHg.

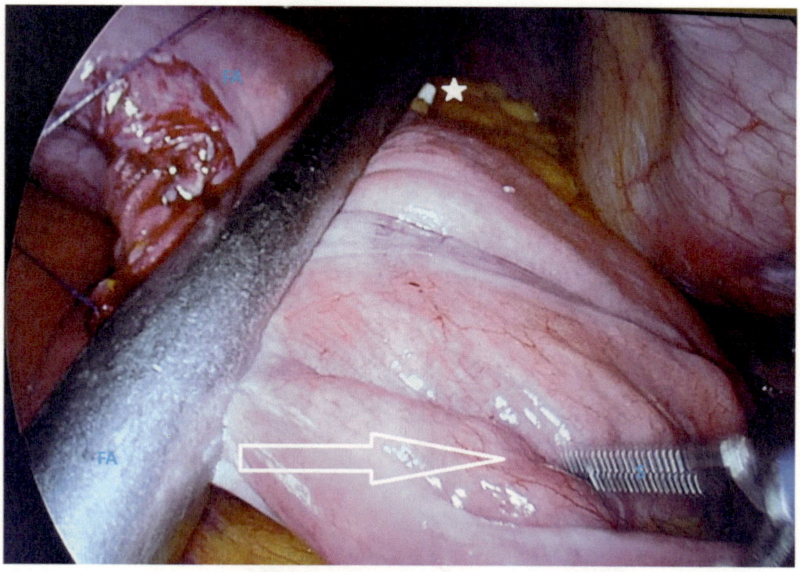

Figure 20.
The enterotomy of the jejunojejunostomy is closed with a linear stapler device (FA: First Assistant). Meanwhile, the FA holds the excess jejunal loop toward the liver, making sure the enterotomy is transected completely (white star). The surgeon (S) verifies the diameter of the entrance of the alimentary limb into the jejunojejunostomy, preventing kinking or obstruction of the food. Minimal diameter should be equal to or more than the length of an opened grasper (2.8 mm).

3.6 Closure of mesenteric gaps

Internal hernia can not always be prevented, but closing both mesenteric gaps might certainly help if done in a proper way.

The first assistant holds the mesentery of the alimentary limb with a grasper via the right trocar and gives traction toward the right side of the patient. Subsequently, the enteroenteric mesenteric gap can be easily visualized. This transverse linear gap can be closed with a non-resorbable suture, or in an ergonomic and quick way with a stapling device (Endo Hernia™) through the left medial trocar (**Figure 21**).

The visualization of the Petersen's space is often more difficult. The first assistant (right trocar) has to stretch some appendices epiploica from the medial part of the colon transversum toward the right upper quadrant. The transverse mesocolon is now stretched, allowing a good view at the J-shaped Petersen's space for closure with a stapling device (**Figure 22**). Pushing up the transverse colon and omentum with the Babcock from the left lateral trocar site might sometimes help in case of severe visceral obesity. For closure of this defect with a Filblock™, the same exposure is needed. Exceptionally, in complex cases with severe adhesions, too much traction at the gastroenterostomy, or poor visualization, the mesenteric defects are left open.

3.7 Methylene blue test at the gastrojejunostomy

The orogastric tube is positioned at the level of the gastrojejunostomy, and leakage risk is checked by forcefully injecting a full syringe of 60 mL of methylene blue and 60 mL of air while obstructing the alimentary limb distally (**Figure 23**). If at this

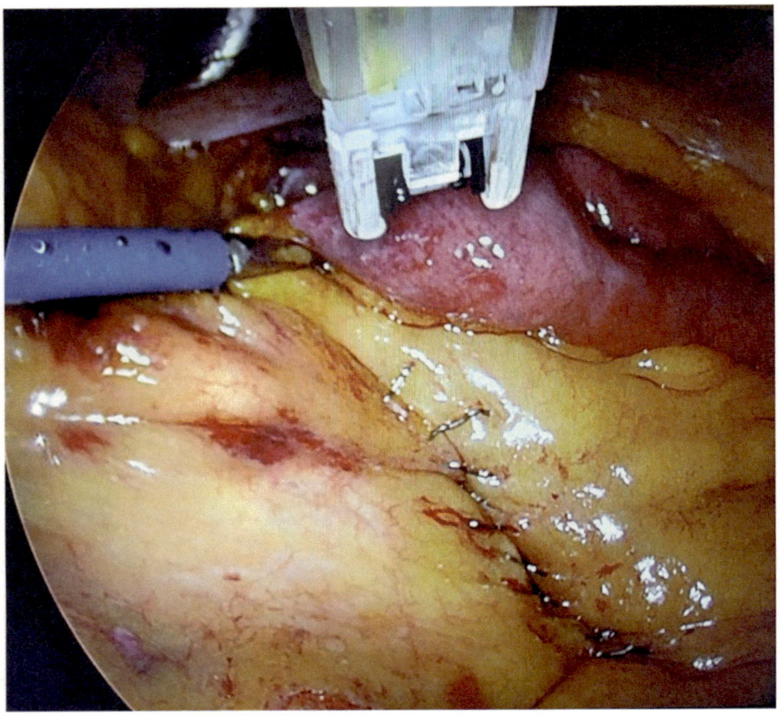

Figure 21.
Closure of the enteroenteric meso gap with a stapling device.

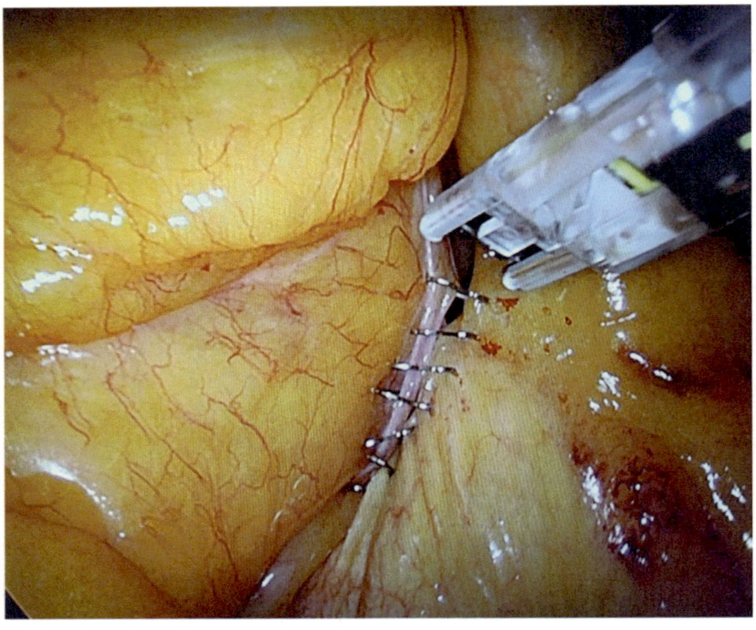

Figure 22.
Closure of the Petersen's space with a stapling device.

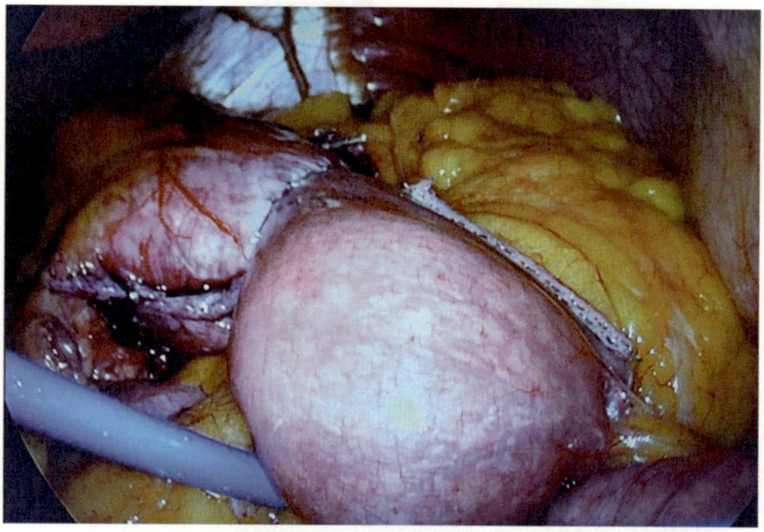

Figure 23.
Methylene blue test.

point any leakage is present or if some traction is detected, the gastrojejunostomy is reinforced with some additional stitches PDS. Using this reliable test, the leak rate of a standard RYGB is zero in our team.

3.8 Hemostasis and closure

Meanwhile, the systolic arterial blood pressure is elevated above 130 mmHg. Now all dissected regions and stapler lines are carefully checked to prevent postoperative intra- or extraluminal bleeding using clips or electrocautery.

The enlarged left lateral trocar port site is closed with one or two stitches with the Endo Close™ trocar site closure device, in order to prevent lateral entrapment or hernia formation (**Figure 24**). No drains are placed in a standard RYGB to prevent postoperative pain and immobilization.

4. Postoperative care

Patients are admitted to the recovery room and are monitored for 1 or 2 hours, and if postoperative nausea is not too bad, a sugar-free popsicle is offered. Thereafter, patients are transferred to the bariatric ward, are stimulated to mobilize a few hours after surgery, and to drink water and eat yogurt. Oral and written information is offered by visits and brochures of the bariatric surgeon, the dietician, and the physiotherapist. After one night of monitoring of pain, hemodynamic parameters, mobilization, and oral intake, patients are dismissed (**Figure 25**).

No liquid, slider food, or ketogenic diet is required after surgery. Normal food rich in proteins is immediately introduced. Upper gastrointestinal imaging is not routinely performed.

To prevent deep venous thrombosis, patients receive subcutaneous thrombosis prophylaxis for 10 days.

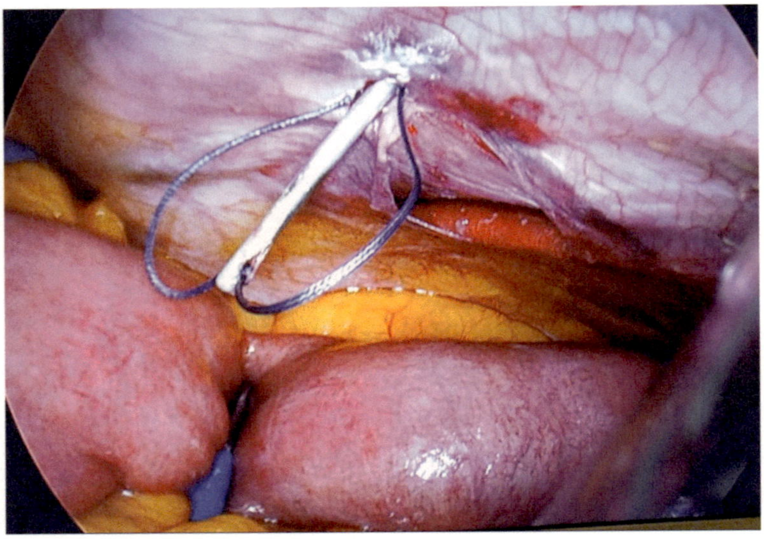

Figure 24.
Closure of the left lateral enlarged trocar site.

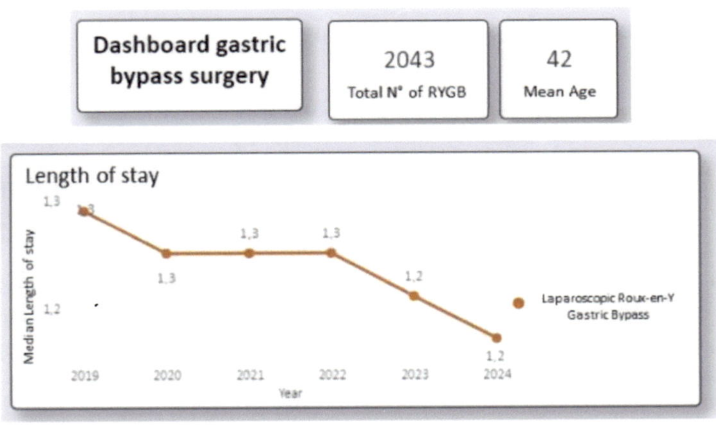

Figure 25.
Between 2019 and 2024 a total of 2043 RYGB operations were performed. Mean age of patients was 42 years old. Mean length of stay is diminishing over the years toward 1.2 days due to a fast track and enhanced recovery protocol.

In standard conditions, proton pump inhibitors are taken for 3 months to prevent marginal ulcer formation. Lifelong or high doses of proton pump inhibitors are advised in patients who smoke or patients on anticoagulants, corticoids, or non-steroidal anti-inflammatory drugs.

Supplementation with bariatric multivitamins and minerals (calcium citrate) is standardized to prevent deficiencies.

Standard postoperative care is scheduled with the dietician and surgeon at 3 weeks, 3 months, 6 months, 12 months, and annually thereafter. A muscle rehabilitation program is offered in our hospital during the first 3 months. Extra psychological support can be added on demand. Patients can have access to extra support using our digital tool, Move Up, with patient information, weight evolution, patient-related outcome measures, questionnaires, training programs, and direct communication with the obesity coordinator.

5. Conclusion

The standardization of the fully stapled Roux-en-Y gastric bypass represents a significant advancement in bariatric surgery. By adhering to uniform protocols for preoperative assessment, intraoperative technique, and postoperative care, healthcare providers can ensure safer procedures, better outcomes, and more efficient training.

The RYGB is associated with good long-term results on weight loss and comorbidity resolution, with minimal operative morbidity and mortality, and can be used even in complex revisional bariatric cases.

As the field of bariatric surgery continues to evolve, ongoing research and refinement of these standards will be essential to maintain and improve the quality of care for patients undergoing RYGB.

6. Summary

The standardized fully stapled Roux-en-Y gastric bypass

- Is a safe procedure with quick recovery and minimal postoperative morbidity and mortality
- Shows better outcomes of long-term results on weight loss and comorbidity resolution
- Allows more efficient training and can be used even in complex revisional bariatric cases

Acknowledgements

Thanks are due to my mentor, Dr. Bruno Dillemans, bariatric surgeon, AZ Sint-Jan Bruges, Belgium.

Conflict of interest

The authors declare no conflict of interest.

Author details

Isabelle Debergh
Department of General Abdominal, Thoracic and Oncological Surgery, AZ Delta Hospital, Roeselare, Belgium

*Address all correspondence to: isabelle.debergh@azdelta.be

References

[1] Mason E, Ito C. Gastric bypass in obesity. The Surgical Clinics of North America. 1967;**47**(6):1345-1351. DOI: 10.1016/s0039-6109(16)38384-0

[2] Dillemans B, Sakran N, Van Cauwenberge S, Sablon T, Defoort B, Van Dessel E, et al. Standardization of the fully stapled laparoscopic roux-en-Y gastric bypass for obesity reduces early immediate postoperative morbidity and mortality: A single center study on 2606 patients. Obesity Surgery. 2009;**19**(10):1355-1364

[3] Agrawal S. Impact of bariatric fellowship training on perioperative outcomes for laparoscopic Roux-en-Y gastric bypass in the first year as consultant surgeon. Obesity Surgery. 2011;**21**(12):1817-1821

[4] Dillemans B, Deylgat B. LRYGB: The fully stapled technique. In: Agrawal S, editor. Obesity, Bariatric and Metabolic Surgery—A Practical Guide. 1st ed. Springer International Publishing; 2016. Chapter 22. ISBN: 9783319345260

[5] Dillemans B, Deylgat B, Viskens S. Laparoscopic Roux-en-Y gastric bypass: The standardized technique. In: Agrawal S, editor. Obesity, Bariatric and Metabolic Surgery—A Comprehensive Guide. 2nd ed. Springer Nature Switzerland; 2023. pp. 337-346. DOI: 10.1007/978-3-030-60596-4_22

[6] Vasas P, Dillemans B, Van Cauwenberge S, De Visschere M, Vercauteren C. Short- and long-term outcomes of vertical banded gastroplasty converted to Roux-en-Y gastric bypass. Obesity Surgery. 2013;**23**(2):241-248

[7] Khewater T, Yercovich N, Grymonprez E, Debergh I, Dillemans B. Conversion of both versions of vertical banded gastroplasty to laparoscopic Roux-en-Y gastric bypass: Analysis of short-term outcomes. Obesity Surgery. 2019;**29**(6):1797-1804

[8] Khewater T, Yercovich N, Grymonprez E, Horevoets J, Mulier JP, Dillemans B. Twelve-year experience with Roux-en-Y gastric bypass as a conversional procedure for vertical banded gastroplasty: Are we on the right track? Obesity Surgery. 2019;**29**(11):3527-3535

[9] Debergh I, Defoort B, De Visschere M, Flahou S, Van Cauwenberge S, Mulier JP, et al. A one-step conversion from gastric banding to laparoscopic Roux-en-Y gastric bypass is as safe as a two-step conversion: A comparative analysis of 885 patients. Acta Chirurgica Belgica. 2016;**116**(5):271-277

[10] Handojo K, Ismaeil A, Van Huele A, Van Neste C, Debergh I, Dillemans B. Roux-enY gastric bypass as conversion procedure of failed gastric banding: Short-term outcomes of 1295 patients in one single center. Obesity Surgery. 2023;**33**(10):2963-2972

Chapter 8

A New Articulating Laparoscopic Instrument in Bariatric Surgery

Nicola Perrotta, Marta Celiento, Alessandro Troisi,
Roberta Russo and Pasquale Campagna

Abstract

Recent literature confirms an increasing use of robotic surgery in the field of bariatrics. However, recent meta-analyses do not to show the advantages of robotics compared to traditional laparoscopy in terms of complications, reoperations, and hospital stays, despite significantly longer operative times and costs. In this context, articulated laparoscopic instruments can be a valid alternative to the more modern robotic technology in bariatric surgery. In the last 3 years, we have introduced ArtiSential® Articulating Laparoscopic Instruments (LIVSMED, Seongnam, Republic of Korea). This new Multi-DOF (Degree of Freedom) laparoscopic instrument provides undeniable advantages due to its extreme flexibility, thanks to the double distal articulation, which consent 360° of movement at the surgical site. In this chapter, we report our experience with the use of ArtiSential® instruments (scissors, graspers, dissectors, needle holders) during bariatric surgery procedures, analyzing their advantages and applications.

Keywords: bariatric surgery, sleeve gastrectomy, gastric bypass, ArtiSential, articulated instruments

1. Introduction

Obesity is a worldwide chronic disease with an associated high numbers of costly disorders [1]. All over the world, the number of obese and superobese people is growing, and bariatric surgery is performed more frequently to avoid serious complications related to obesity. Lots of therapies could be chosen for patients with obesity (e.g., drugs, dietary therapies, physical exercise, etc.), but their effect was unobvious for compliance and not effective in the long term [2]. Nowadays, bariatric surgery is a validated option performed all around the world with different standardized procedures. The effectiveness of bariatric surgery is a significant and sustained weight loss related to an improvement of the comorbiditys. Patients can in fact lose 50% or more of their excess weight [3]. Bariatric surgery has been shown to improve type 2 diabetes, high blood pressure, sleep apnea syndrome, hyperlipidaemia, and GERD (GastroEsophageal Reflux Disease) [4].

There were lots of bariatric procedures that can be applied in clinical practice, including restrictive and malabsorptive ones (Sleeve Gastrectomy, Gastric Bypass,

One Anastomosis Gastric Bypass, Adjustable Gastric Band, etc.) [5–6]. All these types of surgeries are performed using either laparoscopic or robotic surgery. Both methodologies obtained minimally invasive techniques, high-definition vision, and precise operation [7], but robotic bariatric surgery may acquire more advantages for both patients and surgeons in the long run.

With the advent of robotic surgery, an increasing number of centers in the world have challenged their bariatric laparoscopic procedure in robotic and, nowadays, robotic surgery is extremely diffused. The robotic system has been the most ergonomic instrument with the widest range of motion, but operative time was showed longer in robotic bariatric surgery (RBS) and length of hospital stay was not significantly different between RBS and laparoscopic bariatric surgery (LBS). Moreover, estimated blood loss was reported no significant difference in RBS. Reoperation within 30 days, leaks, strictures, pulmonary embolism, and overall complications show no significant difference between LBS and RBS. RBS may be not inferior to LBS during different periods for weight loss assessed by Excess Weight Loss (EWL%) and Body Mass Index (BMI) loss.

Since its introduction, price and costs represent a critical problem of the robotic system, as well as the low cost-effectiveness [8, 9]. The small quantity of units for the institution, the need for an operating theater designated for robotic surgery, and an expert staff to prepare the console constitute further limits to the diffusion of this technology.

Robotic bariatric surgery has also demonstrated that ergonomics has become an important issue in terms of surgeons' fatigability. Based on these problems, a bridge can be obtained by articulated instrument introduction. Through time, some articulating laparoscopic devices with increased freedom of movement have been proposed

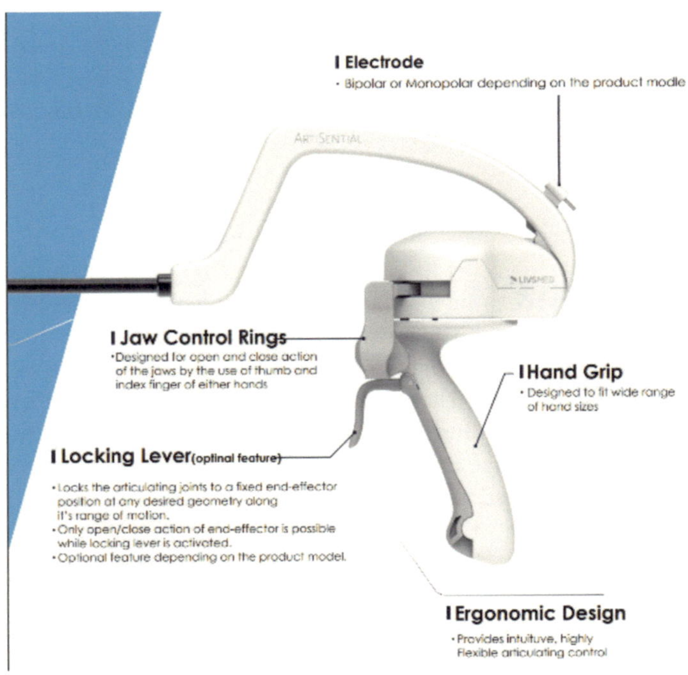

Figure 1.
Handle of the instruments.

in the market. However, most of them have been unsuccessful [10]. ArtiSential® is the first mechanical laparoscopic instrument with the widest angle of motion (360°), that perfectly mimics the movements of the robotic joint (**Figure 1**).

2. ArtiSential® articulating laparoscopic instruments

Straight laparoscopic instruments are limited because the end terminal is aligned on the same axis as the laparoscope. This can lead to a collision between instruments, named also "sword fighting," which hampers free manipulation during the operation. To overcome such limitations, several flexible instruments with articulation have been introduced to overcome the restrictions of maneuverability and for use in laparoscopic surgery. One of these is the new device with multi-degree-of-freedom (DOF) articulation, the ArtiSential, a wide line of single-use articulated instruments.

In the last 3 years we have introduced in our experience ArtiSential® Articulating Laparoscopic Instruments (LIVSMED, Seongnam, Republic of Korea). It has a multi-joint structure that works with a pulley mechanism, whereas the end tool of the conventional laparoscopic instrument has no joint. This structure allows the end tool of ArtiSential® to move 90° up, down, left, and right. The thumb and index finger go into the two holes of the handle (**Figure 2**). The free manipulation provides intuitive movement of the end tool that perfectly matches the movement of the user's fingers and wrists (**Figure 3**). The rest of the fingers grab the main handle for support. On the main handle, there is a lever to activate the "hold" mode. The "hold" mode can fix the end effector at any angle (like a conventional instrument) and allow the insertion of the instrument into the trocars (**Figure 1**).

Several different effectors are available, like Fenestrated Forceps, Bipolar Fenestrated Forceps, Maryland Dissector, Bipolar Maryland Dissector, Bipolar Precise Dissector, Bipolar Curved Dissector, Needle Holder, Precise Needle, Holder Clip Applier Medium Large, Monopolar Spatula, and Monopolar Hook. In commerce there

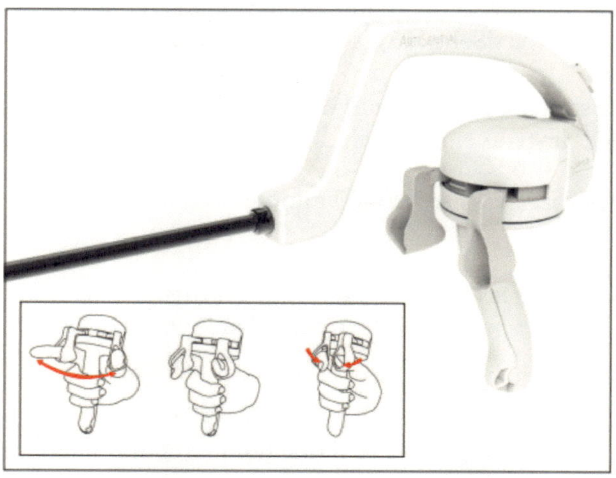

Figure 2.
ArtiSential instrument handle. The thumb and index finger, mainly used for grabbing, go into the two holes on the handle. The movement of this handle and the end tool show identical motion.

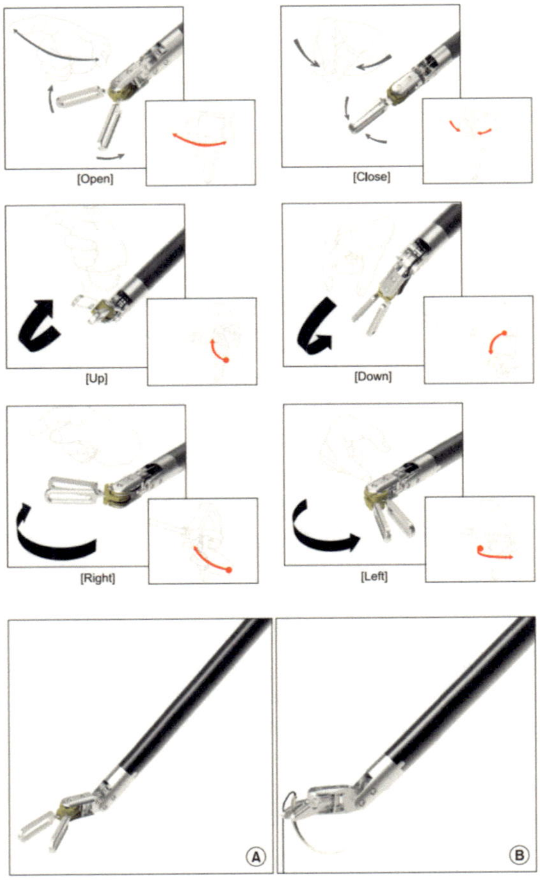

Figure 3.
Instrument hand-end tool coordination. The movement of the thumb, index finger, and wrist perfectly match the movement of the end tool.

are 8 mm diameter instruments with monopolar/bipolar connection, and also 5 mm diameter instruments (ArtiSential 5), both in standard (38 cm shaft length) and short (30 cm) versions.

Like in robotic surgery, Artisential® needs a learning curve, necessary to adapt to the new multi-DOF instruments, which can be easily divided by time [11]:

- In the first approach we need 30–60 minutes to understand the motion of the instruments;
- The next step requires from 4 to 8 hours in the dry lab to begin confident with the motion. This phase is variable in accordance with the experience of the surgeon;
- After achieving the motion, it is safe to step to the patient with a single instrument at a time, choosing and alternating dominant or nondominant hand. Also, in this phase would be necessary up to 10 consecutive procedures to adjust the process and master the use;

- When surgeons are confident with the use of the single instrument, it is time to introduce the use of ArtiSential® in both hands;

- The last phase of the learning curve is the introduction of the needle holder which has more complex movements and needs an initial attitude to articulated instruments suturing.

The learning curve is easily satisfied in a short while and the ability of the surgeon can improve fast case by case.

ArtiSential allows for meticulous dissection with two instruments in the smallest possible space without collision and with maximum control and optimal tactile feedback.

With this instrument, it is possible to reduce tissue trauma generated from the lateral traction of standard laparoscopic instruments by a perpendicular grip of the ArtiSential grasper. A gentle and direct grip is allowed without tension or traction. The articulation consents to a wider variety of surgical maneuvers than stray-fixed laparoscopic instruments.

The experienced laparoscopic surgeon can achieve difficult suturing tasks with the ArtiSential, similar to the robotic system. Another advantage of the ArtiSential is it easily usable during every operation, like any other laparoscopic traditional instrument, also in emergency settings, by simply opening the package [12].

A particular attention merits the control part of the instrument, for the cumbersome appearance that can limit the movements between the camera and the hands of the surgeon. Sometimes we need to modify a little the trocar position to avoid conflicts (**Figure 4**).

Surgeons, in the first procedures, can experience physical stress from the heavier and bigger instruments compared to conventional ones. This is a temporary drawback that will disappear with the use and the exercise. Also, surgeons with small

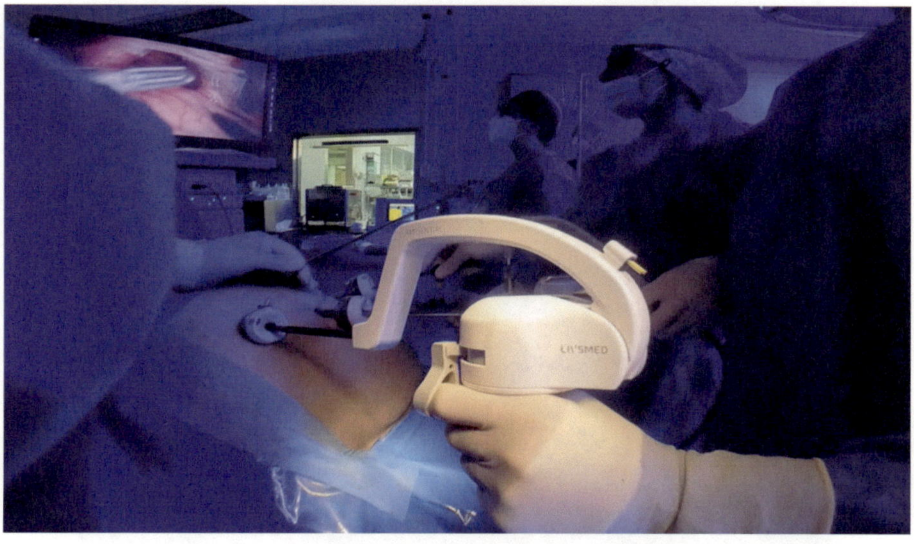

Figure 4.
External vision during surgery.

hands could have difficulties using it, but, actually, there are adjustable Velcro straps attached to the handle rings to fit the user's fingers.

3. Tips and tricks with articulated instruments

In our experience, bariatric surgery is an optimal field of application of articulated instruments, for multiple dissections, manipulations, and gastrointestinal sections and sutures.

3.1 Sleeve gastrectomy

- *Entrance and set up*: Pneumoperitoneum with Verres needle in the left subcostal quadrant. Pneumoperitoneum of 14 mmHg. Positioning of the optical trocar and four other operating trocars (1 of 10 mm; 2 of 5 mm; 1 of 15 mm).

- *Mobilization of the greater curvature*: Incision of the Bertelli peritoneal reflection and asportation of the gastric fundus fat. Dissection of the grater curvature begins by dividing the greater omentum 6 cm proximal to the pylorus. The gastroepiploic vessels are coagulated and sectioned using an energy device for all of the greater curvature toward the short gastric vessels. This dissection is continued to completely divide the gastrophrenic ligament and mobilize the angle of His to identify the left crus of the diaphragm. In this phase, ArtiSential® can provide a better grip on tissue, with less trauma and with easy movements in little space, like during mobilization of the His Angle (**Figure 5**). It is also very useful during diaphragmatic pillar dissection in hiatal hernia repair, frequently performed during all bariatric procedures due to the small space of work (**Figure 6**).

- *Posterior mobilization*: After gaining access into the lesser sac the stomach is lifted anteriorly, sectioning all the adhesions, until all the posterior gastric wall.

- *Bougie placement*: We insert a 40 French bougie under laparoscopic visualization in the stomach directed to the initial divided omental attachments.

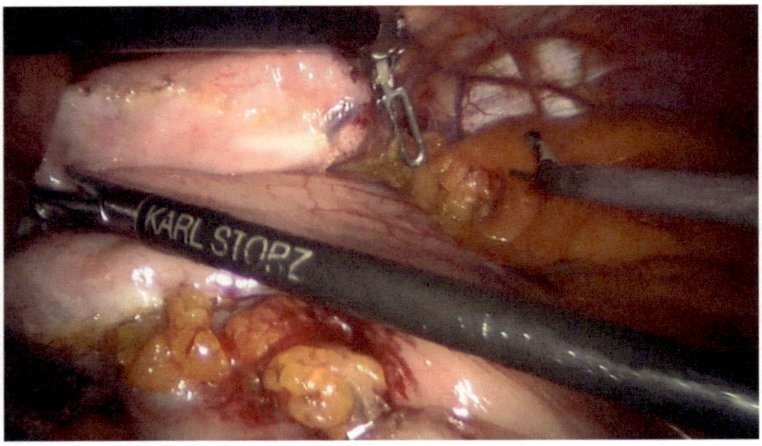

Figure 5.
Mobilization of the angle of his during sleeve gastrectomy.

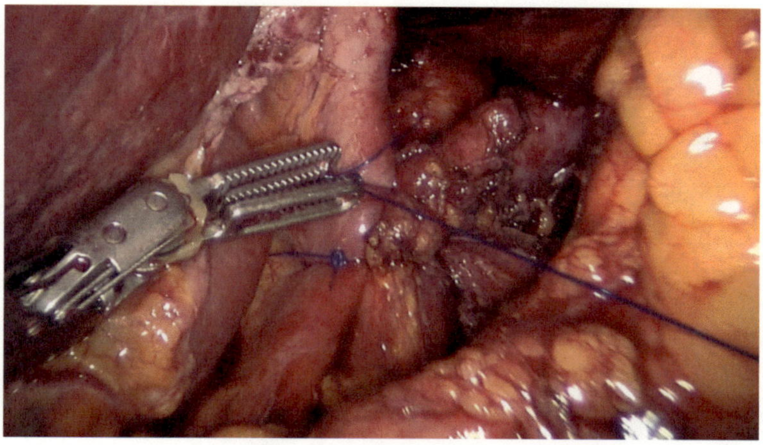

Figure 6.
Suture of the diaphragmatic pillars during hiatal hernia repair.

- *Creation of a stapled sleeve gastrectomy*: A 60 mm endoscopic stapler is inserted in the 15 mm trocar and is used for the gastric section. The first firing is begun to 6 cm to the pylorus along the bougie and parallel to the lesser curvature. Correct ArtiSential grasper traction on the margin of the greater curvature is fundamental to avoid sleeve spiralization. The staple lines are sequentially fired along the bougie, remaining 3–4 cm to the angular notch dividing the fundus at a distance of 1–2 cm lateral to the esophagus at the angle of His. The resected stomach is then removed through the 15 mm port.

- *Closure*: A fascial closure is done at the 15 mm port site, and skin closure is done at all sites.

3.2 Laparoscopic gastric bypass

- *Set up*: Pneumoperitoneum with Verres needle, in left under costal quadrant, of 15 mmHg. Positioning of a supraumbilical optical trocar and other four trocars (2 of 10 mm; 2 of 5 mm).

- *Preparation of the stomach pouch*: To preserve the left gastric artery, a retro gastric tunnel is formed starting at 5–6 cm below the gastroesophageal junction from the lesser curvature in a "peri-gastric" fashioning. With ArtiSential is easy to perform the dissection at the angle of His and entering the lesser sac. Using a linear stapler the stomach pouch is formed with the bougie as calibration. The insertion of the stapler is facilitated by using the end effector of the grasper to take up the posterior wall of the stomach.

- *Fashioning the gastrojejunostomy*: After the omental split, the jejunum measuring is started from the Treitz ligament to 60–70 cm, measuring along the grasper and the bowel is transported antecolic near the stomach. Counting appears easily with the use of ArtiSential atraumatic grasper. The bowel it is opened antimesenterically, and a linear stapler is inserted in the proximal direction. The small end of the stapler is inserted into the gastric pouch, and a side-to-side 3 cm gastrojejunostomy is fashioned to create a small enterostomy. The suture is performed

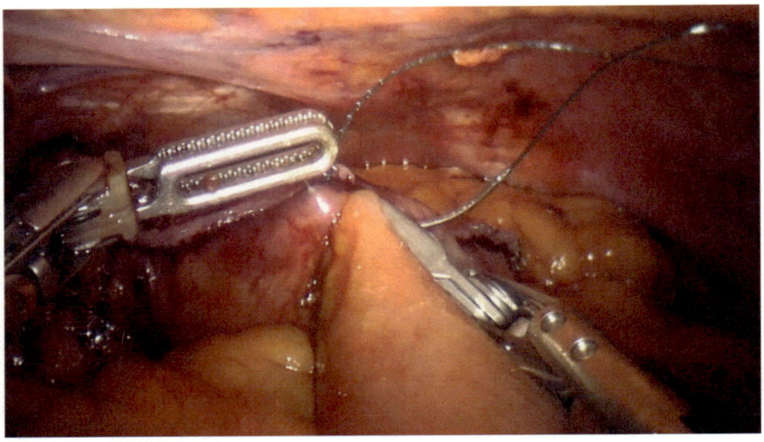

Figure 7.
Gastrojejuno anastomosis during laparoscopic gastric bypass.

rapidly with the ArtiSential device (**Figure 7**). For completing this anastomosis, enterotomy is closed with continuous seromuscular suture. A methylene blue test is performed. Starting from the right side of the enterotomy, a running suture completes the anastomosis.

- *Fashioning the jejunojejunostomy*: Again, measuring of the jejunum is started from the ligament of Treitz to 120–150 cm. The jejunum is opened antimesenterically, and a side-to-side 60 mm jejunojejunostomy is created using a linear stapler. The enterotomy is closed using a double suture in a seromuscular running technique. Proximal to the anastomosis, the jejunum is separated by a linear stapler, converting the omega loop into a Roux-en-Y Gastric Bypass. The ArtiSential needle holder is useful in this operation (with double anastomosis) because consent to the surgeon to maintain the same position during all the procedures.

- *Drainage and closure*: A drainage is placed side to the gastric pouch. All trocars are retrieved under view.

3.3 Laparoscopic OAGB (one anastomosis gastric bypass)

- *Entrance and set up*: Pneumoperitoneum with Verres needle, in left under costal quadrant, of 15 mmHg. Positioning of a supraumbilical optical trocar and other four trocars (2 of 10 mm; 2 of 5 mm)

- *Preparation of the stomach pouch*: The pouch is started under the Crow's Foot (the junction of the body and antrum of the stomach) along the small gastric curvature. Like in laparoscopic gastric bypass, ArtiSential can help perform better and easier dissection and gastric manipulation while performing the retro gastric tunnel (**Figure 8**). A 20 cm gastric tube is fashioned with multiple 60 mm staple firings along a 40 Fr. bougie for gastric calibration tube.

- *Gastrojejunostomy*: After omental split, the measuring of the jejunum is started from the ligament of Treitz to 180–200 cm, according to the Body Mass Index (BMI), measured using the grasper and transported antecolic. Counting seems

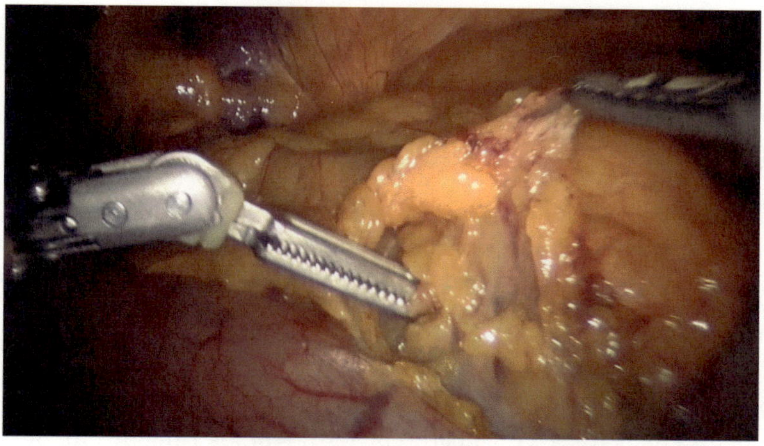

Figure 8.
One anastomosis gastric bypass (OAGB): performing the retro gastric tunnel.

to be easier with the use of ArtiSential. A side-to-side gastrojejunostomy, with a length of 4–5 cm, is created on the anterior gastric wall. The enterotomy is closed with a continuous seromuscular suture. A methylene blue test is performed. A running suture complete the anastomosis.

- *Drainage and closure*: A drainage is placed side to the gastric pouch. All trocars are retrieved under view.

4. Methods

In this retrospective vision, we performed above 70 surgery procedures with ArtiSential® between 2022 and 2024, including bariatric, general, and oncologic surgeries. Especially, 46 patients with bariatric conditions, 14 patients with diverticular stenosis, 11 patients with colorectal cancer, and three patients with stomach cancer are operated on with the ARTISENTIAL® articulated instruments. In this study, we will focus on bariatric patients, analyzing perioperative and short-term postoperative data.

All patients are chosen and preoperatively studied according to the Società Italiana di Chirurgia dell'OBesità (SICOB) e delle malattie metaboliche Guidelines 2023 and the choice to use ArtiSential® is completely random for trying to understand the several limitations of the application of the instruments. Retrospectively, we evaluated the data of patients like age, sex, Body Mass Index (BMI), postoperative stays, numbers of conversion, intraoperative bleeding, and postoperative complications.

In our excellent bariatric center Società Italiana di Chirurgia dell'OBesità (SICOB), two surgeons were implicated in this study, both with experience in the use of ArtiSential® and with a large experience in bariatric surgery. They performed 17 Sleeve gastrectomies, 25 Gastric Bypass, and four One Anastomosis Gastric Bypass (OAGB). All procedures were performed laparoscopically with ArtiSential® grasper, needle holder, and bipolar forceps.

All procedures are performed with a multi-port technique with five trocars. In the sleeve gastrectomy, the surgeon stays between the legs of the patients and operates with an energy device in his dominant hand and the ArtiSential® in his nondominant hand. Instead, we used ArtiSential® instruments in both hands to perform gastric bypass and One Anastomosis Gastric Bypass (OAGB), without using any energy device (such as ultrasounds or radio frequencies).

5. Results

In total 46 patients (17 males/29 females) were operated on with the ArtiSential® device. In the ArtiSential® group, the patients had a median age of 38 years (range 23–55 years) and a median Body Mass Index of 48 kg/m^2 (range 36–59 kg/m^2) (**Table 1**).

There were no intraoperative complications, and estimated intraoperative bleeding was less than 30 ml. No cases of conversion laparotomy and no switch to using a standard laparoscopic instrument. Surgical time is similar due to procedures that we carry out on a daily basis with laparoscopic straight instruments, for Sleeve Gastrectomy the median surgical time was 39′, for the Gastric Bypass the median time was 76′ and for the One Anastomosis Gastric Bypass (OAGB) was of 65′. On 46 surgical interventions, there was no intraoperative mortality. In all patients no drain was placed (**Table 2**).

Only one patient, gastric bypass operated, was complicated by bleeding from the trocar access, treated with a conservative cure, and dismissed on the 5th day of stay. The median length of stay was 3 days (range 2–4 days). There was not any other immediate postoperative general complication, and all patient was dismissed with a liquid diet for the first month. There was no unrelated readmission with no mortality (**Table 3**).

Demographics	Mean ± SD
No. (Male/Female)	46 (17/29)
Age (years)	38 ± 11.2
Height (cm)	161.6 ± 9.3
Weight (kg)	125.2 ± 23.2
Body Mass Index (BMI) (kg/m^2)	48 ± 8.0
EW (kg)	54.6 ± 21.3
Median ASA score	II

Table 1.
Preoperative data undergoing bariatric surgery with the use of ArtiSential.

Operative Time Sleeve Gastrectomy (minutes) ± (SD)	37.78 ± 6.62
Operative Time Laparoscopic Gastric Bypass (minutes) ± (SD)	76.32 ± 9.43
Operative Time OAGB (minutes) ± (SD)	64.97 ± 12.64
Rate of conversions to open surgery number (%)	0 (0%)
Intraoperative Bleeding number (%)	0 (0%)
Intraoperative Mortality (%)	0 (0%)

Table 2.
Intraoperative data.

	No. of cases (%)
Grade I	1 (0.46%)
Grade II	0
Grade III	0
Grade IIIb	0
Grade IV	0
Grade IVa	0
Grade Ivb	0
Length of stay (days)	3.45 ± 1.29

Table 3.
Postoperative data. Postoperative complication sorted by Clavien-Dindo classification: Grade I: Any deviation from the normal postoperative course without the need for pharmacological treatment, or surgical, endoscopic, and radiological interventions. Allowed therapeutic regimens are: drugs as antiemetics, antipyretics, analgetics, diuretics and electrolytes, and physiotherapy. This grade also includes wound infections opened at the bedside. Grade II: Requiring pharmacological treatment with drugs other than such allowed for grade I complications. Blood transfusions and total parenteral nutrition are also included. Grade III: Requiring surgical, endoscopic, or radiological intervention Grade III intervention not under general anesthesia. Grade IIIb: Intervention under general anesthesia. Grade IV: Life-threatening complication (including central nervous system complications) requiring IC/ICU management. Grade Iva: Single organ dysfunction (including dialysis). Grade Ivb: Multiorgan dysfunction Grade V Death of a patient.

In the follow-up to a 1 month, there were no gastric leaks, and the overall late complication rate was 0%.

The mean cost of the surgical material for ArtiSential® is 650 € and it is single-use, higher than the laparoscopic straight instruments, which can be also reusable, but significantly lower than the robotic set up. Wristed instruments could represent a standpoint for surgeons wanting a benefit from the advantages of robotic surgery from a cost-sensitive perspective.

6. Conclusion

This study has several limitations. First the small number of patients selected, this study has a descriptive nature and for this reason is impossible for us to compare the standard laparoscopy to the articulated one. This study shows that ArtiSential® in bariatric surgery can be safe and feasible, but comparative and randomized trials are needed to elaborate more on the results of this work.

Nowadays, articulated instruments are used not only in bariatric but in every field of abdominal surgery.

The new laparoscopic articulating devices are safe and feasible options that do not increase operative time, length of hospital stay, and intraoperative bleeding.

In our experience, ArtiSential® is helpful for performing otherwise difficult tasks in confined anatomical spaces, with lesser trauma on tissue and good tactile feedback. Moreover, these articulated instruments are readily available under any circumstance and can be used in everyday surgical practice, including emergency settings.

The learning curve of ArtiSential® is limited to a few hours in the dry lab and few operative cases. Also, the literature does not report a difference in learning between experts and young surgeons.

Articulated laparoscopic instruments, associated with 3D laparoscopy (like in our experience), can be a valid alternative to the more expensive robotic technology. A robotic center can also reduce the costs of surgery for procedures with a low cost-effectiveness ratio, returning from the robotic to laparoscopic articulated surgery.

Nowadays, more study needs to be published with a wider sample and prospective view and this is a wider field for research.

Author details

Nicola Perrotta*, Marta Celiento, Alessandro Troisi, Roberta Russo and Pasquale Campagna
Azienda Ospedaliera Regionale San Carlo, Potenza—Division of General Surgery, Italy

*Address all correspondence to: nicola.perrotta73@gmail.com

References

[1] Ng M, Fleming T, Robinson M, et al. Global, regional, and national prevalence of overweight and obesity in children and adults during 1980-2013: A systematic analysis for the Global Burden of Disease Study 2013. Lancet. 2014;**384**:766-781

[2] Courcoulas AP, Christian NJ, Belle SH, et al. Weight change and health outcomes at 3 years after bariatric surgery among individuals with severe obesity. JAMA. 2013;**310**(22):2416-2425

[3] Mingrone G, Panunzi S, De Gaetano A, et al. Bariatric–metabolic surgery versus conventional medical treatment in obese patients with type 2 diabetes: 5 year follow-up of an open-label, single-centre, randomized controlled trial. Lancet. 2015;**386**:964-973

[4] Schauer PR, Bhatt DL, Kirwan JP, et al. Bariatric surgery versus intensive medical therapy for diabetes—3-year outcomes. The New England Journal of Medicine. 2014;**370**:2002-2013

[5] Puzziferri N, Roshek TB III, Mayo HG, et al. Long-term follow-up after bariatric surgery a systematic review. JAMA. 2014;**312**(9):934-942

[6] Li K, Zou J, Tang J, et al. Robotic versus laparoscopic bariatric surgery: A systematic review and meta-analysis. Obesity Surgery. 2016;**26**(12):3031-3044

[7] Close A, Robertson C, Rushton S, et al. Comparative cost-effectiveness of robot-assisted and standard laparoscopic prostatectomy as alternatives to open radical prostatectomy for treatment of men with localised prostate cancer: A health technology assessment from the perspective of the UK National Health Service. European Urology. 2013;**64**:361-369

[8] Zhang Z, Miao L, Ren Z, Li Y. Robotic bariatric surgery for the obesity: A systematic review and meta-analysis. Surgical Endoscopy. Jun 2021;**35**(6):2440-2456

[9] Fan G, Zhou Z, Zhang H, et al. Global scientific production of robotic surgery in medicine: A 20-year survey of research activities. International Journal of Surgery. 2016;**30**:126-131

[10] Kim HI, Han SU, Yang HK, et al. Multicenter prospective comparative study of robotic versus laparoscopic gastrectomy for gastric adenocarcinoma. Annals of Surgery. 2016;**263**:103-109

[11] Kim A, Lee CM, Park S. Is it beneficial to utilize an articulating instrument in single-port laparoscopic gastrectomy? Journal of Gastric Cancer. Mar 2021;**21**(1):38-48

[12] Jin HY, Ibahim AM, Bae JH, Lee CS, Han SR, Lee IK, et al. Initial experience of laparoscopic complete mesocolic excision with D3 lymph node dissection for right colon cancer using Artisential®, a new laparoscopic articulating instrument. Journal of Minimal Access Surgery. Apr-Jun 2022;**18**(2):235-240

Chapter 9

First Experience with Robot-Assisted Bariatric Surgery Using the Senhance® System in the Treatment of Morbidly Obese Patients

Alexander G. Khitarian, Arut V. Mezhunts, Kamil S. Veliev, Denis A. Melnikova, Arutyun A. Abovian and Alexander A. Rogut

Abstract

Laparoscopic bariatric surgery is the most effective and long-term treatment for obesity. The results of robot-assisted bariatric surgery are studied using the new Senhance system in the treatment of morbidly obese patients. The optimal trocar placement and robotic arm positioning were analyzed, and the duration of the intervention and the amount of intraoperative blood loss were assessed. In the postsurgery period, we studied the number of recurrences, the number of complications, and their severity according to the Clavien-Dindo scale, as well as the severity of pain syndrome according to the VAS scale. Seventy-four patients were included in the study. According to the immediate results of surgical treatment analysis, the average duration of robot-assisted longitudinal gastric resection was 87 [67, 120] min; robot-assisted Roux bypass-116 [78, 139] min; and robot-assisted mini-bypass surgery-96 [79, 125] min. The mean time of robot-assisted revision surgeries was 141 [112, 184] min. There were no complications requiring surgical treatment, as well as complications related to the cardiovascular system or other. Robotic-assisted bariatric surgery using the Senhance system is feasible and safe for the patient. However, considerable experience is required, as well as cost-benefit analysis, to assess the feasibility of robotic systems in bariatric surgeries.

Keywords: morbid obesity, bariatric surgery, robotic surgery, Senhance robot, sleeve gastrectomy

1. Introduction

Obesity is a serious chronic disease accompanied by a complex of metabolic disorders that increase the risk of severe complications and death. The sharp increase in obesity prevalence has become a huge global health problem and requires urgent attention from country leaders, health systems, and the medical community. If ongoing trends continue, it is estimated that by 2030, 57.8% of the world's adult population will be overweight or obese [1]. Bariatric surgery is the most effective and long-term treatment for obesity [2]. Laparoscopy has been the standard of bariatric surgery for many years due to shorter length of hospital stay, faster recovery, and lower incidence of postoperative complications compared to open bariatric surgery [3, 4]. In order to overcome some technical disadvantages of laparoscopic surgery, such as the lack of three-dimensional (3D) images and restriction of freedom of movement due to the small articulation of laparoscopic instruments, robotic surgical systems were introduced in 1997 [5]. According to a significant number of studies, robot-assisted bariatric surgery is a safe and effective alternative to traditional laparoscopic techniques and demonstrates similar anatomical and functional outcomes at long-term follow-up [6–8]. Although some authors have reported no significant benefits in terms of patient outcomes with robotic bariatric surgery [9], several articles have reported better clinical outcomes after robotic surgery, especially for revision bariatric surgeries [10, 11].

For a long time, robotic surgery has been paired with the only system available, the DaVinci® (Intuitive Surgical, Sunnyvale, CA, USA). Among the alternative technical solutions, The Senhance® Surgical System ® Asensus Surgical US, Inc. (Durham, North Carolina, USA), a robotic surgical system, became available in 2016. This is a modular robotic system, the main differences of which are improved ergonomics for operator, fast docking, improved safety (the optimal point of trocar rotation in the abdominal wall is calculated by each robot arm—fulcrum point, which avoids rough, traumatic manipulations, bruising); Eye-Motion Control technology and haptic feedback, reusable instruments that significantly reduce the cost of surgical treatment, advanced artificial intelligence that allows real-time tissue recognition and marking on the monitor. Additionally, the system allows using a wide range of video systems from different manufacturers and the same accesses and instruments as for manual laparoscopy. This enables the system to be integrated more easily into the daily work of the operating theater.

2. Purpose of study

The purpose of this study was to examine our own results of robot-assisted bariatric surgery using the new Senhance system in the treatment of morbidly obese patients.

3. Materials and methods

The present study is a prospective cohort research including patients who underwent bariatric surgeries using the Senhance digital laparoscopy system at the Surgical Department of Private Healthcare Institution "Clinical Hospital 'RZhD-Medicine'" in the period from January 2022 to May 2023. We performed a total of 74 surgeries. Of these, 12 patients underwent robot-assisted Sleeve Gastrectomy (RA-SG), 20 patients underwent robot-assisted Roux-en-Y Gastric Bypass (RA-RYGB), 36 patients underwent robot-assisted one anastomosis/mini-bypass surgery (RA-OAGB), and 6 patients underwent revisional surgical treatment.

The indications for surgical treatment were indications for standard bariatric surgery according to the National Clinical Guidelines for the Treatment of Obesity in Adults [12], namely Obesity Stage 3 (BMI $\geq$ 40 kg/m^2) or Obesity Stage 2

(BMI ≥ 35 kg/m^2) with obesity-related diseases that can be influenced by weight reduction (type 2 diabetes mellitus, cardiovascular disease, joint disease, obstructive sleep apnea syndrome). All surgeries were performed by a surgical team trained and proficient in this robotic system and with considerable experience in bariatric surgery. Contraindications were acute gastric and duodenal ulcers, the existence of unresectable cancer or if less than 5 years had passed since radical treatment, mental illness, and severe irreversible changes in vital organs.

The standard algorithm of examination of an obese patient included the following range of tests: general blood analysis, blood lipid spectrum (total cholesterol, high-density lipoprotein, low-density lipoprotein, and triglycerides); fasting blood glucose, HbA1c, ALT, AST, gamma glutamine transferase, uric acid, urea, creatinine, bioimpedanceometry, ultrasound of abdominal organs, ultrasound of lower limb veins, echocardiography (ECG), and cardiologist and endocrinologist advice.

We collected data on the duration of surgery, duration of docking, placement of trocars and robotic arms and the need to move them during the intervention, the incidence of intraoperative complications and the need for conversion to laparoscopic surgery, as well as the amount of intraoperative blood loss and early postoperative complications, the severity of pain syndrome on the first day after surgery according to VAS. To capture the data, we used the TRUST Registry protocol (ClinicalTrials.gov Identifier: NCT03385109). All data were summarized and structured into one database using MS Excel 16 (MicroSoft, USA). This study was approved by the local ethical committee of the Private Healthcare Institution clinical hospital "RZD-Medicine." All patients gave written voluntary informed consent to participate in the study. The clinical performance of the patients is summarized in **Table 1**.

The mean weight in patients undergoing primary bariatric surgery was 127.2 ± 26.7 kg, the mean BMI was 45.2 ± 10.2 kg/m^2, and the mean age of the patients was 47.5 years (31–68, [39,55]). The presence of type 2 diabetes mellitus features varied in each patient group; the maximum number of patients with type 2 DM in

Parameter	Type of surgical intervention				
	RA-SG, n = 12	**RA-RYGB, n = 20**	**RA-OAGB, n = 36**	**RA-revis. n = 6**	**Total, N = 74**
Women	11	18	33	6	68
Men	1	2	3	–	6
Age, years, Me [Q_1;Q_2]	47,5 [39;60]	48 [42;53]	47,5 [41;55]	48 [42;55]	47,75
Weight, kg, Me [Q_1;Q_2]	127,5 [113;147,5]	110 [106;148]	123,5 [109;147,5]	92 [84;115]	
BMI, kg/m^2, Me [Q_1;Q_2]	47,6 [37,8;53,5]	42,6 [38,3;47,3]	43,5 [38,2;50,9]	34,1 [28,7;39,4]	
Type 2 diabetes mellitus	2	11	13	–	
Obstructive sleep apnea syndrome	7	6	11	–	
Arterial hypertension	5	12	20	–	

Table 1.
Clinical and demographic parameters of patients.

relation to the total number of patients was observed in the group of patients who underwent RA-RYGB and amounted to 11 patients (55%).

4. Statistical data analysis

Data were collected and the electronic database was formed using a PC and MS Excel 16 software (USA). Statistical processing of data was performed using SPSS Statistica 26.0 (USA) and MS Excel 16 (USA). At the initial stage of statistical analysis, all quantitative data were tested for conformity to the normal distribution law (NDL) according to the Shapiro-Wilk and Kolmagorov-Smirnov criteria, at $p < 0.05$—the sample does not conform to NDL, at $p > 0.05$—the sample conforms to NDL. In groups where samples were distributed according to NDL, it is reasonable to present descriptive data in the form of M ± SD, where M is the mean and SD is the standard deviation. In groups where samples were not distributed according to the NDL, descriptive data are better presented as median (Me), lower and upper limits of the interquartile range (range, IQR) as Q1 and Q2 quartile values (or 25 and 75% percentiles). Minimum and maximum values are also presented for all samples. For nominal and categorical data, descriptive statistics were presented in the form of absolute (number of people) and relative (percentage, %) values.

4.1 Surgical intervention technique

All surgeries were performed under endotracheal anesthesia in the Fowler's position with table rotation to the right side of about 15^0. The height of the operating table location before docking was 105 ± 9 cm, and varied depending on the anatomical features of the patient and the thickness of the anterior abdominal wall.

The following stages can be conventionally distinguished in robot-assisted bariatric surgery:

5. Installing ports and instruments

Port positioning during robot-assisted bariatric surgeries is practically the same as standard laparoscopy, and the convenience of work is in creating a comfortable angle of the robot arms movement, ensured by the use of instruments of different lengths. We used five ports as standard: 1 x 12, 3 x 10, and 1 x 5 mm, and arranged them as shown in **Figure 1**.

We used the following instruments to perform bariatric surgeries: 3D camera with an angle of 30° Olympus VISERA ELITE II (Olympus Corporation, Japan);

Robotic—atraumatic grasper, needle holder, scissors, ultrasound scalpel (ultrasonic), monopolar hook, if necessary—bipolar dissector;

Laparoscopic—Eshelon Flex linear stapling device with 60 mm cassettes in green, yellow and blue colors; atraumatic Babcock clamp; atraumatic intestinal clamps, grasper, monopolar hook.

5.1 Gastric mobilization

When performing RA-SG, gastric large curvature mobilization was performed in a standard way, 2 cm from the pylorus to the angle of His with the use of an ultrasonic

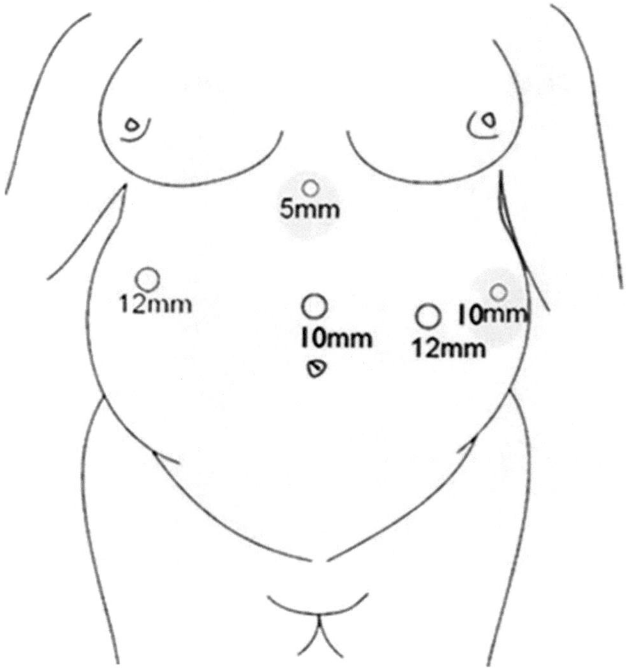

Figure 1.
Schematic diagram of trocar placement.

scalpel. When performing RA-RYGB, we proceeded to form a tunnel in the hepatic-gastric ligament at the level of 2–3 branches of the left gastric artery. In the case of RA-OAGB, the tunnel on the small gastric curvature was formed 2–3 cm below the gastric angle (Crow's foot of the left nerve of Latarjet). The ultrasonic scalpel was used to isolate the gastric vessels and create a posterior gastric space.

5.2 Formation of stomach with linear stapling device

Gastric formation for any type of bariatric surgery, whether RA-SG, RA-RYGB, or RA-OAGB was performed in a robot-assisted fashion through standard 12 mm trocars from the right and/or left subcostal region.

5.3 Robotic intracorporeal suture

In robot-assisted sleeve gastrectomy, robotic intracorporeal suturing consisted of strengthening the stapler suture line. In robot-assisted variants of Roux-en-Y Gastric Bypass and One Anastomosis Gastric Bypass, a manual robotic gastrojejunostomy was formed.

The robotic manipulator arms were positioned at the operating table, as shown in **Figure 2**, after which they were not required to be moved during the surgical procedure.

According to our own previous experience with the new Senhance robotic system, as well as to the literature findings, the system allows us to ergonomically perform some phases of surgical intervention with robotic assistance and others—laparoscopically, depending on the convenience and preferences of the surgeon. Thus, during the

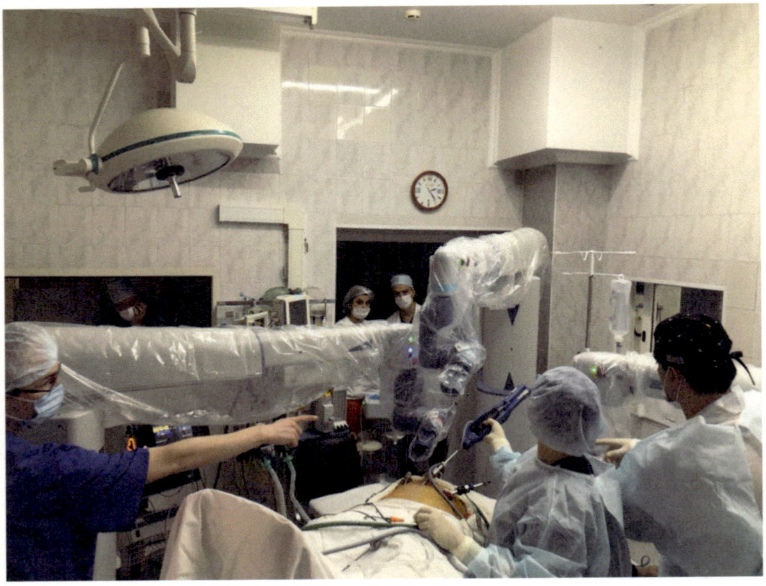

Figure 2.
Arrangement of the robot "arms".

surgical intervention, the planned conversion to a laparoscopic approach to perform individual steps, and vice versa, without loss of time and the need to change instruments, was carried out during the surgical intervention.

Switching of robotic instruments on the robot's "manipulator arms" was performed by the assistant if necessary. The process of switching instruments took a fairly short time, about 45–70 seconds. The surgical control unit of the robotic system is located in the far corner of our operating theater, which allows the surgeon,

Surgery	Robotic phase	Laparoscopic phase
Sleeve Gastrectomy	1—Gastric body and fundus mobilization along the greater curvature; 3—Robotic intracorporeal stapler line oversewing	2—Gastric resection with a linear stapling device
One Anastomosis Gastric Bypass	1—gastric mobilization; 4—formation of manual robotic gastrojejunostomy	2—forming the small pouch with a linear stapler 3—measuring the small intestine loop, its positioning
Roux-en-Y Gastric Bypass	1—gastric mobilization; 3—formation of manual robotic gastrojejunostomy	2—forming the small pouch with a linear stapler; 4—positioning of biliary and alimentary loops of small intestine, their isolation, length measurement; placement of hardware jejunojejunostomy
Revisional surgery	1—Viscerolysis; gastric stump mobilization 3—formation of manual robotic gastrojejunostomy	2—forming the small pouch with a linear stapler 4—positioning of biliary and alimentary loops of small intestine, their isolation, length measurement; placement of hardware jejunojejunostomy

Table 2.
Robotic-assisted and laparoscopic phases of bariatric surgeries.

controlling the manipulators and the camera, to have a good view of everything going on in the operating room, near the table, surrounded by the robot manipulator arms.

We believe that the unique advantages of robotic support are most important when performing dissection at the cardioesophageal junction (angle of His), manual intracorporeal suturing, and working within the same anatomical region. The technique of using the Senhance system when performing robot-assisted phases of surgical intervention and performing the planned conversion is summarized in **Table 2**.

6. Results

According to the immediate surgical treatment results analysis, the average duration of robot-assisted sleeve gastrectomy was 87 [67, 120] min; RA-RYGB-116 [78, 139] min; RA-OAGB-96 [79, 125] min; the mean time of robot-assisted revisional operations was 141 [112, 184] min. We separately recorded the time required for docking and other phases of robot-assisted surgeries. The duration of each phase of surgery is summarized in **Table 3**.

The volume of intraoperative blood loss was less than 50 ml. There were no complications requiring surgical treatment, as well as complications related to the cardiovascular system, respiratory organs or other complications within 1 month. The immediate results of surgical treatment of patients are summarized in **Table 4**.

In the early postoperative period, the patients stayed in the intensive care department until complete stabilization of vital functions within 2 hours, after which they were transferred to the ward of the specialized department. Oral fluid intake was started on the first day, and liquid food intake—on the second day. On the first day after surgical treatment, we evaluated the degree of pain syndrome severity using the visual-analog scale. The average duration of hospitalization after robot-assisted bariatric surgery was 5.4 (4–7) days.

During the work with the system, it became necessary in one case to convert from robot-assisted to manual laparoscopic surgery when performing revision surgery in a patient with severe adhesions in the area of the gastric tube.

7. Discussion

The Senhance robotic system for digital laparoscopy has several technical advantages, such as haptic feedback, a camera guidance system by operator gaze, ergonomics for the surgeon, and reusable instruments compatible with conventional laparoscopic

Time, min	RA-SG	RA-RYGB	RA-OAGB	RA-revis.
Total surgery time, Me [Q_1;Q_2]	87 [67, 120]	116 [78, 139]	96 [79, 125]	141 [112, 184]
Mean docking time, min. (min-max)	7 (6–9)	9 (8–10)	9 (8–10)	10 (9–12)
Mean time at the console, min. (min-max)	56 (51–68)	84 (75–103)	78 (66–94)	100 (87–123)
Mean time of surgery completion—from the moment of robot shutdown to skin closure, min. (min-max)	11 (10–16)	12 (10–18)	11 (9–15)	13 (10–16)

Table 3.
Duration of robot-assisted bariatric surgeries using the Senhance system.

Results	RA-SG	RA-RYGB	RA-OAGB	RA-revis.
Mean volume of intraoperative blood loss, ml	Less than 50	Less than 50	Less than 50	Less than 50
Intraoperative complications	–	–	–	–
Frequency of unplanned conversions to open/ laparoscopic surgery, %	0	0	0	1
Length of stay at anesthesiology and ICU, hours	2	2	2	2
Postoperative complications, according to Clavien-Dindo	–	–	–	–
Postoperative lethality, %	–	–	–	–
Pain syndrome on the first day, according to VAS, mm	22,5 (8–31)	22,5 (8–31)	22,5 (8–31)	25,5 (16–33)

Table 4.
Summarized results of robot-assisted bariatric surgeries using the Senhance system.

instruments, which significantly reduces the cost of treatment and simplifies the integration of the system into the operating room. At the time of publication of this article, we found only two studies in the available literature on bariatric surgery using the Senhance system. One of them was our article published in November 2023, where we described in detail our experience of using this system in bariatric surgery [13]. Tran et al. described their experience; however, they only analyzed the surgical technique of sleeve gastrectomy [14]. A number of researchers have reported the application of this robotic system in colorectal surgery, mainly in the treatment of cancer. For example, Spinelli et al. First reported a successful single-center experience with the Senhance system, safety and efficacy in various types of surgeries, including colorectal surgeries [15]. Samalavicius et al. reported on 13 cases of surgical treatment of colorectal cancer using a new robot-assisted laparoscopy and concluded that the system is convenient and comparable in results with traditional laparoscopy [16]. In June 2023, Vivianda Menke led a publication on the use of this teleoperation robotic system in performing robot-assisted fundoplication in patients with gastroesophageal reflux disease. The authors concluded that the use of the Senhance system demonstrated the safety, efficacy, and methodological superiority of robotic fundoplication [17].

The present study demonstrated the practical feasibility of performing bariatric surgery with the Senhance robotic system through first-hand experience.

The study has a number of limitations, in particular, the small number of cases and the lack of in-house experience with other robotic systems to allow direct comparison between them and comparison with traditional laparoscopy. Once a significant amount of experience has been accumulated, it is planned to demonstrate the comparative advantages of bariatric surgery using the Senhance system, comparing it with classical laparoscopic techniques.

8. Conclusions

Performing robot-assisted bariatric surgery using the Senhance system is feasible and safe for the patient. The immediate results of robotic access are comparable to laparoscopic access. However, significant experience and cost-benefit analysis is required to evaluate the feasibility of robotic systems in bariatric surgery.

Author details

Alexander G. Khitarian[1,2], Arut V. Mezhunts[1,2*], Kamil S. Veliev[1,2], Denis A. Melnikova[1,2], Arutyun A. Abovian[1,2] and Alexander A. Rogut[2]

1 Department of Surgical Diseases, Federal State Budgetary Healthcare Institution of Higher Education, Rostov State Medical University, Rostov-on-Don, Russia

2 Private Healthcare Institution, Clinical Hospital "RZhD-Medicine", Rostov-on-Don, Russia

*Address all correspondence to: arut.mezhunts@mail.ru

References

[1] Kelly T, Yang W, Chen C-S, Reynolds K, He J. Global burden of obesity in 2005 and projections to 2030. International Journal of Obesity. 2008;**32**(9):1431-1437

[2] Schauer PR, Deepak BL, Kirwin JP, et al. Bariatric surgery versus intensivemedical therapy for diabetes—3-year outcomes. The New England Journal of Medicine. 2014;**370**(21):2002-2013

[3] Weller WE, Rosati C. Comparing outcomes of laparoscopic versus open bariatric surgery. Annals of Surgery. 2008;**248**:10-15

[4] Nguyen NT, Goldman C, Rosenquist CJ, et al. Laparoscopic versus open gastric bypass: A randomized study of outcomes, quality of life, and costs. Annals of Surgery. 2001;**234**:279-291

[5] Li K, Zou J, Tang J, Di J, Han X, Zhang P. Robotic versus laparoscopic bariatric surgery: A systematic review and meta-analysis. Obesity Surgery. 2016;**26**(12):3031-3044. DOI: 10.1007/s11695-016-2408-5

[6] Iranmanesh P, Bajwa KS, Felinski MM, Shah SK, Wilson EB. Robotic primary and revisional bariatric surgery. The Surgical Clinics of North America. 2020;**100**(2):417-430. DOI: 10.1016/j.suc.2019.12.011

[7] Fourman MM, Saber AA. Robotic bariatric surgery: A systematic review. Surgery for Obesity and Related Diseases. 2012;**8**(4):483-488. DOI: 10.1016/j.soard.2012.02.012

[8] Wilson EB, Sudan R. The evolution of robotic bariatric surgery. World Journal of Surgery. 2013;**37**(12):2756-2760. DOI: 10.1007/s00268-013-2125-3

[9] Zhang Z, Miao L, Ren Z, Li Y. Robotic bariatric surgery for the obesity: A systematic review and meta-analysis. Surgical Endoscopy. 2021;**35**(6):2440-2456. DOI: 10.1007/s00464-020-08283-z

[10] Tatarian T, Yang J, Wang J, Docimo S, Talamini M, Pryor AD, et al. Trends in the utilization and perioperative outcomes of primary robotic bariatric surgery from 2015 to 2018: A study of 46,764 patients from the MBSAQIP data registry. Surgical Endoscopy. 2021;**35**(7):3915-3922. DOI: 10.1007/s00464-020-07839-3

[11] Dreifuss NH, Mangano A, Hassan C, Masrur MA. Robotic revisional bariatric surgery: A high-volume center experience. Obesity Surgery. 2021;**31**(4):1656-1663. DOI: 10.1007/s11695-020-05174-z

[12] Dedov II, Melnichenko GA, Shestakova MV, et al. National clinical guidelines for the treatment of morbid obesity in adults. Third revision (treatment of morbid obesity in adults). Obesity and Metabolism. 2018;**15**(1):53-70. DOI: 10.14341/omet2018153-70

[13] Khitaryan AG, Mezhunts AV, Veliev KS, Melnikov DA, Abovyan AA, Rogut AA. The first experience of robot-assisted bariatric surgery using the Senhance system in patients with morbid obesity. Pirogov Russian Journal of Surgery. 2023;**11**:82-88. (In Russ.). DOI: 10.17116/hirurgia202311182

[14] Tran T, Irizarry F, Gunda S, Danos D, Cook M. Early experience with the Senhance surgical system in bariatric surgery. JSLS. 2024;**28**(1):e2023.00031. DOI: 10.4293/JSLS.2023.00031

[15] Spinelli A, David G, Gidaro S, Carvello M, Sacchi M, Montorsi M.

Montroni I first experience in colorectal surgery with a new robotic platform with haptic feedback. Colorectal Disease. 2018;**20**(3):228-235. DOI: 10.1111/codi.13882

[16] Samalavicius NE, Janusonis V, Siaulys R, Jasėnas M, Deduchovas O, Venckus R, et al. Robotic surgery using Senhance robotic platform: Single center experience with first 100 cases. Journal of Robotic Surgery. 2020;**14**:371-376

[17] Menke V, Kottmann T, Willeke F, Hansen O. Learning curves and procedural times in Senhance-robotic assisted fundoplication: Results from 237 consecutive patients undergoing robotic fundoplication in a single center as part of the European TRUST Robotic Surgery Registry Study. Surgical Endoscopy. Nov 2023;**37**(11):8254-8262. DOI: 10.1007/s00464-023-10226-3

Chapter 10

Revisional Bariatric Surgery in a Single-Center Experience: Indications and Techniques

Livia Palmieri, Eleonora Rapanotti, Silvia Quaresima, Federica Rizzo, Germana Ginevra Perrone and Alessandro M. Paganini

Abstract

Bariatric surgery is currently considered the most effective treatment of morbid obesity and its comorbidities, including arterial hypertension, diabetes, OSAS and dyslipidemia. However, in a variable percentage of cases, therapeutic success is not achieved with primary bariatric surgery. Therefore, in the event of weight regain, inadequate weight loss, failure to control comorbidities or long-term complications, it is possible to resort to revisional surgery, aimed at relieving weight regain or complications. Revisional bariatric surgery is technically more complex than primary bariatric surgery because it is carried out in an operative field that is hampered by scarring from the first operation and on a modified anatomy. This chapter aims to describe the most common scenarios that may set the indications for revisional bariatric surgery, the surgical techniques employed in the authors experience and the postoperative follow-up.

Keywords: morbid obesity, bariatric surgery, weight regain, inadequate weight loss, complications, revisional bariatric surgery

1. Introduction

Bariatric surgery is approved in the literature as the gold standard treatment for morbid obesity and related comorbidities in patients with severe obesity [1, 2]. The worldwide obesity crisis has led to an exponential rise in the number of bariatric procedures [3]. In the last few years, with the rising demand for bariatric surgery, also revisional bariatric surgery is becoming increasingly necessary. Only in the USA did revisional bariatric surgery increase by 60% from 2011 to 2019 [4], and today it represents around 7 to 15% of the total number of bariatric surgical procedures [5, 6]. In the Swedish Obesity Study, the rate of revisional bariatric surgery in adults reaches 28% [7]; similarly, Shoar et al., in their systematic review, reported this rate up to 23.7% in adolescent patients [8].

Revisional bariatric surgery includes a wide range of procedures either to treat postoperative complications or to address a failure of the initial procedure.

Brethauer et al., in their "Systematic review on reoperative bariatric surgery" [9], define a nomenclature of the procedures:

- Conversion: changing anatomy from one procedure to a different bariatric procedure;
- Corrective: re-exploring the anatomy to address complications of a previous bariatric procedure;
- Reversal: to restore the original anatomy.

Furthermore, revisional bariatric surgery is technically more challenging than primary surgery, with a higher morbidity rate than that recorded for the same procedure performed as primary surgery [10]. Since revisional bariatric surgery is performed on tissues that have had prior surgery and have more adhesions and less vascularity, the higher surgical risks associated with the procedure are readily understood.

2. Indications

Principal indications for revisional bariatric surgery include [11]:

- inadequate weight loss or regain of weight initially lost,
- insufficient resolution or recurrence of a weight-related comorbidity (like type 2 diabetes),
- onset of symptoms and/or complications related to the primary procedure (gastroesophageal reflux disease, bile reflux, fistula, leak, stricture, marginal ulcers, protein malnutrition).

Weight regain or inadequate weight loss are the principal indications for revisional bariatric surgery, accounting for more than 50% of revisional surgeries [11]. Reinhold defined failure of bariatric surgery as loss of <50.0% of the excess weight [12]. More recently, a systematic review by Mann [13] found that losing less than 50% of excess weight following bariatric surgery was the most widely accepted definition for "inadequate weight loss," and less than 25% excess weight loss was the second most common definition.

Depending on the primary bariatric procedure, after surgery, gastroesophageal reflux disease (GERD) can worsen or maybe onset "de novo" [14]. GERD is the principal complication after primary surgery that leads to revisional bariatric procedures [15]. Furthermore, restrictive procedures like sleeve gastrectomy (SG) have a negative impact on GERD, even in patients without preoperative GERD [16], with a high prevalence of de novo GERD evaluated by instrumental exams [17]. Mechanisms that lead to increased intra-abdominal pressure and consequently to the onset or worsening of GERD, and even to Barrett's esophagus, include hypotension of the lower esophageal sphincter, blunting of the angle of His, and increased intraluminal pressure [18]. So, GERD is an important problem for many bariatric patients who cannot control symptoms by medical treatments alone, suffer a worsening quality of life and only have to recur to re-surgery.

Finally, revisional bariatric surgery is often the only possible treatment for technical complications after primary surgery such as fistula, leak, stricture, or marginal ulcers.

3. Preoperative study

Before revisional surgery, all patients need to undergo a multidisciplinary evaluation that includes:

- behavioral and psychosocial assessment,
- nutritional status investigation, with correction of any deficit,
- laboratory, radiologic, and endoscopic studies.

4. Revisional surgery

4.1 Revisions after adjustable gastric banding

Laparoscopic adjustable gastric band (LAGB) placement is the procedure with the lowest morbidity among surgeries for the treatment of morbid obesity. Nevertheless, this technique has shown poor results in weight loss and a complication rate of up to 30% [19]. The most frequent complication after LAGB positioning is device slippage (3–10%), followed by reservoir-related complications (1–5%) and gastric necrosis/perforation (0.1–0.7%) [20–22]. Moreover, patients often report dysphagia and maladaptive eating. The morbidity rate appears to increase by 3–4% for each year the device remains in place, and up to a 40% rate of major complications has been observed ten years after LAGB implantation [22]. Consequently, discharge of the device and revisional surgery, as well as performing another surgical technique, such as Sleeve Gastrectomy (SG) or Roux-en-Y gastric bypass (RYGB), becomes necessary in a large number of patients. At the moment, LAGB is the procedure that most commonly requires conversion, with variable rates from 30–60% [7]. The surgical revision procedure, in addition to higher morbidity [19, 23], is often also difficult to define both with regard to the most suitable surgical technique to choose and with regard to the correct timing indication for revisional surgery (removal of the LAGB and revisional surgery in a single stage or in two stages deferred from each other). In a recent survey by Mahawar et al. [11], RYGB emerged as the commonest revisional procedure after LAGB, followed by SG and One Anastomosis Gastric Bypass (OAGB), and more than half of participants said to prefer a one-stage procedure. All these reasons justify the fact that the number of LAGB procedures has gradually but dramatically decreased in the last two decades because of its short and long-term failure rates.

4.2 Revisions after sleeve gastrectomy

Due to its great diffusion, to date, SG is the most-performed bariatric procedure in the world [5]. However, SG increasingly needs to be converted into other bariatric procedures. The main causes of SG conversion are inadequate weight loss, worsening of GERD, or appearance of de novo GERD [6, 16]. Various surgical techniques are now used in revisional surgery after SG [24]; however, some of these, such as re-sleeve and sleeve plication, have given poor results [25] and therefore today, they only have a marginal role. The most commonly performed surgical procedures in revisional surgery after SG include RYBG or OAGB [24], with excellent long-term results both in terms of excess weight loss and in comorbidities resolution [26]. One of the most recently introduced procedures in bariatric surgery, which is increasingly spreading also as revision surgery after SG, is represented by the Single-Anastomosis Duodenoileal Bypass with Sleeve Gastrectomy (SADI-S) [27]. In their survey, Mahawar et al. [11] reported that RYGB was the preferred procedure by the majority of surgeons, followed by OAGB and SADI-S. Biliopancreatic diversion/duodenal switch (BPD/DS) and re-sleeve are, on the other hand, the procedures of choice by a minority of surgeons.

4.3 Revisions after Roux-en-Y gastric bypass

Although a minimal rate of RYGB requires revisional surgery, RYGB appears to be the most commonly adopted revisional procedure after almost all bariatric procedures [11]. In the few cases in which it is necessary to correct an RYGB, the most commonly performed procedure is pouch reduction [11]. This procedure can be performed either *via* a surgical or an endoscopic procedure, and it is often associated with the concomitant revision of the gastrojejunal anastomosis. In some cases reported in the literature [28], the positioning of a "salvage banding" is described to reduce the size of the gastric pouch and to promote weight loss. In other cases, corrective surgery is indicated to treat complications after RYGB, such as gastrogastric fistula or marginal ulcer.
In the survey by Mahawar et al. [11], bariatric surgeons declared that in revisional surgery after RYGB, they preferred surgical pouch reduction or secondary banding, followed by stoma size reduction and prolongation of the biliopancreatic limb, lastly endoscopic stoma and/or pouch size reduction or conversion to BPD/DS.

5. Surgical techniques

Bariatric surgical procedures can be classified into three main categories based on their functions: restrictive, combined (restrictive and hypoabsorptive), and primarily hypoabsorptive [29]. These procedures aim to achieve weight loss through different mechanisms. The same applies to revisional bariatric procedures.

Restrictive revisional bariatric procedures include laparoscopic re-sleeve (RLSG) after Sleeve Gastrectomy (SG), which reduces the previously created gastric tube, bringing it back to about approximately 60–120 mL in size, extending from the esophagus to the duodenum. In the SG primary procedure, almost 80% of the stomach is removed, leading to a lower amount of hunger-related hormone ghrelin produced, appetite reduction and post-prandial early satiety [30]. However, weight regains or inadequate weight loss may be observed after SG at medium to long-term follow-up, as well as complications such as gastroesophageal reflux disease (GERD), setting the indications for revisional procedures.

Combined restrictive and hypoabsorptive procedures performed in our center are Roux-en-Y gastric bypass (RYGB) and Single-Anastomosis Duodenoileal Bypass with Sleeve Gastrectomy (SADI-S). These surgical techniques combine stomach reduction with alterations to the small intestine's path aiming to reduce absorptive loop length by joining the upper gastrointestinal tract (stomach or duodenum) to the distal small intestine. RYGB has evolved significantly since its inception in the late 1970s [31]. Nowadays, the gastric pouch has been steadily reduced, and the Roux-en-Y complex (biliopancreatic limb, alimentary limb, and common channel) is made up of different lengths of the small intestine. While the small gastric pouch and relatively narrow gastrojejunal stoma size represent the restrictive features, hypoabsorption is guaranteed by the fact that part of the stomach, duodenum, and the upper jejunum are bypassed [32].

Laparoscopic Single-Anastomosis Duodenoileal Bypass with Sleeve Gastrectomy (SADI-S) is a procedure that has been gaining some popularity in recent years, since it has been shown to have a long-lasting and significant impact on weight loss and remission of comorbidities. When performed as a revisional procedure, it involves a previously created Sleeve Gastrectomy, in which the gastric tube may need to be resized if it is substantially dilated, and includes a duodenum transection after the pylorus, at the level of the gastroduodenal artery (GDA), and the creation of a termino-lateral, hand-sewn omega-loop duodenoileal anastomosis. Due to the complex hand-sewn anastomosis and the delicacy necessary when handling the duodenum, this procedure should be reserved for experienced bariatric surgeons in specialized centers [33] and even though it causes significant weight reduction, it is linked to greater risks of complications, such as malabsorption, protein malnutrition, vitamin and mineral deficiencies, anemia, osteoporosis, and anastomotic ulceration (**Table 1**).

5.1 Roux-en-Y gastric bypass (RYGB)

Roux-en-Y gastric bypass is a combined restrictive-hypoabsorptive procedure that was introduced in 1966 by Mason. It accounted for over 60 to 70% of all bariatric operations in the United States since 2003.

5.1.1 Equipment

Equipment for a laparoscopic RYGB include:

- Orogastric tube
- Liver retractor (Nathanson StrongArm® Complete Systems – Mediflex Surgical Products)
- 30-degree laparoscope with light source, monitor and gas insufflation equipment
- Laparoscopic trocars: 5, 10 to 12 mm ports

Patients' selection criteria for revisional RYGB	Patients' selection criteria for revisional SADI
Weight regain/inadequate weight loss	Weight regain/inadequate weight loss after SG
Sweet-eating after SG	Planned two-step's procedure
SG-related GERD	Contraindications are Barrett's esophagus and severe GERD

Table 1.
Shows patients' selection criteria for revisional RYGB and revisional SADI.

- bowel-safe graspers and needle holder
- Laparoscopic ultrasonic/radiofrequency dissector
- Laparoscopic suction irrigator
- Laparoscopic clips
- Laparoscopic linear cutting stapler (Endo GIA™ Universal Staplers | Medtronic; ECHELON™ Stapler by ETHICON™ | J&J MedTech)

5.1.2 Surgical technique

Laparoscopic techniques vary among surgeons since there is no established standardization. The steps of RYGB include gastric pouch creation, creation of the biliopancreatic limb, gastrojejunostomy and jejunojejunostomy creation (**Figure 1**).

Under general anesthesia, the patient's positioning is in a supine split legs position. The lead operating surgeon stands between the patients' legs once the patient is prepped and draped, and the monitor is positioned above the patient's head, behind the left shoulder.

To establish a 12–13 mmHg pneumoperitoneum, we commonly use open access and an optical trocar inserted at about 12 cm from the xiphoid process above the

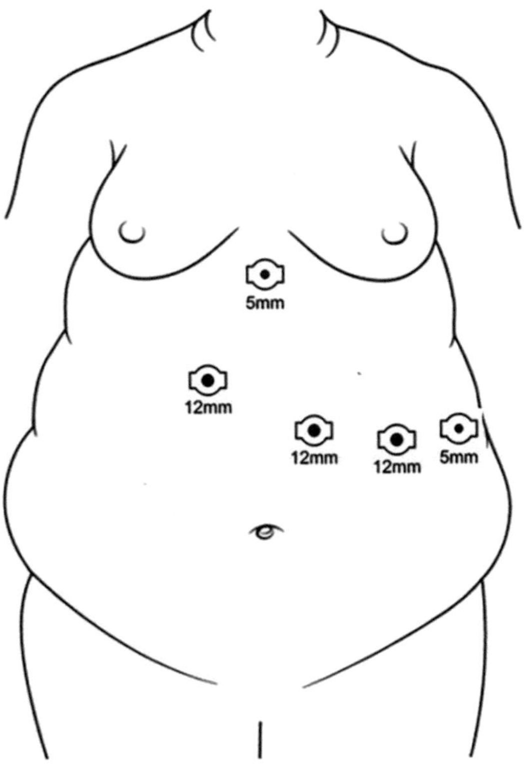

Figure 1.
Trocar placement in RYGB.

umbilicus and on the left of the midline. Two more 12 mm ports are inserted, respectively, in the left and in the right upper quadrants, and two 5 mm ports, just below the xiphoid process for liver retraction and in the left lumbar region for the assistant.

5.1.2.1 Step 1: Gastric pouch creation

Adequate exposure of the gastroesophageal junction is essential, which can be facilitated by placing the patient in reverse Trendelemburg position and by retracting the left lobe of the liver using a Nathanson retractor (Nathanson StrongArm® Complete Systems – Mediflex Surgical Products).

After the incision of the phrenogastric peritoneal reflection with a monopolar electrocoagulation hook near the angle of His, and having exposed the left diaphragmatic crus and the gastrohepatic ligament, the dissection begins by opening the peritoneal reflection along the lesser curvature of the stomach between the second and third branch of the perigastric vascular arch, using a radiofrequency device (LigaSure, Medtronic, Minneapolis, Minnesota, USA or Enseal, Ethicon Endo-Surgery, Johnson & Johnson, Cincinnati, Ohio, USA), to gain access to the bursa omentalis. Once the retrogastric window is obtained, the gastric pouch is created by using a linear stapler, which is initially directed transversely, tacking a 45 mm bite and then fired vertically toward the angle of His, maintaining a distance from 0.5 to 1 cm from this, guided by an orogastric tube. MacLean et al. demonstrated that the optimal gastric pouch must be 20 to 30 cc in volume [34]. A small opening is then created on the posterior wall of the gastric pouch, again guided by the presence of the orogastric tube (**Figure 2**).

5.1.2.2 Step 2: Creation of the biliopancreatic limb and of the Gastrojejunostomy

The biliopancreatic limb, also known as the afferent limb, includes the duodenum and proximal jejunum tract that remains in continuity with the excluded stomach.

The length of the biliopancreatic loop is measured at 100 to 150 cm, starting from the ligament of Treitz. At this level, a small opening is created on the antimesenteric side of the bowel loop. A branch of a linear stapling device with a 3.5 mm staple height is introduced inside the bowel loop, it is closed, and the bowel loop is transposed in antecolic, antegastric position in order to be anastomosed to the posterior wall of

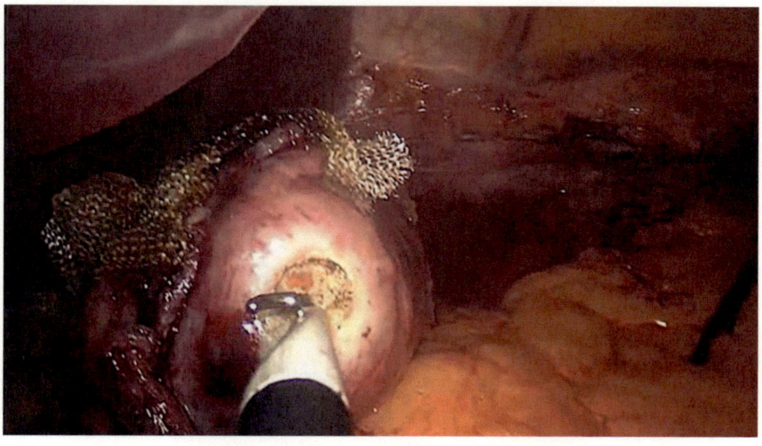

Figure 2.
Creation of a small opening on the posterior wall of the gastric pouch.

the gastric pouch. The size of the gastrojejunal anastomosis should be no larger than 2.5 cm. The remaining opening is hand-sewn with an absorbable continuous suture in two layers to close the anterior defect (**Figure 3**).

The biliopancreatic afferent limb contains digestive enzymes secreted from the stomach, from the hepatobiliary tract, and from the pancreas.

5.1.2.3 Step 3: Creation of the Jejunojejunostomy

The length of the alimentary limb is measured at 100–150 cm from the gastrojejunostomy in order to be anastomosed to the biliopancreatic limb with a side-to-side jejunojejunostomy (JJ) anastomosis using a mechanic vascular cartridge. The remaining opening is hand-sewn with an absorbable continuous suture in a single layer to close the anterior defect (**Figure 4**).

It is essential to recognize and close, with a non-absorbable suture, the transverse mesocolon defect (Petersen's space) and the mesenteric defect that could be potential sites of internal herniation of intestinal loops.

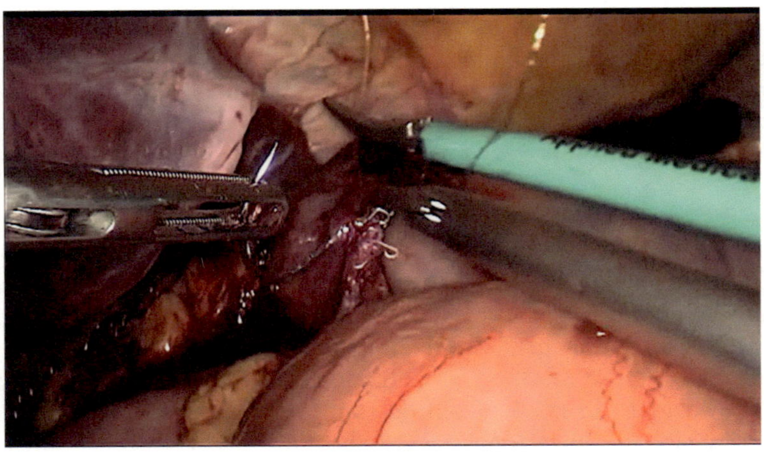

Figure 3.
Creation of the gastrojejunostomy.

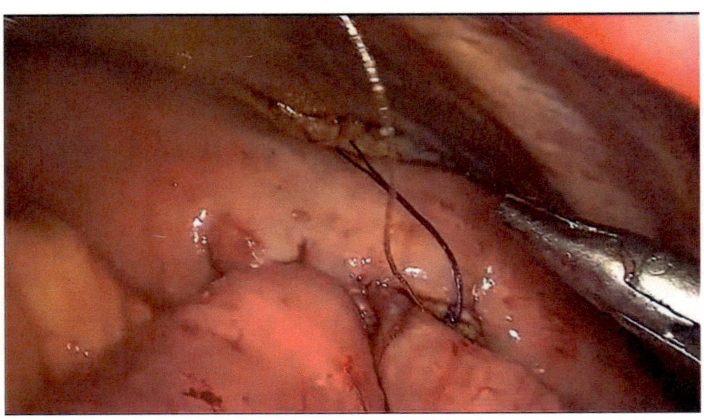

Figure 4.
The Jejunojejunostomy.

5.1.2.4 Leak test

Before completing the procedure, a leak test of both anastomoses is performed while keeping both in view. After positioning a nasogastric tube, and after creating a mechanical occlusion downstream of both anastomoses, 150 ml of methylene blue dye with saline solution is administered by the anesthesiologist through the nasogastric tube in order to check for any possible leakage.

To create the Roux-en-Y configuration, the biliopancreatic afferent loop is then divided with a vascular 60 mm cartridge after opening the mesentery immediately proximal to the gastrojejunal anastomosis, in order to avoid the so-called "candy-cane" effect.

5.2 Single-anastomosis duodenoileal bypass with sleeve gastrectomy (SADI-S)

Sánchez-Pernaute et al. proposed in 2007 the single-anastomosis duodenoileal bypass with sleeve gastrectomy (SADI-S), describing it as a technical simplification of the duodenal switch (DS), to reduce its complexity, morbidity and mortality maintaining the same weight loss and comorbidities resolution results [35].

5.2.1 Equipment

Equipment for a laparoscopic SADI-S include:

- Orogastric tube
- Liver retractor (Nathanson StrongArm® Complete Systems – Mediflex Surgical Products)
- 30-degree laparoscope with light source, monitor and gas insufflation equipment
- Laparoscopic trocars: 5, 10 to 12 mm ports
- bowel-safe graspers
- Laparoscopic ultrasonic/radiofrequency dissector
- Laparoscopic suction irrigator
- Laparoscopic needle holder
- Laparoscopic clips
- Laparoscopic linear cutting stapler.

5.2.2 Surgical tecnique

The proposed technique consists of a sleeve gastrectomy followed by an omega-loop duodenoileal anastomosis with a 250–300 cm efferent limb, as measured in a retrograde fashion starting from the ileo-cecal valve (**Figure 5**).

Under general anesthesia, the patient positioning is in supine, split leg position secured to the operative table by foot tops and belts. The table tilt is changed starting with anti-Trendelemburg and then to a horizontal position, depending on the step of the surgery.

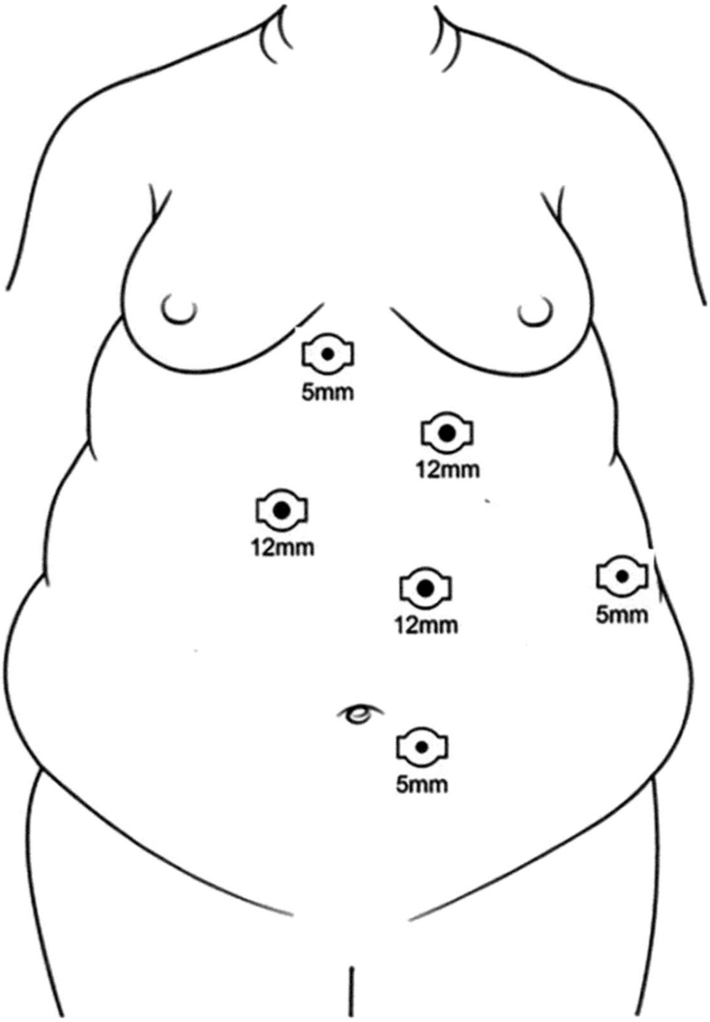

Figure 5.
Trocar placement in SADI-S.

The procedure begins in the same manner as with a SG, with the surgeon standing between the patient's legs.

To establish a 12–13 mmHg pneumoperitoneum, we commonly use open access and an optical trocar placed 2–3 cm to the left of the midline 15 cm caudal from the xiphoid process for the placement of the 30-degree lens. Two 12 mm trocars for both working hands of the surgeon are placed in the right and left hypochondria, the latter close to the costal arch, and two more 5 mm trocars, respectively, on the left upper quadrant along the anterior axillary line and below the xiphoid process for liver retraction. An accessory 5 mm trocar may be added below the umbilicus in left paramedian position during the second phase of the procedure to facilitate bowel measurement and creation of the duodenoileal anastomosis.

5.2.2.1 Step 1: Mobilization of the stomach

This is the first phase of the operation. In the patient who already had a previous SG, followed by weight regain or inadequate weight loss, the surgical procedure starts with the mobilization of the stomach antrum using a radiofrequency device (LigaSure, Medtronic, Minneapolis, Minnesota, USA or Enseal, Ethicon Endo-Surgery, Johnson & Johnson, Cincinnati, Ohio, USA), removing all adhesions in the lesser sac in order to have a complete dissection until the gastroduodenal artery is identified. It is important to exclude the presence of a hiatal hernia. In case this is suspected preoperatively, the esophageal hiatus should be explored, and the herniated stomach should be reduced in the abdomen together with at least 3 cm of the abdominal esophagus and a hiatoplasty should be performed.

5.2.2.2 Step 2: Duodenal dissection preserving the right gastric artery

The dissection of the first portion of the duodenum is continued from the pylorus distally after identification of the gastroduodenal artery. The assistant retracts the antrum upwards to facilitate the dissection of the posterior face of the first part of the duodenum. The posterior dissection is carried close to the duodenal wall with the aim of preserving the right gastric artery in order to guarantee the duodenal blood supply. A peritoneal window is created between the first portion of the duodenum and the infundibulum of the gallbladder, and an elastic tape is passed around the duodenum with an upward traction by the assistant in order to complete the preparation of the duodenum. When 2.5–3 cm of the duodenum distal to the pylorus have been prepared, the duodenum can be safely divided with a 60 mm linear stapler cartridge and 3.5 mm staple heights (Endo GIA™ Tri-Staple™ technology – Medtronic; ECHELON™ Stapler by ETHICON™ | J&J MedTech).

5.2.2.3 Step 3: Bowel mobilization and duodenoileal anastomosis

The second phase of the operation starts with placing the operative table in a horizontal position and with the surgeon and camera assistant moving to the left of the patient and a sixth 5 mm trocar which can be optionally placed. The bowel measurement starts from the ileocecal valve and proceeds in a retrograde direction after intravenous administration of Hyoscine butylbromide 20 mg, to obtain bowel relaxation, until 250–300 cm of ileum are counted and marked in preparation for an end-to-side anastomosis with the duodenum. It is important that the distal bowel should be left at the right iliac fossa to avoid torsion of the bowel during creation of the anastomosis. The double-layer duodenoileal anastomosis is created end-to-side using an absorbable barbed suture (V-Loc™ – Medtronic; STRATAFIX™ - J&J MedTech).

5.2.2.4 Leak test

The final check of the anastomosis is performed with a methylene blue test and a drain is placed in the left upper quadrant of the patient and in the perianastomotic area.

6. Risk stratification for revisional surgery

In our experience with revisional surgery: male gender, a higher BMI, T2DM and postoperative complications after primary surgery were associated with higher risk of complications (like bleeding, leakage, obstruction, stenosis, trocar site hernia, deep vein thrombosis, pulmonary embolism).

7. Postoperative care protocols

In our center postoperative care protocol includes:

- Upper Gastrointestinal Contrast Study in POD 1
- Blood test analysis (e.g., blood count and inflammatory indices)
- At discharge patients follow a stiff dietary regimen divided into three steps (liquid, semiliquid and solid diet), each one 3 weeks long-lasting, with protein, vitamins and minerals supplementations according to the type of procedure
- Enoxaparin treatment for 4 weeks
- Proton-pump inhibitor for 6 months for the prevention of marginal ulcers
- Treatment with ursodeoxycholic acid during the weight loss phase to prevent gallstone formation (at least 6 months)

8. Outcomes

Outcomes of revisional bariatric surgery are critically important for both patients and surgeons to understand, as these procedures often come with the potential for significant benefits but are also at increased risk. Many studies [9, 36, 37] have shown that while the complication rates after revisional surgery are generally higher than those following primary bariatric surgery, the resultant improvements in weight loss and reduction in comorbid conditions can be substantial. This section will examine the specific outcomes related to different types of reoperative procedures, including those addressing failed weight loss and weight regain, as well as those aimed at treating acute and chronic complications.

As previously mentioned, one of the procedures that nowadays often requires conversion is the laparoscopic adjustable gastric banding (LAGB), for its innate potential failure due to insufficient and unstable weight loss at mid-term follow-up, especially if compared to other primary restrictive procedures like Sleeve Gastrectomy (SG) and the need to manage complications like hardware related issues, dysphagia and maladaptive eating [38]. Ibrahim et al. reported a high reoperation rate, with nearly 1 in 5 patients requiring at least one additional gastric band-related surgical procedure, and consequently a considerable rise in health costs [39].

The main conversion procedures are laparoscopic sleeve gastrectomy (LSG) and Laparoscopic Roux-en-Y Gastric Bypass (LRYGB): both have good outcomes in terms of weight loss with a maximum of excess weight loss (EWL) of 74% at 36 months follow-up reported by Hii et al. [40], but clearly there is a higher complications' rate if compared to primary SG and RYGB, due to the scarred tissue of the stomach and also a higher reoperation rate. However, LRYGB seems to have better long-term results than LSG [41] in terms of weight loss. Anyway, LAGB is progressively disappearing [42], so further investigations are beyond our aim.

The other most often revised primary bariatric procedure is SG, for the reasons previously described, and RYGB represents the most frequent conversion procedure after SG. First, it is the most common bariatric procedure performed globally [42] and, secondly, up to 30% of the cases require revisional surgery for inadequate weight loss, weight regain, and/or the development of severe upper gastrointestinal symptoms (especially GERD) [43]. In particular, most patients experience significant symptom improvement post-revision, especially when converted to Roux-en-Y gastric bypass (RYGB) [44], which is, in fact, the procedure of choice in case of GERD symptoms [45] and weight issues.

Outcomes in terms of weight loss after revisional RYGB are poor if compared to primary RYGB, regardless of the index surgery. Dardamanis et al. found a non-statistically significant difference in terms of BMI between both groups after 5 years of follow-up (33.1 kg/m^2 for revisional versus 31.5 kg/m^2 for primary procedures) and in terms of % EBMIL (revisional operations had 60.5% of % EBMIL versus 72% for primary operations) after 5 years of follow-up, demonstrating comparable effects on weight loss at the price of increased operative time, duration of hospitalization and conversion rate in the revisional group [46].

Pędziwiatr [47] et al. report a reduction in terms of %EWL from primary to revisional RYGB; on the other hand, they highlight no substantial differences between the two groups in terms of comorbidity remission rate (diabetes mellitus and hypertension), but a higher mortality rate, complications' rate and operative time in the revisional group.

Better results in terms of weight loss come from the conversion of SG to Single-Anastomosis Duodenoileal Bypass (SADI)14 or Biliopancreatic Diversion with Duodenal Switch (BPD-DS) [48].

Dijkhorst et al. [49] report a statistically significant difference in terms of total weight loss (%TWL) between revisional SADI and revisional RYGB (21.8 ± 11.7 vs. 7.2 ± 12.5; $p < .001$) with comparable outcomes in postoperative micronutrient deficiencies, complications' rate, and quality of life (QOL) scores and they do not recommend conversion from an SG into an RYGB as a preferred procedure unless GERD or functional problems related to the SG are the primary indications for revisional surgery.

Osorio et al. [48] demonstrate that DS, which was meant to be the original surgical step following SG, is slightly better than SADI in weight control, but at the price of nutritional issues: patients in fact need extra supplementations in order to compensate, vitamin and nutrient deficiencies, so this type of conversion is limited to those patients with high-grade obesity and persistent diabetes/hypertension who are committed to a strong adherence to follow-up instructions.

Therefore, revisional bariatric surgery is an effective adjuvant therapy in weight recidivism, especially with the aim to stabilize weight loss, but in general, results do not exceed those obtained with primary surgery (**Table 2**) [52].

One crucial point of bariatric surgery efficacy is the resolution or the improvement of obesity-related comorbidities.

If the metabolic effect is hugely demonstrated for primary bariatric surgery [53], the same effect is achievable with revisional surgery in case of relapse after initial remission or persistence of metabolic conditions like type 2 diabetes mellitus (T2DM) after primary surgery.

Primary Procedure	Revisional SG	Revisional RYGB	Revisional SADI
LAGB	%EWL: 55.4 [50] %TWL: /	%EWL: 60.7 [50] %TWL: /	/
SG	/	%EWL: 69.13 [51] %TWL: 29.45 [51]	%EWL: 87.6 [51] %TWL: 38.7 [51]

Table 2.
The comparative outcomes of different revisional procedures at 36 months follow-up.

Patients with persistent or relapsed T2DM after bariatric surgery can significantly improve glucose control and use of diabetes medications, when eligible for revisional surgery, despite the type of index procedure and the type of conversion [54].

Koh et al. [37] demonstrate that revision to duodenal switch (r-DS) had the highest proportion of T2DM improvement at 100%, followed by the revision to Sleeve Gastrectomy (r-SG) at 98.0%, revision to Roux-en-Y gastric bypass (r-RYGB) at 94.0% and pouch/gastrogastric fistula revision after previous Roux-en-Y gastric bypass (PGGF) at 76.0%. Similarly, for remission of T2DM, r-DS had the highest proportion of 69.0%, followed by r-RYGB at 62.0%, r-SG at 33.0%, and lastly, PGGF at 20%. r-DS had the highest proportion of hypertension (HTN) improvement at 91.0%, followed by PGGF at 84.0%, r-RYGB at 83.0% and r-SG at 56.0%. For remission of HTN, r-DS had the highest proportion at 44.0%, followed by r-RYGB at 40.0%, PGGF at 20.0% and finally r-SG at 18.0%. Similarly, they state that the hyperlipidemia and Obstructive Sleep apnea syndrome (OSAS) remission rates are 37% and 86%, respectively, even if a subgroup analysis by type of revision was not possible because of a limited number of studies exploring these issues.

Another important issue is the management of complications after primary surgery: in fact, complications may be the reason for revisional surgery – in terms of corrective and reversal procedures.

The SOReg is one of the most important national registries related to bariatric surgery. Axer et al. conducted the largest survey that reports a higher statistically significant complications' rate in terms of both intraoperative and early and late postoperative complications after revisional RYGB [55].

The MBSAQIP Data Registry [56] is another data registry that estimates that the incidence of at least one complication requiring reoperation or intervention within 30 days following revisional SG (RSG) is twice as high as compared to primary SG (PSG) (1.9 and 2% for RSG vs. 0.9 and 1.1% for PSG respectively, $p < 0.05$). Length of stay and 30-day mortality rates for primary and revisional SG are the same. 30-day readmission rate of revisional gastric bypass (RGBP) as compared to primary gastric bypass (PGBP) was 8.3 vs. 6.3% ($p < 0.05$). Also, the incidence of at least one complication requiring reoperation or intervention following RGBP was 3.9 and 4%, respectively, versus 2.4 and 2.7% for PGBP ($p < 0.05$). In addition, readmission rates and unplanned admission rates to the ICU were significantly higher for RGBP as compared to RSG (8.3 and 2% for RGBP vs. 4.1 and 0.9% for RSG, respectively, $p < 0.05$). The incidence of at least one reoperation or one intervention following RGBP was also significantly higher compared to RSG (3.9 vs. 1.9% and 4 vs. 2%, respectively, $p < 0.05$).

Management of early and late complications offers several different options, including conservative treatment (like percutaneous drainage, supportive therapy, and fasting) to endoscopic treatment to surgery: the choice depends on the general conditions of the patients, that is, whether the patient is stable or not, the type of primary intervention (each procedure has specific issues to deal with) and the grade of the complexity of the complication itself [9].

Protein caloric malnutrition is a critical issue for revisional bariatric surgery: symptoms are diarrhea and/or steatorrhea, muscle wasting, edema, and excessive weight loss [44]. It can occur after every bariatric surgery, especially when the patient's compliance to nutritional supplementation therapy is not excellent, but it is more common after hypoabsorptive procedures, where there is an altered biliary and pancreatic anatomy, resulting in digestion/absorption problems. This complication may be observed, for example, in up to 38% of patients after One Anastomosis Gastric Bypass (OAGB) [44] and other hypoabsorptive conditions.

9. Conclusion

Revisional bariatric surgery plays a vital role in managing persistent obesity, comorbid diseases, and complications, achieving sustained weight loss in patients who have undergone primary bariatric procedures. While these surgeries are associated with higher risks, the overall outcomes in terms of symptom resolution and quality of life improvement are positive, although the success rate in terms of weight loss is not as high as after primary surgery. Greater efforts should be made in optimizing patient selection so as to select the right procedure for the right patient, in order to enhance the efficacy and safety of every bariatric surgery.

Author details

Livia Palmieri[1], Eleonora Rapanotti[2], Silvia Quaresima[2], Federica Rizzo[2], Germana Ginevra Perrone[2] and Alessandro M. Paganini[2]*

1 General and Endocrine Surgery Unit, Santa Maria Hospital, Terni, Italy

2 Department of General Surgery and Surgical Specialties, Sapienza University of Rome, Rome, Italy

*Address all correspondence to: alessandro.paganini@uniroma1.it

References

[1] Golzarand M, Toolabi K, Farid R. The bariatric surgery and weight losing: A meta-analysis in the long- and very long-term effects of laparoscopic adjustable gastric banding, laparoscopic roux-en-Y gastric bypass and laparoscopic sleeve gastrectomy on weight loss in adults. Surgical Endoscopy. 2017;**31**(11):4331-4345. DOI: 10.1007/s00464-017-5505-1

[2] Buchwald H et al. Bariatric surgery: A systematic review and meta-analysis. JAMA. 2004;**292**(14):1724-1737. DOI: 10.1001/jama.292.14.1724

[3] Colquitt JL, Pickett K, Loveman E, Frampton GK. Surgery for weight loss in adults. Cochrane Database of Systematic Reviews. 2014;(8):CD003641. DOI: 10.1002/14651858.CD003641.pub4

[4] English WJ et al. American Society for Metabolic and Bariatric Surgery 2018 estimate of metabolic and bariatric procedures performed in the United States. Surgery for Obesity and Related Diseases. 2020;**16**(4):457-463. DOI: 10.1016/j.soard.2019.12.022

[5] Angrisani L et al. IFSO worldwide survey 2016: Primary, endoluminal, and revisional procedures. Obesity Surgery. 2018;**28**(12):3783-3794. DOI: 10.1007/s11695-018-3450-2

[6] Clapp B et al. Trends in revisional bariatric surgery using the MBSAQIP database 2015-2017. Surgery for Obesity and Related Diseases. 2020;**16**(7):908-915. DOI: 10.1016/j.soard.2020.03.002

[7] Hjorth S et al. Reoperations after bariatric surgery in 26 years of follow-up of the Swedish obese subjects study. JAMA Surgery. 2019;**154**(4):319-326. DOI: 10.1001/jamasurg.2018.5084

[8] Shoar S et al. Long-term outcome of bariatric surgery in morbidly obese adolescents: A systematic review and meta-analysis of 950 patients with a minimum of 3 years follow-up. Obesity Surgery. 2017;**27**(12):3110-3117. DOI: 10.1007/s11695-017-2738-y

[9] Brethauer SA et al. Systematic review on reoperative bariatric surgery: American Society for Metabolic and Bariatric Surgery Revision Task Force. Surgery for Obesity and Related Diseases. 2014;**10**(5):952-972. DOI: 10.1016/j.soard.2014.02.014

[10] Inabnet WB et al. Comparison of 30-day outcomes after non-LapBand primary and revisional bariatric surgical procedures from the longitudinal assessment of bariatric surgery study. Surgery for Obesity and Related Diseases. 2010;**6**(1):22-30. DOI: 10.1016/j.soard.2009.10.007

[11] Mahawar KK et al. Practices concerning revisional bariatric surgery: A survey of 460 surgeons. Obesity Surgery. 2018;**28**(9):2650-2660. DOI: 10.1007/s11695-018-3226-8

[12] Reinhold RB. Critical analysis of long term weight loss following gastric bypass. Surgery, Gynecology & Obstetrics. 1982;**155**(3):385-394

[13] Mann JP, Jakes AD, Hayden JD, Barth JH. Systematic review of definitions of failure in revisional bariatric surgery. Obesity Surgery. 2015;**25**(3):571-574. DOI: 10.1007/s11695-014-1541-2

[14] Felinska E et al. Do we understand the pathophysiology of GERD after sleeve gastrectomy? Annals of the New York Academy of Sciences.

2020;**1482**(1):26-35. DOI: 10.1111/nyas.14467

[15] Chiappetta S, Lainas P, Kassir R, Valizadeh R, Bosco A, Kermansaravi M. Gastroesophageal reflux disease as an indication of revisional bariatric surgery-indication and results-a systematic review and metanalysis. Obesity Surgery. 2022;**32**(9):3156-3171. DOI: 10.1007/s11695-022-06183-w

[16] Balla A et al. Does sleeve gastrectomy worsen gastroesophageal reflux disease in obese patients? A prospective study. Surgical Innovation. 2022;**29**(5):579-589. DOI: 10.1177/15533506211052745

[17] Balla A et al. Manometric and pH-monitoring changes after laparoscopic sleeve gastrectomy: A systematic review. Langenbeck's Archives of Surgery. 2021;**406**(8):2591-2609. DOI: 10.1007/s00423-021-02171-3

[18] Peng B-Q, Zhang G-X, Chen G, Cheng Z, Hu J-K, Du X. Gastroesophageal reflux disease complicating laparoscopic sleeve gastrectomy: Current knowledge and surgical therapies. Surgery for Obesity and Related Diseases. 2020;**16**(8):1145-1155. DOI: 10.1016/j.soard.2020.04.025

[19] Berende CAS, de Zoete J-P, Smulders JF, Nienhuijs SW. Laparoscopic sleeve gastrectomy feasible for bariatric revision surgery. Obesity Surgery. 2012;**22**(2):330-334. DOI: 10.1007/s11695-011-0501-3

[20] Chevallier J-M et al. Complications after laparoscopic adjustable gastric banding for morbid obesity: Experience with 1,000 patients over 7 years. Obesity Surgery. 2004;**14**(3):407-414. DOI: 10.1381/096089204322917954

[21] Gagner M, Milone L, Yung E, Broseus A, Gumbs AA. Causes of early mortality after laparoscopic adjustable gastric banding. Journal of the American College of Surgeons. 2008;**206**(4):664-669. DOI: 10.1016/j.jamcollsurg.2007.11.014

[22] Suter M, Calmes JM, Paroz A, Giusti V. A 10-year experience with laparoscopic gastric banding for morbid obesity: High long-term complication and failure rates. Obesity Surgery. 2006;**16**(7):829-835. DOI: 10.1381/096089206777822359

[23] Langer FB et al. Inadequate weight loss vs secondary weight regain: Laparoscopic conversion from gastric banding to roux-en-Y gastric bypass. Obesity Surgery. 2008;**18**(11):1381-1386. DOI: 10.1007/s11695-008-9479-x

[24] Switzer NJ, Karmali S, Gill RS, Sherman V. Revisional bariatric surgery. The Surgical Clinics of North America. 2016;**96**(4):827-842. DOI: 10.1016/j.suc.2016.03.004

[25] De Angelis F, Avallone M, Albanese A, Foletto M, Silecchia G. Re-sleeve gastrectomy 4 years later: Is it still an effective Revisional option? Obesity Surgery. 2018;**28**(11):3714-3716. DOI: 10.1007/s11695-018-3481-8

[26] Andalib A, Alamri H, Almuhanna Y, Bouchard P, Demyttenaere S, Court O. Short-term outcomes of revisional surgery after sleeve gastrectomy: A comparative analysis of re-sleeve, roux en-Y gastric bypass, duodenal switch (roux en-Y and single-anastomosis). Surgical Endoscopy. 2021;**35**(8):4644-4652. DOI: 10.1007/s00464-020-07891-z

[27] Sánchez-Pernaute A, Rubio MÁ, Pérez N, Marcuello C, Torres A, Pérez-Aguirre E. Single-anastomosis duodenoileal bypass as a revisional or second-step operation after sleeve

gastrectomy. Surgery for Obesity and Related Diseases. 2020;**16**(10):1491-1496. DOI: 10.1016/j.soard.2020.05.022

[28] Irani K, Youn HA, Ren-Fielding CJ, Fielding GA, Kurian M. Midterm results for gastric banding as salvage procedure for patients with weight loss failure after roux-en-Y gastric bypass. Surgery for Obesity and Related Diseases. 2011;**7**(2):219-224. DOI: 10.1016/j.soard.2010.09.024

[29] Tsenteradze T et al. Navigating bariatric surgery: Understanding and managing short-term and long-term complications. Cureus. 2024;**15**(11):e48580. DOI: 10.7759/cureus.48580

[30] Arias E, Martínez PR, Li VKM, Szomstein S, Rosenthal RJ. Mid-term follow-up after sleeve gastrectomy as a final approach for morbid obesity. Obesity Surgery. 2009;**19**(5):544-548. DOI: 10.1007/s11695-009-9818-6

[31] Faria GR. A brief history of bariatric surgery. Porto Biomedical Journal. 2017;**2**(3):90-92. DOI: 10.1016/j.pbj.2017.01.008

[32] Mitchell BG, Gupta N. Roux-en-Y Gastric Bypass. In: StatPearls. Treasure Island (FL): StatPearls Publishing; 2024. Consultato: 24 giugno 2024. [Online]. Disponibile su: http://www.ncbi.nlm.nih.gov/books/NBK553157/

[33] Eichelter J et al. Surgical technique of single anastomosis Duodeno-Ileal bypass with sleeve gastrectomy (SADI-S). Surgical Technology International. 2022;**41**:sti41/1571. DOI: 10.52198/22.STI.41.GS1571

[34] Christou NV, Look D, MacLean LD. Weight gain after short- and long-limb gastric bypass in patients followed for longer than 10 years. Annals of Surgery. 2006;**244**(5):734-740. DOI: 10.1097/01.sla.0000217592.04061.d5

[35] Sánchez-Pernaute A et al. Proximal duodenal-ileal end-to-side bypass with sleeve gastrectomy: Proposed technique. Obesity Surgery. 2007;**17**(12):1614-1618. DOI: 10.1007/s11695-007-9287-8

[36] Mahawar KK et al. The first consensus statement on revisional bariatric surgery using a modified Delphi approach. Surgical Endoscopy. 2020;**34**(4):1648-1657. DOI: 10.1007/s00464-019-06937-1

[37] Koh ZJ et al. Metabolic outcomes after revisional bariatric surgery: A systematic review and meta-analysis. Surgery for Obesity and Related Diseases. 2020;**16**(10):1442-1454. DOI: 10.1016/j.soard.2020.05.029

[38] Mirkin K, Alli VV, Rogers AM. Revisional bariatric surgery. The Surgical Clinics of North America. 2021;**101**(2):213-222. DOI: 10.1016/j.suc.2020.12.008

[39] Ibrahim AM, Thumma JR, Dimick JB. Reoperation and medicare expenditures after laparoscopic gastric band surgery. JAMA Surgery. 2017;**152**(9):835-842. DOI: 10.1001/jamasurg.2017.1093

[40] Hii MW, Lake AC, Kenfield C, Hopkins GH. Laparoscopic conversion of failed gastric banding to roux-en-Y gastric bypass: Short-term follow-up and technical considerations. Obesity Surgery. 2012;**22**(7):1022-1028. DOI: 10.1007/s11695-012-0594-3

[41] Coblijn UK, Verveld CJ, van WagensveldBA,LagardeSM.Laparoscopic roux-en-Y gastric bypass or laparoscopic sleeve gastrectomy as revisional procedure after adjustable gastric band--A systematic review. Obesity Surgery. 2013;**23**(11):1899-1914. DOI: 10.1007/s11695-013-1058-0

[42] Angrisani L et al. IFSO worldwide survey 2020-2021: Current trends for bariatric and metabolic procedures. Obesity Surgery. 2024;**34**(4):1075-1085. DOI: 10.1007/s11695-024-07118-3

[43] Saliba C, El Rayes J, Diab S, Nicolas G, Wakim R. Weight regain after sleeve gastrectomy: A look at the benefits of Re-sleeve. Cureus. 2018;**10**(10):e3450. DOI: 10.7759/cureus.3450

[44] Khalaj A et al. Revisional bariatric surgery due to complications: Indications and outcomes. Obesity Surgery. 2023;**33**(11):3463-3471. DOI: 10.1007/s11695-023-06832-8

[45] Kichler K, Rosenthal RJ, DeMaria E, Higa K. Reoperative surgery for nonresponders and complicated sleeve gastrectomy operations in patients with severe obesity. An international expert panel consensus statement to define best practice guidelines. Surgery for Obesity and Related Diseases. 2019;**15**(2):173-186. DOI: 10.1016/j.soard.2018.11.006

[46] Dardamanis D, Navez J, Coubeau L, Navez B. A retrospective comparative study of primary versus revisional roux-en-Y gastric bypass: Long-term results. Obesity Surgery. 2018;**28**(8):2457-2464. DOI: 10.1007/s11695-018-3186-z

[47] Pędziwiatr M et al. Revisional gastric bypass is inferior to primary gastric bypass in terms of short- and long-term outcomes-systematic review and meta-analysis. Obesity Surgery. 2018;**28**(7):2083-2091. DOI: 10.1007/s11695-018-3300-2

[48] Osorio J, Lazzara C, Admella V, Franci-León S, Pujol-Gebellí J. Revisional laparoscopic SADI-S vs. duodenal switch following failed primary sleeve gastrectomy: A single-center comparison of 101 consecutive cases. Obesity Surgery. 2021;**31**(8):3667-3674. DOI: 10.1007/s11695-021-05469-9

[49] Dijkhorst PJ et al. Single anastomosis duodenoileal bypass or roux-en-Y gastric bypass after failed sleeve gastrectomy: Medium-term outcomes. Obesity Surgery. 2021;**31**(11):4708-4716. DOI: 10.1007/s11695-021-05609-1

[50] Sharples AJ, Charalampakis V, Daskalakis M, Tahrani AA, Singhal R. Systematic review and meta-analysis of outcomes after revisional bariatric surgery following a failed adjustable gastric band. Obesity Surgery. 2017;**27**(10):2522-2536. DOI: 10.1007/s11695-017-2677-7

[51] Balamurugan G et al. Comparison of efficacy and safety between roux-en-Y gastric bypass (RYGB) vs one anastomosis gastric bypass (OAGB) vs single anastomosis duodeno-ileal bypass with sleeve gastrectomy (SADI-S): A systematic review of bariatric and metabolic surgery. Obesity Surgery. 2023;**33**(7):2194-2209. DOI: 10.1007/s11695-023-06602-6

[52] Mora Oliver I, Cassinello Fernández N, Alfonso Ballester R, Cuenca Ramírez MD, Serrano JO. Revisional bariatric surgery due to failure of the initial technique: 25 years of experience in a specialized unit of obesity surgery in Spain. Cirugía Española (Engl Ed). 2019;**97**(10):568-574. DOI: 10.1016/j.ciresp.2019.07.012

[53] Ji Y et al. Effect of bariatric surgery on metabolic diseases and underlying mechanisms. Biomolecules. 2021;**11**(11):1582. DOI: 10.3390/biom11111582

[54] Aleassa EM, Hassan M, Hayes K, Brethauer SA, Schauer PR, Aminian A. Effect of revisional bariatric surgery

on type 2 diabetes mellitus. Surgical Endoscopy. 2019;**33**(8):2642-2648. DOI: 10.1007/s00464-018-6541-1

[55] Axer S, Szabo E, Agerskov S, Näslund I. Predictive factors of complications in revisional gastric bypass surgery: Results from the Scandinavian obesity surgery registry. Surgery for Obesity and Related Diseases. 2019;**15**(12):2094-2100. DOI: 10.1016/j.soard.2019.09.071

[56] El Chaar M, Stoltzfus J, Melitics M, Claros L, Zeido A. 30-day outcomes of revisional bariatric stapling procedures: First report based on MBSAQIP data registry. Obesity Surgery. 2018;**28**(8):2233-2240. DOI: 10.1007/s11695-018-3140-0

Chapter 11

Endoscopic Treatment for Obesity

Bonifacio García Ramos, Monica Angulo Trejo, César David Quiróz Guadarrama, Victor García Ramos, José Antonio Angulo Trejo, Edgar Alejandro Ibáñez Cruz and Alberto Rodríguez Gallardo

Abstract

Obesity is a very important pathology worldwide, as it is related to heart disease, stroke, and type 2 diabetes mellitus. Its treatment is based on comprehensive management by a multidisciplinary team with the aim of improving the nutritional status of the patients. Various forms of surgical treatment have existed for years, with a high risk of complications. Currently, endoscopic bariatric therapies have had a great increase and have been innovative tools for the treatment of obesity. They are generally based on restrictive mechanisms, through a reduction in gastric volume, size restriction, and, in some cases, gastric bypasses, even with little accessibility to them in routine practice. However, these techniques have the potential to reduce adverse events, hospital costs, and post-surgical recovery times. The following chapter aims to explain the different current and future endoscopic bariatric therapies in order to disseminate knowledge about this currently important topic.

Keywords: obesity, endoscopic bariatric therapies, bariatric surgery, nutrition, multidisciplinary team

1. Introduction

Obesity is defined according to the World Health Organization (WHO) as an abnormal or excessive accumulation of fat that presents a significant health risk and is closely related to long-term complications. Another definition is when there is a Body Mass Index (BMI) greater than 30 kg/m^2 [1]. This pathology affects more than 650 million adults worldwide [2], generating multiple complications such as type 2 diabetes mellitus, high blood pressure, hepatic steatosis, and cardiovascular diseases [3].

From 1991, when the first guidelines of the National Institutes of Health on gastrointestinal surgery for obesity were published, bariatric surgery was the only option available as a management for severe obesity [4]; however, it was not available for all patients, hence the importance of promoting new therapeutic options with the aim of improving the quality of life and avoiding complications.

Currently, there are several therapeutic options for this pathology such as lifestyle modification, pharmacological treatment, and endoscopic (metabolic and bariatric)

therapies, which offer greater efficacy (10–25%) and are less invasive than bariatric surgeries.

Bariatric endoscopic therapies (EBT) are defined as a spectrum of minimally invasive techniques and devices that use endoscopic access for weight control and resolution or improvement of comorbidities associated with obesity [2].

The main objective of endoscopic treatments is to combine the effect of weight loss with an improvement in metabolic complications, since they exert both a restrictive and metabolic effect, significantly decreasing morbidity in patients.

These procedures have gained relevance in the medical field, becoming the most effective and lasting option for the treatment of obesity, especially in moderately obese patients with a BMI of 30–35 kg/m^2 or in patients with BMI >40 kg/m^2 who do not want or are not candidates for surgical procedures [2]. They usually involve the stomach; however, there are also procedures that remodel the duodenum or small intestine.

The first endoscopic bariatric therapy was the Garren Edwards Bubble, developed in 1985; it was discontinued due to its high rate of complications and low efficacy; however, it was the impetus for the development of intragastric balloons [5].

In 2015, the American Society of Gastrointestinal Endoscopy (ASGE) and the American Society of Metabolic and Bariatric Surgery (ASMBS) defined the safety and efficacy of these therapies with a success ≥25% weight loss at 12 months and a low rate of complications ≤5% [3, 5].

Later, in 2024, the European Society of Gastrointestinal Endoscopy (ESGE) and the ASGE recommended the use of endoscopic bariatric therapies (EBMT) in adults with obesity, in combination with lifestyle changes, for patients with a BMI greater than 30 kg/m^2 or between 27 and 29.9 kg/m^2 with at least one obesity-related comorbidity. Since EBMT can be used both as primary therapy and as a bridge before bariatric surgery, it was concluded not to establish an upper BMI limit for consideration [5].

In this same guideline, decreases in total body weight loss (TBWL) of 11.9% (95% CI, 7.7–16.0) were observed for subgroups with a BMI of 27.0 to 29.9 kg/m^2. For patients with class I and II obesity, TBWL percentages ranged from 5.0 to 18.6%. In the case of class III obesity, the total weight loss was 13.1% (95% CI, 10.8–15.4) at 12 months [6].

Bariatric endoscopic procedures can be classified into four groups: (1) procedures that reduce gastric volume, (2) procedures that delay gastric emptying, (3) referral procedures, and (4) other procedures.

Another classification is depending on the organ of the gastrointestinal tract in gastric and intestinal. Gastric interventions induce weight loss and those of the intestine have direct effects on metabolic conditions.

Endoscopic therapies work through one of the following mechanisms: the first is through the restriction or reduction of gastric capacity, either through the use of sutures or endoscopic plicature or the installation of devices that generate a decrease in gastric volume; the second by prolonging satiety by delaying gastric emptying; the third by reducing the absorption of calories through the postprandial emptying of food ingested from the stomach before reaching the intestine; and the fourth is focused on the small intestine with the aim of preventing food passage through the duodenum through a deviation of the gastrointestinal tract, preventing food from mixing with bile and pancreatic acids (blocking metabolic effects) [7].

The most relevant procedures and some examples will be explained below.

2. Procedures that reduce gastric volume

The two main approaches to achieving gastric restriction is by filling the stomach with a balloon, which limits the space available for food or dividing the size of the stomach by using sutures to achieve a decrease in space for food, inducing early satiety and decreasing calorie intake [7].

2.1 Intragastric balloons (IGB)

Its goal is to reduce gastric volume. The mechanism of action is the stimulation of the mechanoreceptors in the stomach, which then stimulate the vagus nerve by sending signals to the hypothalamus that subsequently induces the feeling of satiety and decreases gastric emptying.

The first gastric balloon was placed in 1982 by Nieben and Harboe in Denmark [8]. There are different shapes and sizes; however, most are round or oval, made of silicone, which limits the injury of the gastric mucosa and have an approximate volume of 400–700 ml. They can be filled with liquid (saline solution with methylene blue), gas, or both, demonstrating greater weight loss in those patients in whom they were filled with liquid. Its placement is under endoscopic control, either with the patient sedated, or it can be swallowed in the form of a capsule, being able to be in the body for up to 6 months, and even up to 12 months (Orbera 365). A decrease of up to 13.2% in total body weight loss at 6 months and 11.3% per year [9] has been demonstrated.

The new guideline from ASGE and ESGE indicates that, according to a meta-analysis, nine randomized clinical trials addressed the TBWL during IGB removal (at 6 and 12 months), with a sample size of 779 individuals. A significant improvement of 10.7% in total weight loss (95% CI, 4.1–9.7) was recorded compared to approximately 3.4% associated with lifestyle changes [6].

IGBs can be used as primary therapy in patients with overweight or mild to moderate obesity, with a decrease in total body weight of 10–12% [10].

The most common and studied intragastric balloon is the Orbera, being the only device that has met the standards of Preservation and Incorporation of Valuable Endoscopic Innovations established by the ASGE (**Figure 1**) [2].

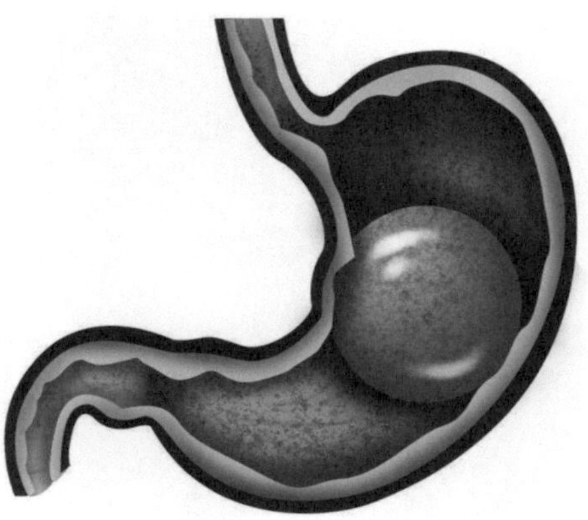

Figure 1.
Schematic representation of intragastric balloon.

There are some adaptive symptoms that can occur after the placement of a balloon such as persistent nausea, vomiting, pain, and generalized abdominal discomfort and symptoms of reflux; in case of persistence of obstructive symptoms, it may require the early removal of the balloon, which occurs in less than 5% of cases [11]. The serious adverse effects reported are mucosal injury, gastric or esophageal perforation, balloon migration, obstruction of the outflow, and infections due to excessive growth of bacteria in the fluid that fills the balloon.

A risk associated with balloon removal is the possibility of recurrent weight gain. Initially, the mechanism of action of IGB for weight loss was thought to be primarily due to the restriction provided by the balloon. However, subsequent analyses of gastric emptying have shown that the effects are also partly due to a reduction in gastric emptying rate. Therefore, upon balloon removal, not only is the restriction lost, but gastric emptying is also restored, emphasizing the need for lifestyle and dietary changes [6].

The absolute contraindications for its placement are: presence of gastric, duodenal, and esophageal ulcers, regardless of the presence or not of active bleeding, previous gastric surgery, gastric and esophageal varicose veins, hiatal hernia >5 cm, and the use of anticoagulants [12].

2.2 Transpiloric ferry (TPS)

It consists of a silicone balloon that is anchored in the region of the pylorus, is attached to a silicone catheter that is inserted into the duodenum, and has a smaller oval balloon at its tip. It is released endoscopically and placed in the stomach; it is designed to remain for up to 12 months; after release, peristalsis takes the smallest balloon beyond the pylorus, causing an intermittent obstruction of the gastric outlet, delaying gastric emptying [13].

Among its advantages are that the filling of the balloon is faster and the gastric emptying slower.

It is mainly indicated for obese patients with a body mass index of 30–40 kg/m^2 (**Figure 2**).

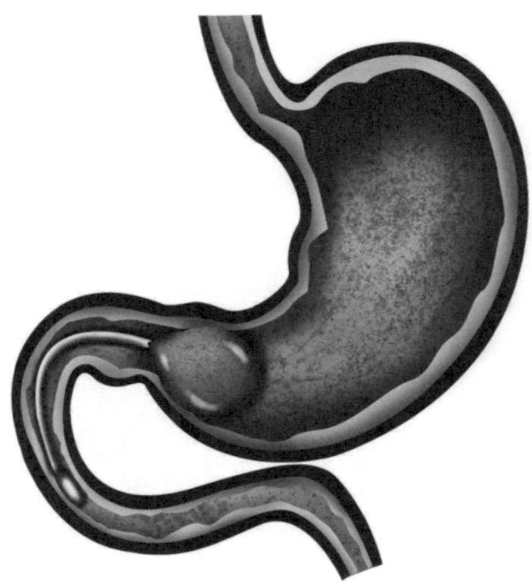

Figure 2.
Schematic representation of transpiloric ferry.

2.3 Satiesfera

It is a device consisting of a nitinol guide with oval polyethylene terephthalate balls. It is implanted in the pylorus and duodenum endoscopically. Its principle of action lies in the decrease in food intake associated with the delay in food transit through the duodenum.

3. Procedures that reduce gastric volume

3.1 Endoscopic sleeve gastroplasty (ESG)

This procedure was described in 2013 by Abu Dayyeh [14] and is performed with the OverStich system. Its objective is to imitate surgical gastrectomy, which leads to the reduction of gastric volume and the induction of early postprandial fullness. It also seems to have a metabolic effect, since it has been shown that there is a significant decrease in liver enzymes, glycosylated hemoglobin (HbA1c), triglyceride level, and systemic blood pressure [15]. Another advantage is that it is a reversible method. The main indications are patients with mild to moderate obesity.

A suture device is placed at the tip of the double-channel endoscope, which is equipped with a curved needle guide that allows continuous or interrupted sutures along the major curvature of the stomach. The total weight loss reported at 12 months was 68.3% [16].

According to the ASGE and the ESGE, when considering the results of the TBWL at 12 months in seven randomized studies with more than 340 subjects, a loss of 10.5% was observed, representing 4.4 times more compared to lifestyle changes alone [6].

Additionally, the results of the meta-analysis from four randomized controlled trials with a minimum of 6 months of follow-up reported a percentage of serious adverse events of 3.2%. Selected examples of these events included abdominal abscess (0.76%), upper gastrointestinal bleeding (0.76%), malnutrition (0.76%), extraluminal bleeding (0.45%), hepatic abscess (0.45%), and abdominal pain, nausea, or vomiting requiring prolonged hospitalization (4.07%) [6].

Several studies have been carried out that compare the efficacy and adverse effects of this procedure with respect to surgical treatments, with a lower TBWL at 12 months compared to surgery (17 vs. 30.5%) but with a lower adverse effect rate of 2.9 vs. 11.8% [17].

Procedure with authorization in force by the Food and Drug Administration (FDA) since 2022 (**Figure 3**).

3.2 Primary endoluminal surgery for obesity (POSE)

It is a bariatric method that uses a flexible endoscope and a minimally invasive surgical approach. The operating system is used without incisions. It is a more complex device, equipped with a 54 Fr (Transport)-controlled tube capable of maneuvering in four directions and has four channels for specialized instruments to grasp the folds of the fabric (g-Lix and g-Prox EZ) to position fabric anchors (g-Cath EZ) and to visualize the light [18–20].

In this procedure, the anchor points are placed at the bottom of the stomach, creating eight to new folds; usually, three to four are placed at the level of the distal body near the antro opposite to the angular incision.

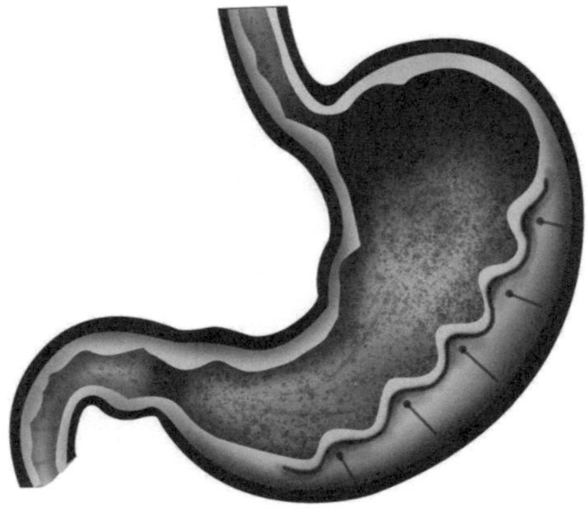

Figure 3.
Schematic representation of endoscopic sleeve gastroplasty.

The total weight loss reported at 12 months was 44.9% [16].

Currently, different variants of plication techniques have been proposed. The López-Nava group modified the POSE technique by performing the plication in the gastric body to alter its motility (POSE-2), demonstrating a TBWL of 15.7% at 6 months, without significant adverse effects [20].

Despite the benefits of non-invasive procedures, neither procedure has been shown to be as effective as laparoscopic sleeve gastrectomy (LSG) with respect to weight loss and BMI; however, a lower rate of complications and a lower in-hospital stay after the procedure have been demonstrated [21].

Authorized in 2006 for tissue apposition in the United States, it is still in clinical trial and currently awaiting approval by the FDA (**Figure 4**).

3.3 Percutaneous gastric aspiration therapy

The AspireAssist system (Aspire Bariatrics, Inc. King of Prussia, PA, USA) was used for obesity grade 2 and 3, approved by the FDA, being even more effective than an intragastric balloon. This procedure consisted of placing a percutaneous endoscopic gastrostomy tube associated with an external device, which aspirated

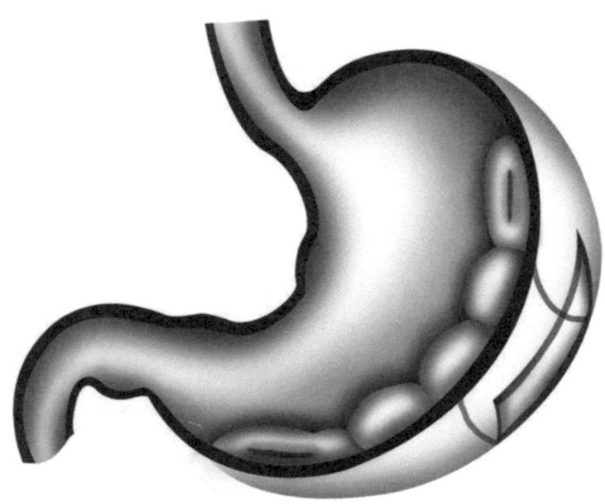

Figure 4.
Schematic representation of primary endoluminal surgery for obesity.

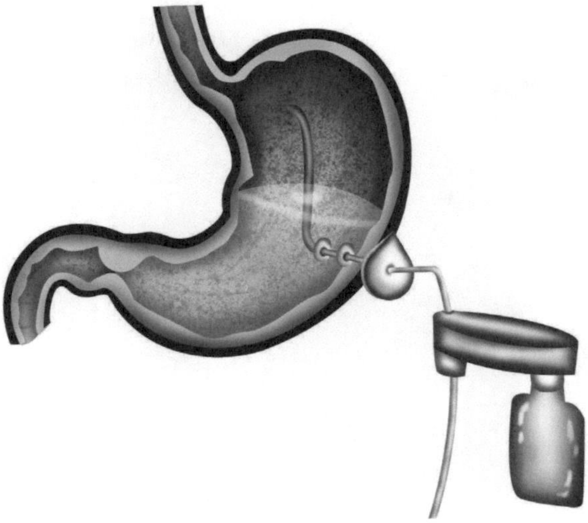

Figure 5.
Schematic representation of percutaneous gastric aspiration therapy (AspireAssist system).

approximately 30% of the gastric content after meals, with a TBWL of 18.3% (12 months) and 18.7% (48 months). In February 2022, it was withdrawn from the market due to lack of funding (**Figure 5**) [22, 23].

4. Endoscopic malabsorption interventions

4.1 Duodenal mucosa resurfacing (DMR)

The duodenal mucosa resurfacing (Fractyl, Lexington, MA) is a catheter-based technique that performs hydrothermal ablation of the duodenal mucosa using a balloon filled with hot water. It consists of introducing through the mouth to the duodenum and is placed distally to the Váter ampule on a guide by fluoroscopy. The 2 cm balloon catheter is designed to isolate the mucosa from the rest of the layers of the duodenum via injection of saline solution to subsequently perform hydrothermal ablation of the mucosa between the Váter ampule and the Treitz ligament.

It has been shown that in patients with type 2 diabetes mellitus, there is a hypertrophy of the duodenal mucosa with a greater number of enteroendocrine cells, which increases the secretion of gastric inhibitory polypeptide (GIP), which increases the level of cyclic AMP in pancreatic β cells by stimulating glucose-dependent insulin secretion [20, 24]. This effect causes a decrease in HbA1c of approximately 1.2% 6 months after the procedure. However, at present, this procedure is only for experimental use (**Figure 6**).

4.2 Duodenal: jejunal bypass sleeve (DJBS)

The duodenal–jejunal bypass sleeve (Endobarrier) (GI Dynamics, Boston, MA, USA. U.S.) is a teflon-coated device that favors the malabsorption process, working similar to a Roux Y gastric bypass, carrying the food through a thin and flexible

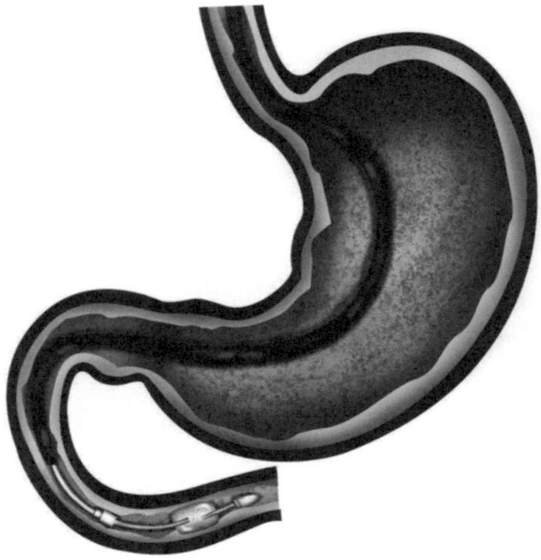

Figure 6.
Schematic representation of duodenal mucosa resurfacing.

tube of approximately 60 cm to the yeyuno without going through the duodenum (duoden-yeyunal bypass), avoiding the absorption of food [20]. The duration of this treatment is up to 12 months.

A success rate has been demonstrated with a TBWL of 12.6–35% and a 1% reduction in glycosylated hemoglobin compared to patients with only changes in the diet [2, 25].

The FDA suspended the approval of this procedure due to a high incidence of liver abscesses; however, there is currently a new STEP-1 trial in the United States that began in February 2019 and ends in 2025 to evaluate the reintroduction of it (**Figure** 7).

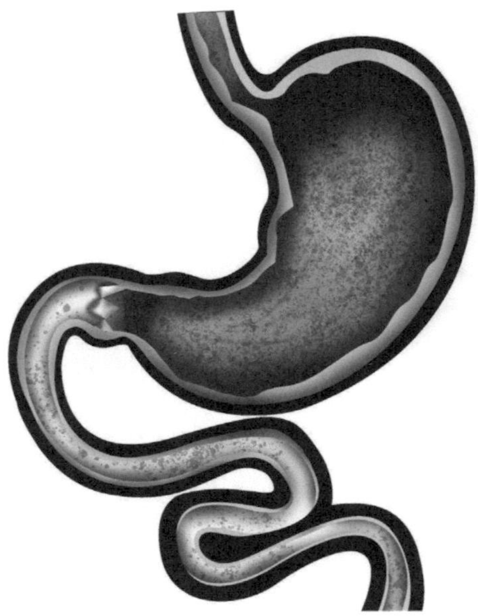

Figure 7.
Schematic representation of duodenal - Jejunal bypass sleeve.

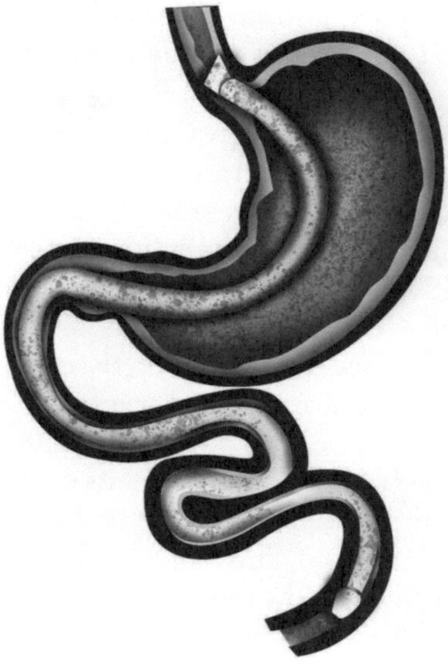

Figure 8.
Schematic representation of Gastroduodeno - Yeyunal bypass.

4.3 Gastroduodeno: yeyunal bypass

Endo Bypass System (ValenTx, Maple Grove, MN, EE. USA) is a 120 cm fluoropolymer device that is anchored to the region of the gastroesophageal junction, with the aim of bringing the food to the small intestine. It remains in the body for up to 12 months, with a total weight loss of up to 35.9%. However, the Endo Bypass system is not yet approved by the FDA and the CE (**Figure 8**) [19, 26].

4.4 The incisionless magnetic anastomosis system

The Incisionless Magnetic Anastomotic System (IMAS), introduced by GI Windows (Westewood, MA, USA) [20], consists of creating an anastomosis without intestinal incisions through the use of two magnets with the aim of diverting nutrients and bile acids into the ileum, causing a malabsorption process. This procedure is performed when a magnet is placed by enteroscopy at the level of the proximal yeyunus and terminal ileum through a colonoscopy simultaneously to create an anastomosis by means of local tissue necrosis. The magnets are removed approximately 2 weeks later through the feces [20, 27].

A TBWL of 14.6% has been demonstrated within 12 months of its completion, in addition to a reduction in glycosylated hemoglobin of 1–1.9% in patients with type 2 diabetes mellitus [28].

The drawback is that anastomosis is not reversible, and there are still no studies that report the consequences of long-term malabsorption [20].

5. Complications

There is evidence that complications after bariatric surgeries are rare; however, they can be devastating and even deadly. The mortality rate of the laparoscopic gastric sleeve is 0–1.2%.

Complications can be classified into early (leaks (0.1%), stenosis (0.1%), and bleeding) and late (stenosis (0.49%) and gastroesophageal reflux disease (GERD) (6%) [29].

Bariatric endoscopic therapies, especially GBIs, are safe but, in some cases, uncomfortable, mainly causing nausea persisting for more than 7 days; in various studies, an early extraction rate of the Orbera IGB of 7% has been demonstrated. Among the most serious complications are migration (1.4%) and gastric perforation (0.1%), emphasizing that 50% of patients had undergone previous gastric surgeries.

In the AspireAssist, up to 4.1% of adverse effects have been reported; minor complications include the presence of granulation tissue in the stoma (40.5%) and infection of the stoma (14.4%), and among the severe (3.6%) are gastric ulcers and peritonitis [22].

The EndoBarrier has an extraction rate of 18.7%; its main complications are migration (4.9%), gastrointestinal hemorrhage (3.86%), obstruction of the device (3.4%), hepatic abscesses (0.12%), cholangitis (0.12%), and esophageal perforation (0.12%) [30].

With respect to IMAS, it shows a low rate of complications, mainly related to post-procedure diarrhea.

The ESSENTIAL trial showed a complication rate for POSE of 4.7% including extra-gastric bleeding (0.4%), hepatic abscess (0.4%), chest pain, and fever [31].

6. Conclusions

Currently, a multidisciplinary team must offer endoscopic bariatric therapies, lifestyle modifications, and appropriate nutritional counseling as a fundamental tool in the treatment of obesity. There is sufficient evidence of the effectiveness of these procedures for the treatment of obesity, as well as certain comorbidities (type 2 diabetes mellitus).

It is also important to mention that although their effectiveness is usually slightly lower than surgical procedures (laparoscopic gastric sleeve), they have the advantage of being safer, less invasive, and reversible therapies.

However, despite the fact that there is a wide range of endoscopic therapies available, some are still not approved by the FDA for reproduction, in addition to the fact that there is a deficiency in training programs by endoscopist doctors, which has limited their dissemination and use, hence the importance of knowing this topic for the application and dissemination of knowledge and generating interest in new therapeutic strategies for this complex pathology that requires a multidisciplinary management with the aim of reducing morbidity and mortality in our patients.

Author details

Bonifacio García Ramos[1*], Monica Angulo Trejo[1], César David Quiróz Guadarrama[2], Victor García Ramos[3], José Antonio Angulo Trejo[4], Edgar Alejandro Ibáñez Cruz[1] and Alberto Rodríguez Gallardo[3]

1 Mexican Institute of Social Security, Monterrey, Mexico

2 NewCity Hospital, Tijuana, Mexico

3 Mexican Institute of Social Security, Veracruz, Mexico

4 Mexican Institute of Social Security, Queretaro, Mexico

*Address all correspondence to: bonifacio_bonice@hotmail.com

References

[1] World Obesity Federation. World obesity Atlas 2023 [Internet]. 2023. Available from: https://data.worldobesity.org/publications/?cat=19 [Accessed: January 11, 2024]

[2] Ibrahim Mohamed BK, Barajas-Gamboa JS, Rodriguez J. Endoscopic bariatric therapies: Current status and future perspectives. JSLS. 2022;**26**(1):1-7. DOI: 10.4293/JSLS.2021.00066

[3] Heymsfield SB, Wadden TA. Mechanisms, pathophysiology, and management of obesity. The New England Journal of Medicine. 2017;**376**:254-266. DOI: 10.1056/NEJMra1514009

[4] National Institutes of Health Gastrointestinal Surgery for Severe Obesity. Consensus Development conference panel. Annals of Internal Medicine. 1991;**115**(12):956-961

[5] Hogan RB, Johnston JH, Long BW, et al. A double-blind, randomized, sham-controlled trial of the gastric bubble for obesity. Gastrointestinal Endoscopy. 1989;**35**(5):381-385. DOI: 10.1016/s0016-5107(89)72839-x

[6] Jirapinyo P, Hadefi A, Thompson C, et al. American Society for Gastrointestinal Endoscopy–European Society of Gastrointestinal Endoscopy guideline on primary endoscopic bariatric and metabolic therapies for adults with obesity. Thieme Endoscopy. 2024;**56**(06):437-456. DOI: 10.1055/a-2292-2494

[7] Shikora S, Sharaiha RZ, White KP, Macedo G, Toouli J, Kow L. Resumen de las directrices de consenso sobre el tratamiento de la obesidad – Una iniciativa conjunta y multidisciplinaria de la Federación Internacional para la Cirugía de la Obesidad y los Trastornos Metabólicos (IFSO) y la Organización Mundial de Gastroenterología (WGO). Gastroenterología Latinoamericana. 2023;**34**(2):1-310

[8] Nieben OG, Harboe H. Intragastric balloon as an artificial bezoar for treatment of obesity. Lancet. 1982;**1**(8265):198-199. DOI: 10.1016/s0140-6736(82)90762-0

[9] Abu Dayyeh B, Kumar N, Edmundowicz SA, et al. ASGE bariatric endoscopy task force systematic review and meta-analysis assessing the ASGE PIVI thresholds for adopting endoscopic bariatric therapies. Gastrointestinal Endoscopy. 2015;**82**(3):425-438. DOI: 10.1016/j.gie.2015.03.1964

[10] Mechanick JI, Apovian C, Brethauer S, et al. Clinical practice guidelines for the perioperative nutrition, metabolic, and nonsurgical support of patients undergoing bariatric procedures - 2019 update: Cosponsored by American Association of Clinical Endocrinologists/American College of Endocrinology, the Obesity Society, American Society for Metabolic & bariatric surgery, obesity medicine association, and American Society of Anesthesiologists - executive summary. Endocrine Practice. 2019;**12**:1346-1359. DOI: 10.4158/GL-2019-0406

[11] Espinet E, Del Pozo AJ, Turró R, et al. Spanish Intragastric balloon consensus statement (SIBC): Practical guidelines based on experience of over 20 000 cases. Revista Española de Enfermedades Digestivas. 2023;**115**(1):22-34. DOI: 10.17235/reed.2022.9322/2022

[12] Neto MG, Silva LB, Grecco E, et al. Brazilian intragastric balloon consensus

statement (BIBC): Practical guidelines based on experience of over 40,000 cases. Surgery for Obesity and Related Diseases. 2018;**14**(2):151-159. DOI: 10.1016/j.soard.2017.09.528

[13] Marinos G, Eliades C, Raman Muthusamy V, Greenway F. Weight loss and improved quality of life with a nonsurgical endoscopic treatment for obesity: Clinical results from a 3- and 6-month study. Surgery for Obesity and Related Diseases. 2014;**10**(5):929-934. DOI: 10.1016/j.soard.2014.03.005

[14] Abu Dayyeh BK, Rajan E, Gostout CJ. Endoscopic sleeve gastroplasty, a possible endoscopic alternative to surgical sleeve gastrectomy for the treatment of obesity. Gastrointestinal Endoscopy. 2013;**78**(3):530-535. DOI: 10.1016/j.gie.2013.04.197

[15] Sharaiha RZ, Kumta NA, Saumoy M, et al. Endoscopic sleeve gastroplasty significantly reduces body mass index and metabolic complications in obese patients. Clinical Gastroenterology and Hepatology. 2017;**15**(4):504-510. DOI: 10.1016/j.cgh.2016.12.012

[16] Gys B, Plaeke P, Lamme B, et al. Endoscopic gastric plication for morbid obesity: A systematic review and meta-analysis of published data over time. Obesity Surgery. 2019;**29**(9):3021-3029. DOI: 10.1007/s11695-019-04010-3

[17] Mohan BP, Asokkumar R, Khan SR, et al. Outcomes of endoscopic sleeve gastroplasty; how does it compare to laparoscopic sleeve gastrectomy? A systematic review and meta-analysis. Endoscopy International Open. 2020;**8**(4):558-565. DOI: 10.1055/a-1120-8350

[18] Espinós JC, Turró R, Mata A, et al. Early experience with the incisionless operating platform™ (IOP) for the treatment of obesity: The primary obesity surgery endolumenal (POSE) procedure. Obesity Surgery. 2013;**23**(9):1375-1383. DOI: 10.1007/s11695-013-0937-8

[19] Telese A, Sehgal V, Magee CG, et al. Bariatric and metabolic endoscopy: A new paradigm. Clinical and Translational Gastroenterology. 2021;**12**(6):1-10. DOI: 10.14309/ctg.0000000000000364

[20] Mauro A, Lusetti F, Scalvini D, et al. A comprehensive review on bariatric endoscopy: Where we are now and where we are going. Medicina (Kaunas, Lithuania). 2023;**59**(3):636. DOI: 10.3390/medicina59030636

[21] Novikov AA, Afaneh C, Saumoy M, et al. Endoscopic sleeve Gastroplasty, laparoscopic sleeve gastrectomy, and laparoscopic band for weight loss: How do they compare? Journal of Gastrointestinal Surgery. 2018;**22**(2):267-273. DOI: 10.1007/s11605-017-3615-7

[22] Thompson CC, Abu Dayyeh BK, Kushner R, et al. Percutaneous gastrostomy device for the treatment of class II and class III obesity: Results of a randomized controlled trial. The American Journal of Gastroenterology. 2017;**112**(3):447-457. DOI: 10.1038/ajg.2016.500

[23] Crothall K. 2022 Aspire bariatrics company update. [Internet]. 2022. Available from: https://www.aspirebariatrics.com/ [Accessed: April 25, 2024]

[24] Seino Y, Fukushima M, Yabe D. GIP and GLP-1, the two incretin hormones: Similarities and differences. Journal of Diabetes Investigation. 2010;**1**(1-2):8-23. DOI: 10.1111/j.2040-1124.2010.00022.x

[25] Rohde U, Hedbäck N, Gluud LL, Vilsbøll T, Knop FK. Effect of the

endobarrier gastrointestinal liner on obesity and type 2 diabetes: A systematic review and meta-analysis. Diabetes, Obesity & Metabolism. 2016;**18**(3): 300-305. DOI: 10.1111/dom.12603

[26] Sandler BJ, Rumbaut R, Swain CP, et al. One-year human experience with a novel endoluminal, endoscopic gastric bypass sleeve for morbid obesity. Surgical Endoscopy. 2015;**29**(11):3298-3303. DOI: 10.1007/s00464-015-4081-5

[27] Reja D, Zhang C, Sarkar A. Endoscopic bariatrics: Current therapies and future directions. Translational Gastroenterology and Hepatology. 2022;**7**(21):1-13. DOI: 10.21037/tgh.2020.03.09

[28] Machytka E, Bužga M, Zonca P, et al. Partial jejunal diversion using an incisionless magnetic anastomosis system: 1-year interim results in patients with obesity and diabetes. Gastrointestinal Endoscopy. 2017;**86**(5):904-912. DOI: 10.1016/j.gie.2017.07.009

[29] Alvarenga ES, Lo Menzo E, Szomstein S, Rosenthal R. Safety and efficacy of 1020 consecutive laparoscopic sleeve gastrectomies performed as a primary treatment modality for morbid obesity. A single-center experience from the metabolic and bariatric surgical accreditation quality and improvement program. Surgical Endoscopy. 2016;**30**(7):2673-2678. DOI: 10.1007/s00464-015-4548-4

[30] Kaplan LM, Jb B, Mullin C, et al. EndoBarrier therapy is associated with glycemic improvement, weight loss and safety issues in patients with obesity and type 2 diabetes on oral antihyperglycemic agents. In: Proceedings of the 76th Scientific Sessions, New Orleans. 2016

[31] Sullivan S, Swain JM, Woodman G, et al. Randomized sham-controlled trial evaluating efficacy and safety of endoscopic gastric plication for primary obesity: The ESSENTIAL trial. Obesity (Silver Spring). 2017;**25**(2):294-301. DOI: 10.1002/oby.21702

Chapter 12

Endoscopic Sleeve Gastroplasty: Technique Evolution

Jimi Izaques Bifi Scarparo and Bruno Sander

Abstract

According to the World Health Organization (WHO), in 2019, 2.3 billion people were overweight worldwide. In Brazil, overweight already affects 52.5% of adults, and this rate has been increasing every year. New weight loss alternatives have emerged, including endoscopic sleeve gastroplasty (ESG), an endoscopic procedure that reduces stomach volume through internal sutures, to demonstrate the safety, efficacy, and durability of ESG in patients undergoing a new endoscopic suturing technique, called Sander-Scarparo Technique, in obese patients. A retrospective study in two different health centers, with participants who underwent the Sander-Scarparo Technique in ESG, compares them to the traditional technique that was performed between July 2017 and December 2019. Participants were distributed into different groups, with follow-up time ranging from 12 to 48 months, depending on the interval between the procedure and data collection. All were at least 18 years old, had a minimum body mass index (BMI) of 30 kg/m2 (grade I obesity), and had no previous bariatric surgery. The variables that may influence the efficacy and durability of ESG were analyzed (suture patterns [U versus U + argon (with or without oversuture)]): "Sander-Scarparo Technique," resuture, number of sutures, number of bites, weight loss (in kilograms), percentage of total body weight loss (%TBWL), percentage of excess weight loss (%EWL), argon plasma electrocautery, and complications and intercurrences, in a follow-up of up to 4 years after the procedure, at 12-month interval.

Keywords: obesity, weight loss, and slimming, bariatric endoscopy, endoscopic suture with overstitch, endoscopic sleeve gastroplasty (ESG), bariatric surgery

1. Introduction

The development of accessories capable of performing plications and sutures that encompass the entire wall of the gastrointestinal tract has made possible the development of techniques for gastric volume reduction. "Endoscopic sleeve gastroplasty (ESG)" is a term that has been neglected in medical circles of Brazil in order to avoid the allusion that this method is bariatric surgery. The most accepted term is endoscopic gastroplasty or gastric endosuture. Endoscopic sleeve gastroplasty (ESG) is a method of gastric volume reduction, both in length and width, performed using a suture device (Overstitch ™) coupled to a single or double-channel endoscope, which allows the creation of suture lines that reach all layers of the gastric wall and aims to reduce gastric volume and, thus, cause early satiety, delayed gastric emptying, and weight loss [1]. It was first introduced in our country in 2017 and, since then, it is estimated that more than 20,000 patients in Brazil have already undergone the method by now (2024). Despite literature showing good results of ESG efficacy, with a literature review of up to 1600 patients [2], multicenter studies [3] even with high-risk patients [4], failures due to insufficient weight loss or regain of lost weight sometime after the procedure were also found. Brunaldi et al. [5], even, demonstrated that the follow-up of these patients has not been well described and, in addition, in some cases there may be ESG failure, with need to review the procedure by means of resuturing [6, 7]. Another study showed the feasibility of ESG, even after failure of gastric plication (POSE) [8]. As for Lopez-Nava et al. [8], it shows that resuturing has been a good alternative in repairing ESG failures, accompanied by weight regain, recommending this option in patients in whom the stomach did not maintain the tubularized shape. Literature on this subject [9–11] has not yet paid attention to the possibility of a relationship between the efficacy and durability of gastric restriction and suture patterns or that a reinforcement of the primary suture with the use of oversuture may influence the maintenance of the tubularized shape of the stomach. Also, it has not been verified, the effect that the number of threads to suture and bites (each point applied to pierce the gastric wall) may have on the formation of fibrosis between the gastric folds and also establishing a link between nutritional and psychological follow-up and the results of ESG.

Another valid question is whether the time elapsed after ESG influences the durability of the tubularized shape, suggesting that gastric volume restriction decreases over the months or whether fibrosis and adhesion between the folds occur, even after the expected loosening of the sutures. Thus, understanding these variables better can contribute to the improvement of suture techniques, and the findings of this study may be of great relevance to the medical and scientific community and to society in general, since the results, conclusions, and all publications arising from them have great potential to indicate changes in the method, with increased safety, efficacy, and durability of ESG.

1.1 Authors' objective

To evaluate the efficacy and safety of ESG, in a 12 to 48-month follow-up, in obese patients who underwent the procedure between July 2017 and August 2020 in a bicentric study.

The specific objectives of this study were:

a. To identify weight loss after ESG, in short and medium term, at intervals of up to 12 months, up to a maximum of 48 months.

b. To indicate the durability of gastric diameter reduction, up to 48 months after the procedure, from endoscopic verification of stomach tubulization maintenance.

c. To demonstrate the efficacy of the Sander-Scarparo Technique on weight loss and the durability of the tubularized stomach shape.

2. Methods

The study was conducted at two independent private Day Hospitals, Sander Medical Center, located in the municipality of Belo Horizonte - MG, and Clinica Scarparo Hospital Dia, located in the municipality of São Paulo - SP. Participants underwent the procedure between July 2017 and August 2020, with data collection up to September 2021. This is a longitudinal and retrospective study to obtain information on the medical procedure called endoscopic gastroplasty, of a clinical trial type. As equipment for performing ESG has already been approved by ANVISA (The National Health Surveillance Agency-Brazil), it is thus called post-market surveillance. The initial population of all patients with obesity (BMI > 30 kg/m^2), over 18 years of age, who underwent the ESG procedure at the research center, between July 2017 and August 2020, with primary objective of obesity control, and who had the more than 12 months of follow-up after the procedure, were included in the study. From this initial population, patients who underwent bariatric surgery or who became pregnant after ESG and those who did not complete the minimum follow-up time of 12 months at the research center were excluded.

2.1 Inclusion criteria

a. Minimum age of 18 years.

b. BMI of 30 kg/m^2 or higher.

c. Having undergone ESG between July 2017 and August 2020;

d. Minimum follow-up time of 12 months, carried out at the participating research center after ESG.

2.2 Exclusion criteria

a. Having undergone bariatric surgery.

b. Having had a pregnancy after ESG.

c. Patients who underwent the procedure, but for whom data collection was not possible.

2.3 Procedures

2.3.1 Pre-intervention

Since ESG is performed under general anesthesia, all patients underwent the protocol established by the anesthesia team at the research center, which consisted of an eight-hour fast, immediately before the procedure, and, previously, laboratory tests (blood count, coagulation test, kidney, liver and thyroid function, blood glucose and glycosylated hemoglobin, electrolyte, and B vitamin levels), imaging tests (chest X-ray and upper digestive endoscopy), spirometry, electrocardiogram and cardiological evaluation, pre-anesthetic evaluation, and other tests that were deemed necessary individually before the procedure. Concomitantly, pre-operative nutritional and psychological evaluations were also carried out. All data were stored in a database.

2.3.2 Intervention

The procedure was performed under general anesthesia, with orotracheal intubation, with the assistance of an anesthesiologist. The patient preparation protocol consisted of:

a. Cardiopulmonary and multiparametric monitoring;

b. Patient in left lateral decubitus position;

c. Endoscopic evaluation of the esophagus-stomach-duodenum to:

- Assess whether the gastric preparation was adequate (stomach without food residues);
- Prior study of the gastric chamber in relation to its morphology;
- Strategic planning of sites for gastric sutures;
- Application and dotted marking with Argon plasma, in all patients, outlining the limits of the area to be sutured, forming an area similar to a right trapezoid, with the following limits: 1. Transition from the gastric body to the antrum, 2. Lesser curvature, 3. Gastric fundus, 4. Greater curvature. The purpose of this marking is to assist in orientation of the sutures throughout the procedure, serving as a reference to the stitches limits.
- From January 2020, we also began applying Argon plasma continuously, longitudinally between the gastric folds, from the greater curvature to the lesser curvature, up to the limits of the suture, from distal to proximal, with an average spacing of 3 centimeters between the application lines, with the aim of increasing fibrosis and improving adhesion between the sutured gastric folds.

Procedure protocol consisted of:

a. Introducing the overtube guided by the dual-channel endoscopic device until it fits into the dental arch.

b. Removing the endoscopic device and coupling the overstitch to the device at its distal tip and to the working arch next to the channel insertion.

c. Introducing a threaded needle holder into the right channel of the device.

d. Introducing the unexposed corkscrew-type helix through the left channel of the device.

e. Testing the suture operation mechanism at least twice before introducing the entire assembly through the overtube.

f. Lubricating the entire assembly with xylocaine gel.

g. Introducing the assembled device through the overtube, up to its distal limit, without passing and with the balloon cuff still deflated.

h. Inflating the balloon cuff with 7–10 mL of air and activating the use of carbon dioxide (CO2) with an appropriate pump.

i. Passing the distal limit of the overtube and heading to the gastric chamber.

j. Starting the gastric sutures, with the first thread, closest to the angularis incision, at the transition from the body to the antrum, with an average interval of about 1 centimeter between the stitches and about 3 centimeters between the suture lines, making a U-shape with each thread, being the "U" top at the beginning and the end of the suture, on the greater curvature, and the "U" base the lesser curvature, in the following sequence of stitches (bites)

   Points 1 to 3: Anterior wall.
   Points 4 to 6: Anterior wall—2 cm distant and distal to point 1.
   Points 7 to 9: Greater curvature.
   Points 10 to 12: Greater curvature – 2–3 cm distant from point 3.
   Points 13 to 14: Posterior wall.
   Points 15 to 17: Posterior wall—2 cm distant and next to point 5.
   Points 18 to 20: Repeat the reverse sequence on the greater curvature of points 3 and 4.
   Points 21 to 22: Close to point 1 and release needle with continuous pressure on the blue button of the needle holder.

k. Performing approaching of the sutured walls with light traction on the suture thread to conform the gastric tube and shape the remaining sutures.

l. Performing controlled cutting of the thread with cinch (appropriate thread cutting device) after all walls have been approached.

m. Reassembling the needle holder with a new suture thread; n) Repeating this suture pattern as many times as necessary (which occurs, on average, four to six times) until the entire body and part of the gastric fundus are completely sutured, preserving only the antrum and the proximal part of the fundus.

n. Applying a new layer of suture over the suture that has already been performed (U pattern + oversuture), in a new reinforcement pattern which we call "Sander Technique" ("Sander Technique" oversuture protocol which started in September 2018, empirically, using two more threads with several bites over the first layer of stitches, with the aim of reinforcing the primary U suture).

o. Removing the entire assembly to the overtube, with the needle locked, after sutures have been completed.

p. Deflating the balloon cuff to remove the assembly.

q. Reintroducing only the endoscopy device after disconnecting the overstitch, for revision of the suture made and cleaning of the gastric chamber, as well as revision of potential hemorrhagic complication.

r. Documenting, by means of photographic images, the entire process and the final status.

s. Removing the device to the distal tip of overtube and removing the entire assembly, evaluating possible esophageal lesions caused by the introduction of the overtube.

t. Placing the patient under anesthesiologist care for anesthetic reversal and post-anesthetic recovery (RPA).

u. Discharging patients from the hospital with an average time of 3 hours after the end of the procedure.

2.3.3 Post-intervention

Discharge was carried out after release by an anesthesiologist, approximately 3 hours after the procedure. Patients received a prescription for a proton pump inhibitor (Dexlansoprazole, 40 mg once a day) for 6 months and symptomatic medications for nausea, vomiting, and abdominal pain. The prescribed diet for the first month was 15 days of liquid diet and 15 days of soft diet, with the solid diet starting only after the 31st day.

2.4 Follow-up, data collection, and processing

All patients were followed up and their data were collected and recorded in the WebClin electronic medical record and in specific and individual anamnesis forms, which are part of the care protocol of the study execution center. Number of patients in each group gradually decreased due to the number of eligible patients in each of the time intervals. Thus, the group that completed 12 months post-procedure included all patients included in the study, that is, those who underwent ESG between July 2017 and August 2020. The 24-month group was composed of those who underwent ESG from July 2017 to September 2019. The 36-month group consisted of patients who underwent ESG from July 2017 to September 2018. Whereas the 48-month group included only those who underwent ESG in July, August, and September 2017, as will be shown below. Thus, the group with the largest number of patients analyzed was the group with 12 months of follow-up, and the group with the smallest number of patients analyzed was the 48-month follow-up group, which included only those who underwent ESG in 3 months of 2017. Therefore, the smaller number of participants in the groups with longer follow-up time does not represent a loss of participants over the course of the study but reflects the smaller number of participants who were eligible to be part of those groups. Weight was analyzed at each time interval, as well as possible post-intervention

Post-procedure period	Physician	Nutritionist	Psycologist
1st year	Monthly	Monthly	Monthly
2nd year	Quaterly	Quaterly	Quaterly
3rd e 4th years	Semi-annual	Semi-annual	Semi-annual
Source: Research data, 2022.			

Table 1.
Details of the multidisciplinary follow-up period after ESG.

complications and intercurrences, clinical and endoscopic follow-up data, both with regular consultations and with upper digestive endoscopy every 12 months, which aimed to evaluate the maintenance of stomach tubulization. This tubulization was verified by insufflating air under supervision in the stomach, with the use of an endoscope, seeking to find a format that mimicked the surgical sleeve ("sleeve-like"), with an approximate visual reduction of more than 40% of the gastric distensibility and diameter, with reduction of its volume. The breakdown of data collection, from the multidisciplinary follow-up, was carried out in the form shown in **Table 1**.

2.5 Main clinical variables studied and measures taken

Suture patterns: These variables, explained in the Intervention topic, refer to the types of sutures used in the primary procedure. The U pattern was used between July 2017 and August 2018. From then on, the U pattern plus oversuture (U + OS pattern - "Sander Technique") was used as a protocol. This change in suture pattern occurred by the personal and empirical choice of the researcher, with the aim of using oversuture to try to apply a reinforcement over the U pattern suture. When analyzing suture patterns in relation to the durability and effectiveness of the procedure, the weight variation of the patients was also compared according to the maintenance of endoscopic tubulization of the stomach, at predefined time intervals (follow-up time), thus allowing the comparison of suture patterns.

Oversuture: From September 2018, the practice of oversuture was used as a protocol in the procedures, empirically, using two more threads and several bites over the first layer of stitches, with the aim of trying to reinforce the primary U suture. This new suture pattern was called the "Sander Technique" and usually makes the gastric diameter even narrower, since a new layer of stitches is applied over the U suture stitches, further reducing the distensibility and storage capacity of the stomach. Therefore, since September 2018, oversuture has been used in most patients, with the exception of those in whom the stomach had already reached a very narrow diameter after the U pattern and oversuture could cause a very significant restriction to the point of negatively affecting the quality of life of these patients or when there were technical difficulties in performing the oversuture, such as the limitation of the device movement in the gastric chamber.

Resuturing: This variable describes the revision of the primary procedure, when there is a failure to maintain the stomach in a tubulized format, allowing it to widen again. Resuturing consists of redoing the suture, as in the primary procedure, with the aim of tightening the stomach again, seeking the permanence of the tubulized format. Resuturing was indicated when the control endoscopy, performed at intervals of 12 months, indicated the dilation of the gastric diameter, with early rupture of stitches, without occurrence of fibrosis between the folds and, consequently, without consolidation of stomach tubulization.

Time elapsed since the primary procedure: Serial control endoscopies were performed every 12 months.

Number of threads: It was defined according to the observed reduction in the stomach diameter as the procedure progressed. The threads are of standard size. As in any other type of suture, the closer the stitches (bites), the more thread will be used, requiring the use of a larger number of threads. At the same time, increase in the number of threads and number of bites also increases the time to perform the procedure, since more time is used to perform a suture with a larger number of stitches.

Number of stitches (bites): An average spacing of 1 cm between one bite, and another was used. A bite was defined as the transposition of the needle with the thread of all layers of the gastric wall (mucosa, muscularis mucosae, submucosa, muscularis, and serosa). Each bite corresponds to a complete stitch and the suture is the sum of all the bites of that thread. To perform ESG, it is necessary to perform several sutures, in the body and stomach fundus, using several threads.

%TBWL (% Total Body Weight Loss): Percentage of total body weight lost. This variable shows, in percentage, the weight lost in relation to the initial weight and serves as a comparison parameter between participants with different initial weights. Thus, a patient with an initial weight of 100 kg who has lost 20 kg has also lost 20% of TBWL, as well as a patient with an initial weight of 90 kg who has lost 18 kg has also lost 20% of TBWL.

%EWL (% Excess Weight Loss): Percentage of excess weight lost. Here is another illustrative example to understand this variable—if the patient initially weighs 100 kg and his ideal weight to reach a BMI of 25 kg/m^2 is 70 kg, then his excess weight is 30 kg. Consequently, if he lost 21 kg, then he lost 70% of his excess weight.

Weight: This variable describes the weight, in kilograms, measured in the patient at each of the evaluations, from the time of ESG.

Absolute weight loss: Measure, in kilograms, of the weight variation, from the largest to the smallest measurement.

Method safety: This variable analyzes complications that occur during the procedure and that determine any type of new intervention, clinical, endoscopic or surgical, or that prevent the patient from being discharged from the hospital on the same day of the procedure. Complications are unfavorable developments, such as a result of a disease or a specific treatment performed, or even the appearance of a new disease that developed as a consequence of the procedure performed. They are not expected events, but rather an eventual risk that depends on the clinical evolution and are persistent unsatisfactory results that may require a complementary surgical procedure. Gastric perforation with acute abdomen, with surgical resolution, is an example of a complication.

Intercurrences: Intercurrences are events that correspond to the occurrences that follow the procedure performed. They are already expected adverse events, relatively uniform and predictable to a certain extent, considering the specificity of the technique and the individual reaction of each patient. As they are the most common findings after gastric manipulation in therapeutic endoscopic procedures, abdominal pain and vomiting were described as intercurrences (adverse events) and were evaluated in a time interval of up to 15 days after the procedure, since most of the intercurrences inherent to the intervention occur in this time interval. Bleeding (upper gastrointestinal hemorrhage - UGIH) is also added as intercurrences, as long as it is self-limiting, without the need for any complementary therapy, since it may occur relatively frequently at the suture sites, due to the transposition of the needle and the superficial laceration of the gastric wall by the helix.

Method effectiveness: Evaluate weight loss and weight loss maintenance. According to the recommendation of the American Dietary Association and the Framingham Heart Study Group49,50, weight loss greater than 10% of initial total body weight or loss of more than 25% of initial excess weight, within 12 months after the procedure, was defined as effective. To avoid the analysis of non-sustained weight loss (with weight regain in the short and medium term), the analysis was divided into time intervals of 12 months, starting 12 months after the procedure up to 48 months after. Sustained weight loss could then also be evaluated.

Method durability: Investigates the procedure's ability to maintain gastric tubulization in the short and medium term. The tubulized format of the stomach, gastric tubulization or tubulized stomach was defined as the visual reduction of gastric distensibility and diameter, by at least 40% of the usual endoscopic pattern, with a reduction in its volume, mimicking the endoscopic appearance of the surgical sleeve ("sleeve-like"), with or without visualization of fibrous bands between the gastric folds. This variable was analyzed by upper gastrointestinal endoscopy performed at predefined times, every 12 months, after ESG (from 12 to 48 months after the procedure). The variable aims to analyze whether ESG can maintain gastric tubulization over time, even after the already expected spontaneous loosening of the threads, which occurs throughout the first year after the procedure.

Argon: Immediately before suturing, since January 2020, argon plasma electrocauterization (WEM Argon2, with the 60 W - 2 L/min setup) was performed between the folds, on the gastric mucosa, in the longitudinal direction, from the greater to the lesser curvature, and with an average interval of 3 centimeters between the cauterizations, expecting to induce greater fibrosis formation after the procedure, facilitating the adhesion of the gastric folds between them. The variable aims to analyze whether argon plasma electrocauterization was a facilitator in the formation of fibrosis between the sutured folds in the ESG procedure, inducing the maintenance of gastric tubulization for a longer time and, therefore, influencing the durability of the method.

3. Results

The initial convenience sample consisted of 208 patients who underwent ESG between July 2017 and August 2020. Of these, 19 were excluded from the analyses, 15 of them because they underwent bariatric surgery after ESG and four others because they became pregnant after the procedure. Additionally, of these 19 patients excluded from the analysis, 18 did not complete the minimum follow-up time of 12 months after the procedure with the multidisciplinary team. Thus, a total of 189 patients were analyzed in this study, 144 women and 45 men, with a mean age of 39 years and an initial mean BMI of 36.08 kg/m^2.

Regarding the follow-up time with multidisciplinary follow-up until data collection, the first group, of 12 months, had 189 patients; the group with 24 months had 149; the group with 36 months had 51; and the group with 48 months had 16 patients. Whereas in relation to patients who underwent control endoscopy every 12 months,

Period of EGD performance	Time interval completed after EGD	Patients with multidiscplinary consultation	Patients with control endoscopy
July 2017 to August 2020	12 months	189	168
July 2017 to September 2019	24 months	149	125
July 2017 to September 2018	36 months	51	48
July, August, and September 2017	48 months	16	12

Source: Research data.

Table 2.
Number of eligible participants in each group, by time interval.

in each of the research periods, in the first group there were 168 participants who underwent endoscopy 12 months after the procedure; in the second group, 125 participants at 24 months; in the third group, 48 at 36 months; and in the fourth group, of the 16 patients who underwent the procedure between July and September 2017, 12 of them underwent the 48-month follow-up endoscopy and four of them did not return to that follow-up endoscopy.

It is observed that the number of patients analyzed decreased gradually, following the inclusion in each group, due to the number of those who were eligible in relation to the minimum required follow-up time, in each of the four groups (**Table 2**).

It was found that 87.8% of patients achieved a loss of more than 10% of their total initial weight; over 25% of excess weight loss was achieved within 12 months and 85.1% of those who underwent control endoscopy at 12 months had a tubularized stomach.

In 14.9% of cases, there was primary procedure failure and the stomach appeared not tubularized and open 12 months after ESG, with visible thread and no fibrosis formation, as revealed by control endoscopy. These patients also reported poor weight loss, less than 10% of total body weight.

3.1 Bivariate analysis results

3.1.1 Sample description and weight measure evolution

Descriptive statistics revealed that women had a lower average initial weight (92.85 kg) than men (121.26 kg). Additionally, women had an average of 27.57 kg of excess weight (extra kilos beyond a BMI of 25 kg/m^2), with an average BMI of 35.60 kg/m^2, whereas men had an average excess weight of 41.29 kg, with an average BMI of 37.93 kg/m^2.

It is noteworthy that the minimum age was 18 years, and the maximum age was 85 years, the lowest and highest BMI values were 30.01 and 46.48 kg/m^2, respectively (**Table 3**).

In general, patients' weight decreased over the months, starting with an overall average weight of 99.37 kg on the day of the procedure and ending with an average of

Patients Gender		N	Mean	Inf LIm 95% méd.	Sup Lim 95% méd.	Mediana	SD	Min.	Max.
Feminine	Initial weight	144	92,85	91,36	94,34	93,50	9,05	70,70	119,00
	Height	144	1,61	1,60	1,62	1,62	0,06	1,50	1,72
	Initial BMI	144	35,60	35,14	36,06	35,75	2,81	30,05	42,04
	Ideal weight	144	65,28	64,47	66,09	65,61	4,92	56,25	73,96
	Excess weight	144	27,57	26,39	28,75	27,49	7,15	13,39	45,90
	Age	144	39,58	37,17	42,00	36,00	14,67	18,00	88,00
Masculine	Initial weight	45	121,26	116,82	125,71	121,40	14,78	92,50	155,00
	Height	45	1,79	1,77	1,81	1,78	0,06	1,62	1,93
	Initial BMI	45	37,93	36,69	39,18	37,30	4,15	30,01	46,48
	Ideal weight	45	79,98	78,31	81,64	79,21	5,54	65,61	93,12
	Excess weight	46	41,29	37,36	45,21	39,68	13,07	16,40	69,60
	Age	45	39,27	35,90	42,64	38,00	11,21	18,00	74,00

SD: standard deviation; min: minimum; max: maximum.
Source: Research data.

Table 3.
Descriptive data of sample by gender.

76.92 kg, with a sustained loss of 21.09% of %TBWL and 70.83% of %EWL, in the 48-month follow-up group. BMI also showed a reduction from 36.08 to 28.66 kg/m^2 (**Table 4**).

3.1.2 Comparison between suture patterns (U versus U + OS)

This variable was measured in patients who underwent control endoscopies at 12 (N = 168) and 24 months (N = 125) after ESG. At 36 and 48 months, there were no patients in the U + OS pattern who had reached this follow-up interval to allow for this comparison. At 12 months, the percentage of gastric tubularization maintenance was observed to be 70.5% in the U pattern versus 97.7% in the U + OS pattern. At 24 months, 94.0% maintained gastric tubularization in the U pattern versus 93.1% in the U + OS Pattern (**Table 5**).

Specifically in patients who had a tubular stomach on the control endoscopy, in terms of %TBWL, the average loss at 12 months in the U pattern was 17.9% versus 18.8% in the U + OS pattern. Whereas at 24 months, this loss was 20.9% (U) versus 21.6% (U + OS). The %EWL, in the 12 months, showed a loss of 64.4% in the U

		Weight		Weight loss		%TBWL		%EWL		BMI	
	N	Average [IC 95%]	Std. Dev	Average [IC 95%]	Std. Dev	Average [IC 95%]	Std. Dev	Average [IC 95%]	Std. Dev	Average [IC 95%]	Std. Dev
Starting time	189	99,37 [97,3; 101,44]	15,82	-	-	-	-	-	-	36,08 [35,66; 36,5]	3,24
12 months	189	82,8 [81,1; 84,5]	11,9	−16,82 [−17,78; −15,87]	6,64	−16,54% [−17,78; −15,87]	4,90%	56,04% [53,30%; 58,78%]	19,10%	30,13 [29,73; 30,52]	2,75
24 months	149	78,52 [76,51; 80,53]	11,35	−20,26 [−21,60; −18,92]	7,57	−20,15% [−21,60; −18,92]	5,31%	69,69% [65,81%; 73,58%]	21,95%	28,67 [28,17; 29,16]	2,78
36 months	51	78,76 [74,79; 82,72]	13,19	−20,11 [−22,73; −17,49]	8,73	−19,77% [−22,73; −17,49]	5,50%	70,54% [64,20%; 76,89%]	21,13%	28,41 [27,63; 29,19]	2,60
48 months	16	76,92 [68,17; 85,66]	13,77	−21,26 [−26,27; −16,24]	7,89	−21,09% [−26,27; −16,24]	3,83%	70,83% [61,25%; 80,42%]	15,08%	28,66 [27,21; 30,10]	2,28
P-value		0,000		0,000		0,000		0,000		0,000	

Source: Research data.

Table 4.
Evolution of patients weight by time period of treatment.

		Suture pattern				
		U pattern		U pattern + Oversuture		P-value
Tubularized stomach—12 months (N = 189)		N	%	N	%	
	No	23	26,4	3	2,9	0,000
	Yes	55	63,2	87	86,3	
	Not evaluated	9	10,3	12	11,8	
Tubularized stomach—24 months (N = 149)	No	4	4,8	4	6,7	0,600
	Yes	63	75,9	54	81,8	
	Not evaluated	16	19,3	8	13,3	
Tubularized stomach—36 months (N = 51)	No	5	9,8	0	0,0	—
	Yes	36	70,6	0	0,0	
	Not evaluated	10	19,6	0	0,0	

Pearson's Chi-squared test.
Source: Research data.

Table 5.
Analysis of gastric tubularization over time, in relation to the absolute number of patients, according to the suture pattern.

pattern versus 60.4% in the U + OS pattern. And in the 24 months, the difference was 77.4% (U) versus 68.1% (U + OS). It is important to note that the mean weight and initial BMI in patients with U + OS pattern (37.7 kg/m^2) was higher than in the U pattern (35.2 kg/m^2), therefore, the initial excess weight was also higher in patients with the U + OS pattern.

Even though the patients did not have a tubular stomach at 12 months, they had a higher %TBWL when submitted to the U + OS pattern (−11.43%) compared to those with the U pattern (−6.58%). Of the 189 patients who completed 12 months of follow-up, 21 (11.1%) could not be evaluated for stomach tubularization because they did not show up for the control endoscopy. And at 24 months, 24 patients (16.1%) of the 149 who completed this time interval also did not perform the control endoscopy (**Figure 1**; **Table 6**).

At 12 and 24 months, mean weight of patients with tubularized stomach was lower in those with the U pattern compared to the U + OS pattern. However, as patients in the U + OS pattern had a higher initial mean weight, the mean absolute weight loss, in kilograms, was greater in this suture pattern, with mean weight loss of 17.96 kg (12 M) and 20.36 kg (24 M) for the U pattern and 19.82 kg (12 M) and 22.70 kg (24 M) for the U + OS pattern (**Table 7**).

As for when analyzing the data on durability and need for resuturing, in the time intervals, according to each suture pattern, in the group of patients who did not need resuturing at 12 months, 82.8% had been sutured with the U pattern and 97.1% with the U + OS pattern (P-value 0.003), demonstrating that the U + OS pattern had a lower percentage of primary procedure failure. Of the 189 patients who reached a follow-up period of 12 months, 18 (9.52%) underwent resuturing at 12 months, because they did not keep the stomach tubularized (failure of the primary procedure), with 83.4% (N = 15) of them having initially undergone the U-shaped suture pattern, and only 16.6% (N = 3) of them having undergone the U + OS pattern (P-value 0.021). In the remaining intervals, after 12 months, the patients required similar resuturing in both suture patterns (**Table 8**).

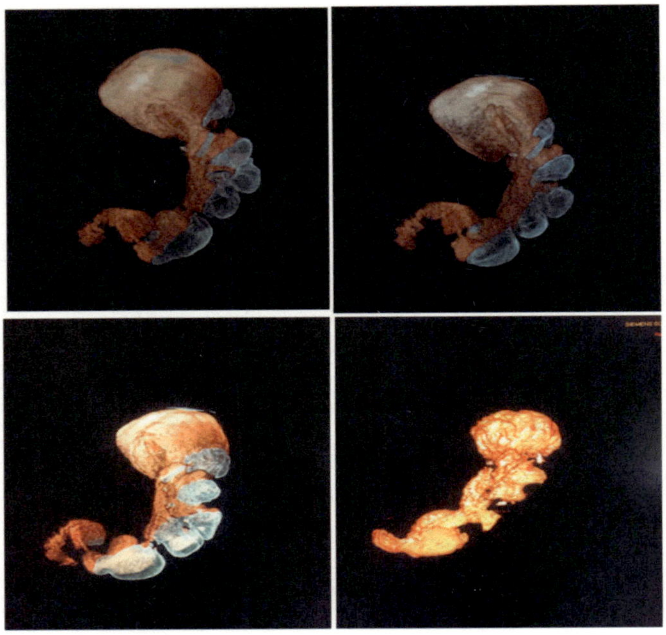

Figure 1.
3D images of a tubular stomach after ESG. Source: Images provided by Dr. Luiz Mattar.

Tubularized Stomach 12 months	Suture pattern					
		U pattern		U pattern + Oversuture		
	Metrics 12 months	Mean	n	Mean	n	P-value
No	Weight	85,3	23	85,5	3	0,615
	Weight loss	−6,09	23	−11	3	0,039
	%TBWL	−6,58%	23	−11,43%	3	0,031
	%EWL	25,23%	23	38,97%	3	0,229
	BMI	32,25	23	32,58	2	0,841
Yes	Weight	81,6	55	83,8	87	0,153
	Weight loss	−17,96	55	−19,82	87	0,028
	%TBWL	−17,91%	55	−18,85%	87	0,035
	%EWL	64,39%	55	60,35%	87	0,194
	BMI	29,22	55	30,02	87	0,026
Not evaluated	Weight	77,7	9	79,5	12	0,669
	Weight loss	−10,83	9	−15,7	12	0,005
	%TBWL	−12,27%	9	−16,42%	12	0,016
	%EWL	47,38%	9	54,59%	12	0,394
	BMI	30,25	9	30,46	12	0,831

Source: Research data.

Table 6.
Comparison of variables by suture pattern at 12 months.

Tubularized stomach—24 months	Suture pattern					
		U pattern		U pattern + Suture		P-value
	Mean 24 months	Média	N	Mean	N	
No	Weight	84,25	4	82,25	4	0,770
	Weight loss	−6,93	4	−12,55	4	0,149
	%TBWL	−7,50	4	−13,20	4	0,149
	%EWL	−25,83	4	40,16	4	0,386
	BMI	31,93	4	32,75	4	0,773
Yes	Weight	76,11	63	80,38	54	0,003
	Weight loss	−20,36	63	−22,7	54	0,124
	%TBWL	77,40	63	−21,58	54	0,457
	%EWL	77,40	63	68,02	54	0,015
	BMI	27,73	63	29,06	54	0,001
Not evaluated	Weight	82,29	16	—	8	—
	Weight loss	−15	16	—	8	—
	%TBWL	−15,26	16	—	8	—
	%EWL	53,49	16	—	8	—
	BMI	30,21	16	—	8	—

Source: Research data.

Table 7.
Comparison of variables by suture pattern at 24 months period.

3.1.3 Analysis of number of bites (stitches) and threads and procedure time

In patients with the U + OS pattern, a greater number of bites and threads were used than those used in patients with the U pattern. In the U pattern, an average of five threads and 95 bites was used, and in the U + OS pattern, an average of seven threads and 154 bites.

Patients with the U + SS pattern required more time than those with the U pattern (113 minutes versus 97 minutes) (**Table 9**).

3.1.4 Analysis of complications and intercurrences

The percentage of complications and intercurrences within 15 days after the procedure was evaluated and each suture pattern was compared in isolation. The data revealed no statistically significant difference between that percentage and the patterns (P-value 0.201) (**Table 10**).

3.1.5 Argon plasma usage

Multivariate analysis over a 12-month period regarding argon usage and its influence on the tubularized stomach demonstrated a positive outcome for maintaining tubularization. However, no significant correlation was found between argon usage and gastric tubularization durability in other time intervals (p-value 0.288).

Tubularized stomach 24 months		Suture pattern				
		U pattern		U + Suture pattern		P-value
	Resuture	N	%	N	%	
12 months	No	63	72,4	87	85,3	0,001
	Yes	15	17,2	3	2,9	
	Not evaluated	9	10,4	12	11,8	
12 ~ 24 months	No	63	75,9	56	84,8	0,000
	Yes	4	4,8	2	3	
	Not evaluated	16	19,3	8	12,2	
24 ~ 30	No	77	97,5	32	94,1	0,377
	Yes	2	2,5	2	5,9	
	Not evaluated	0	0,0	0	0,00	
30 ~ 36	No	49	64,5	0	0,00	
	Yes	2	2,6	0	0,00	
	Not evaluated	25	32,9	0	0,00	
36 ~ 42	No	46	90,2	0	0,00	
	Yes	5	9,8	0	0,00	
	Not evaluated	0	0,0	0	0,00	
42 ~ 48	No	15	93,8	0	0,00	—
	Yes	1	6,3	0	0,00	0
	Not evaluated	0	0,0	0	0,0	0

Source: Research data.

Table 8.
Comparison of number of resutures by suture pattern, in relation to the absolute number of patients who were analyzed in each time interval.

3.2 Multivariate analysis results

3.2.1 Tubularized stomach

There was a significant difference (P = 0.037) in the percentage of patients with a tubularized stomach between 12 and 24 months. When a patient had a tubularized stomach at 12 months, the odds of maintaining it at 24 months were 2.43 times higher than the odds of having a tubularized stomach at 12 months, counting from time zero (procedure completion). There was no significant difference for this variable at other times (**Figure 2**).

a. At 12 months, the odds of a patient with the U + OS pattern having a tubularized stomach were 18 times higher than that of a patient with the U pattern.

b. In the U pattern, the odds of a patient with a tubularized stomach at 12 months maintaining it at 24 months were seven times higher than the odds of reaching 12 months with a tubularized stomach, starting from time zero (procedure date). As for in the U + OS pattern, this correlation was not detected.

			U pattern					U pattern + Oversuture					
			N	Mean	Inf L 95% mean	Sup L 95% mean	Std. Dev	N	Mean	Inf L 95% mean	Sup.L 95% mean	Std. Dev	
P-value	4	*BITES*	30	75,27	72,14	78,39	8,36	0	—	—	—	—	0,000
	5		52	102,00	99,99	104,01	7,22	0	—	—	—	—	
	6		5	129,20	123,76	134,64	4,38	5	127,20	124,98	129,42	1,79	
	7		0	—	—	—	—	52	143,27	141,70	144,84	5,63	
	8		0	—	—	—	—	37	167,84	165,90	169,78	5,82	
	9		0	—	—	—	—	4	195,00	185,11	204,89	6,22	
	4	TIME	30	88,83	86,55	91,12	6,11	0	—	—	—	—	0,000
	5		52	96,92	95,24	98,60	6,04	0	—	—	—	—	
	6		5	115,00	108,79	121,21	5,00	5	102,00	93,67	110,33	6,71	
	7		0	—	—	—	—	52	112,79	110,99	114,58	6,45	
	8		0	—	—	—	—	37	122,97	121,03	124,92	5,83	
	9		0	—	—	—	—	4	143,75	136,13	151,37	4,79	

Source: Research data.

Table 9.
Comparison of bites per number of threads and time in minutes, in each P suture pattern.

c. In other time intervals, there was no significant difference in the percentage of patients with a tubularized stomach between the suture patterns (**Table 11**).

3.2.2 Resuture

When evaluating only patients with the U pattern among themselves, the odds of requiring resuturing up to 12 months were 8.4 times higher than between 12 and 24 months. However, there was no significant difference between times for the U + SS pattern.

a. At 12 months, there was a significant difference (P-value = 0.003) in the percentage of patients with resuturing when comparing the suture patterns. At this time, odds of a patient with U pattern requiring resuturing were 6.7 times higher than those of a patient with U + OS pattern.

		Suture pattern				
		U pattern		**U + Suture pattern**		**P-value**
	Resuture	**N**	**%**	**N**	**%**	
Complications	No	87	100,0	102	100,0	—
	Yes	0	9,9	0	0,0	
Intercurrences	No	82	94,3	92	90,2	0,201
	Bleeding	3	3,4	2	2,0	
	Vomiting up to 15 days	2	2,3	8	7,8	

Pearson's Chi-squared tests.
Source: Research data.

Table 10.
Analysis of complications and intercurrences by suture patterns.

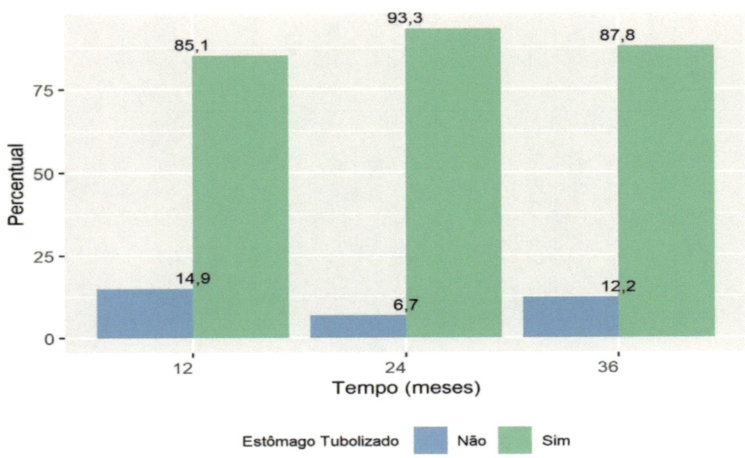

Figure 2.
*Influence of time on the tubularized stomach. Source: Research data **H: Time (months); V: Tubularized stomach.*

Time	OR	CI - 95%	P-value
24/12	2,43	[1,05; 5,58]	0,037
36/12	1,26	[0,45; 3,52]	0,661
36/24	0,52	[0,16; 1,69]	0,275

OR: odds ratio; CI: confidence interval.
Source: Research data.

Table 11.
Influence of time on the tubularized stomach.

b. When evaluating only patients with the U pattern among themselves, the odds of requiring resuturing up to 12 months were 8.4 times higher than between 12 and 24 months. As for the U + OS pattern, there was no significant difference between times.

c. In the 24-month follow-up and beyond, there was no significant difference (P-value >0.050) in the analysis of resuturing and its relationship between suture patterns.

d. Resuturing did not show a statistical difference in safety when compared to the primary procedure. However, in terms of weight loss efficacy, results were similar to those already seen in the primary procedure at 12 and 24 months.

3.2.3 Number of bites and threads

a. At 12 months, there was a significant influence (P-value = 0.000) of the number of bites on the percentage of patients with a tubularized stomach. For each additional unit in the number of bites, odds of patient having a tubularized stomach increased by 1.04 times.

b. Statistical tests revealed that, from 98 bites onward, there was a significant difference (P-value = 0.001) in the percentage of patients with a tubularized stomach between 12 and 24 months. After the stomach was tubularized at 12 months, odds of it remaining so at 24 months were 4.71 times higher than those of having it tubularized at 12 months from time zero, when that number of bites was used. There was no significant difference in the percentage of patients with a tubularized stomach between the other times (**Figure 3**).

Upon examining the influence of time and number of sutures on tubularized stomach, it was observed that:

a. For each suture thread unit added to the number of threads, odds of the patient having a tubularized stomach at 12 months increased by 2.48 times. However, there was no significant influence for 24 and 36 months.

b. When five sutures were used, the odds of a patient with a tubularized stomach at 12 months maintaining it at 24 months were 4.13 times higher than their odds of having a tubularized stomach at 12 months.

c. For six threads to suture or more, there was no significant difference in the percentage of patients with a tubularized stomach between the time intervals.

d. When analyzing the number of threads to suture and bites in relation to safety, no direct statistical relationship was found between these variables.

e. In relation to efficacy and durability, increasing the number of threads to suture and bites showed a direct relationship with the maintenance of stomach tubulization and weight loss (**Figure 4**).

3.2.4 Argon plasma usage

Due to a lack of data, the analysis was only performed on patients who had undergone the procedure 12 months before. During this period, the use of Argon resulted in a 16.1% increase in the percentage of patients with a tubularized stomach (**Figure 5**).

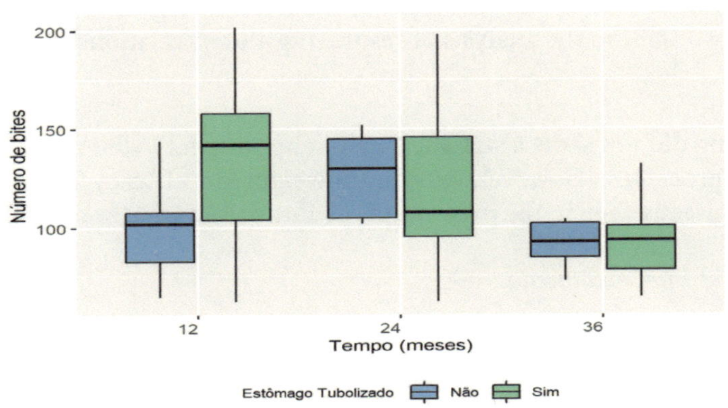

Figure 3.
Influence of time and number of bites on tubularized stomach. Source: Research data. V: Number of bites H1: Time (months); H2: Tubularized Stomach – No – Yes.

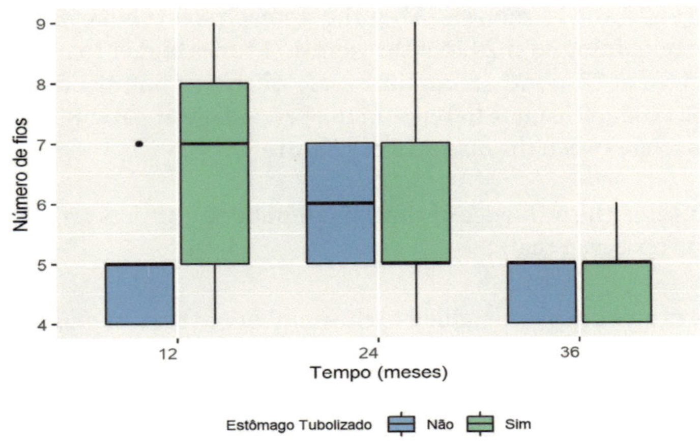

Figure 4.
Influence of time and number of threads on the tubularized stomach. Source: Research data. V: Number of threads; H1: Time (months); H2: Tubularized Stomach – No – Yes.

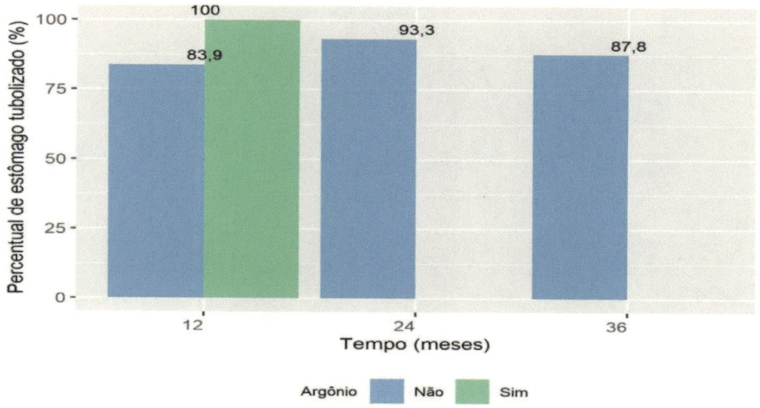

Figure 5.
Influence of time and argon on the tubularized stomach. Source: Research data. V: Percentage of tubularized stomach; H1: Time (months); H2: Argon – No – Yes.

3.2.5 Other variables related to weight loss and stomach tubularization

a. At 6 months, patients had lost an average of 11.5 kg (54% of the total weight lost over 48 months), at 12 months they had lost an average of 17 kg (79% of the total weight lost over 48 months), and at 18 months they had lost an average of 20.2 kg (94% of the total weight lost over 48 months). Whereas in the 48-month group, patients had a sustained average weight loss of 22.4 kg. Weight loss was greater among men than among women.

b. Most patients who reached 12 months with a tubularized stomach reported, at time zero a mean weight of 10 kg less than those who reached 12 months without a tubularized stomach, indicating a lower initial BMI. There was no significant difference in weight between the levels of this variable at other time points.

c. Patients who adhered to nutritional and psychological follow-up had a higher average initial weight than those who did not follow up, with those who sought nutritional counseling having an average of 9 kg higher and those who sought psychological counseling having an average of 6 kg higher.

d. Patients who did a follow-up with a nutritionist and psychologist in the first 12 months had a greater mean weight loss than patients without follow-up, up to the 30-month interval. There was no significant difference (P-value >0.050) in weight loss from 36 months onward.

e. There was a significant difference (P-value <0.050) in weight loss between the suture patterns up to 24 months, with patients with the U + OS pattern having greater weight loss than those with the U pattern.

f. Patients with a tubularized stomach showed greater weight loss than those without a tubularized stomach (18 versus 8% %TBWL at 12 months) (**Figure 6**).

g. The odds of a patient under nutritional follow-up having their stomach tubularized at 12 months were 52 times higher than a patient without this support.

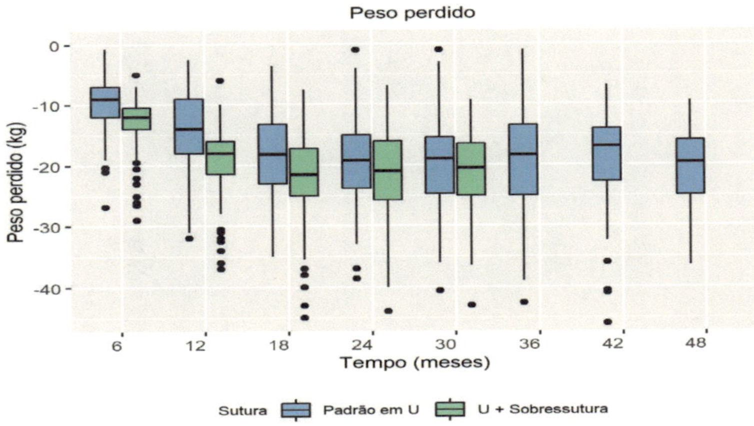

Figure 6.
Influence of time and suture patterns on weight loss. Source: Research data. H: Weight loss (kg); H1: Time (months); H2: Suture, U-pattern, U + SS pattern.

h. The odds of a patient without a nutritionist who achieved tubularized stomach at 12 months maintaining it at 24 months were 24 times greater than the odds of them having achieved tubularized stomach in the first 12 months. In turn, the odds of this patient without a nutritionist, who achieved tubularized stomach at 12 months, maintaining it at 36 months were 21 times greater than the odds of them having achieved tubularized stomach in the first 12 months;

i. Odds of a patient with a nutritionist, who reached 12 months with a tubularized stomach, of maintaining a tubularized stomach at 36 months was 0.18 times lower than the odds of having a tubularized stomach in the first 12 months;

j. The odds of a patient with psychological counseling having their stomach tubularized at 12 months were 62 times higher than those of a patient without psychological counseling.

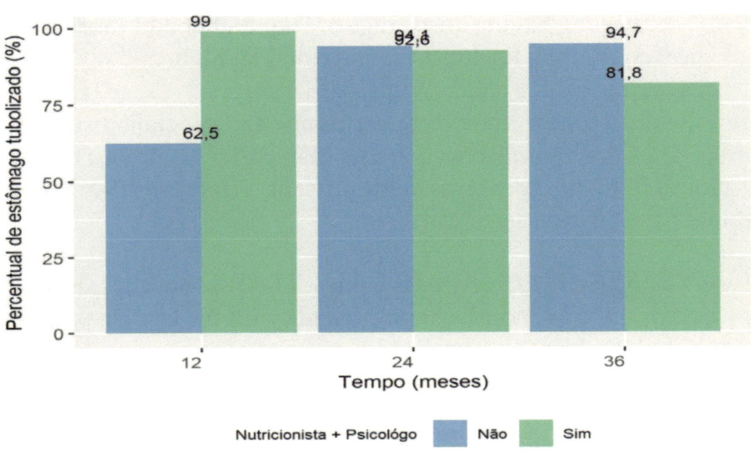

Figure 7.
Influence of nutritionist and psychologist on tubularized stomach. Source: Reseach data. V: Percentage of tubularized stomach; H1: Time (months); H2: Nutritionist + Psychologist – No – Yes.

k. Odds of a patient without psychological counseling who achieved stomach tubularization at 12 months maintaining that tubularization at 24 months were nine times higher than the odds of having the tubularization in the first 12 months, while at 36 months, this odds since the first 12 months was 11 times higher than the odds the patient had of having the tubularization in the first 12 months.

l. Odds of a patient with psychological counseling who had stomach tubularization at 12 months maintaining this condition at 36 months were 0.04 times lower than the odds of having their stomach tubularization in the first 12 months (**Figure** 7).

4. Discussion

The initial sample of this study appears to reflect the general profile of patients seeking weight loss procedures. When analyzed for excess weight and initial BMI, men generally had higher values in these variables. The pattern of these patients seems to be reflected in other aspects of the sample, with women having a lower average excess weight (27.57 kg above the BMI 25 kg/m^2) and lower initial BMI (average BMI of 35.60 kg/m^2), compared to men. Men also had higher values (average excess weight of 41.29 kg above the BMI 25 kg/m^2 and average BMI of 37.93 kg/m^2). A remarkable observation in this study was the gradual decrease in the number of analyzed participants, by time intervals. This decrease was due to the minimum time required from the procedure to data collection, which reduced the number of eligible participants for follow-up in each of the four groups. Thus, a reduction in the number of analyzed participants was observed, compared to the initial sample, starting with N = 189 in the 12-month follow-up group (100%), N = 149 (78.8%) at 24 months, N = 51 (27%) at 36 months, and N = 16 (8.5%) at 48 months. Regarding the number of patients who underwent control endoscopies at the pre-established times, this decrease compared to the number of patients in each group was slightly higher, being 88.9% (N = 168) at 12 months, 66.2% (N = 125) at 24 months, 25.4% (N = 48) at 36 months, and 6.35% (N = 12) at 48 months. However, the sample loss in the first three time groups was small (less than 20%) when considering the number of patients eligible for those groups, based on the time elapsed since the procedure. In the 12-month group, the sample loss was 11.1% (21 of 189), in the 24-month group it was 16.1% (24 of 149), in the 36-month group it was 5.9% (3 of 51), and in the 48-month group it was 25% (4 of 16). Statistical analysis showed that, for the samples of this study, up to the 36-month time group, there was a maximum test power of 95% regarding the significance level of the sample size and the power of the test. For the 48-month time, a test power of 85%.

Despite ESG procedure being recognized as effective in obese patients [12, 13], high-risk patients [14], morbidly obese patients [15] and even in comparison with other methods [16], meeting the recommendations of health institutions, management of patients who have not achieved success still requires further analysis by new studies. In addition, in some patients there is evidence of revision need, due to failure of the primary procedure, through resuturing, in addition to the importance of constant review of procedures for technical improvement [6]. In this way, this study has brought several findings that can contribute in this matter, when considering the improvement of procedure for the benefit of the technique, in general, and for patients, in addition to bringing suggestions for changes in suture patterns.

One of the findings brought up by this study was the effectiveness in weight reduction, with an average initial weight of 99.37 kg and a final weight of 76.92 kg (in the 48-month group), in addition to a reduction in BMI (from 36.08 to 28.66 kg/m^2) and an average loss of 21.09% of total initial weight (%TBWL), and 70.83% of excess weight (%EWL).

An additional and original finding of this research on durability and effectiveness of the technique was the reapproching of the primary procedure through resuturing, as well as the analysis of suture pattern, when comparing the U versus U + OS patterns. The analyses showed that U + OS pattern was more effective in weight loss in the first 12 months after the intervention. This pattern also showed greater durability (tubularized stomach) up to 12 months. In addition, regardless of the suture pattern used, when the stomach was already tubularized at 12 months, it tended to remain tubularized after this time interval. When the U + SS pattern was used, tubulization occurred more effectively. Additionally, the data show that the U + SS pattern provided better markers in the first 12 months, such as weight loss, %EWL, and %TBWL.

When analyzing the variable related to the need for resuturing, the use of the U + OS pattern was also more effective, since, in both the first 12 months and subsequent times, participants in the U pattern research had a greater need for resuturing than those with the U + OS pattern. This data is likely also related to the greater number of threads and bites used in the U + OS pattern. However, it takes longer to perform the procedure.

Regarding the impossibility of establishing a statistical correlation between the types of suture patterns and the percentage of complications within 15 days, further research focused on this variable is suggested to investigate this relationship more thoroughly. In addition, another finding that needs further investigation is the use of argon plasma electrocautery and its interference in the procedure durability and the need for resuturing. While the present study cannot confirm these hypotheses, multivariate analysis showed that there may be some influence of argon use on stomach tubulization up to 12 months post-procedure.

In general, it is known that fibrosis (mucosa x mucosa and serosa x serosa) occurs within 12 months. Tubularization occurs during this period, and thus, the stomach is unlikely to open up later, except in cases of repeated dietary excesses that increase intragastric pressure to the point of undoing the adhesions between the folds caused by fibrosis. As observed in this study, the percentage of patients with a maintained tubularized stomach was 85.1% at 12 months and tends to remain so when compared to other time intervals. This reinforces the hypothesis that after the consolidation of the tubularized stomach shape for up to 12 months, with fibrosis formation, the suture pattern used in the primary procedure no longer has relevance to the durability of this tubularization. Among the analyzed patients, in the 12- to 24-month period, maintenance of stomach tubularization, which was already tubularized, was 2.43 times greater than the odds of the stomach reaching a tubularized shape between 0 and 12 months. This confirms that if the fibrosis process occurs within 12 months, the odds of stomach opening up after this time tend to decrease. The importance of the first 12 months for the subsequent durability in maintaining the tubularized shape of the stomach then becomes clear.

Based on the 12-month time frame, it was observed that chances of a patient with U + OS pattern having a tubularized stomach were 18 times greater than those of a patient sutured with only U pattern, something not observed at 24 months, since tubularization occurs within the first 12 months. It is inferred that the U + OS pattern was more effective in stomach tubularization formation.

When analyzing the time elapsed since the procedure, a significant difference was observed in the percentage of patients with a need for resuturing, comparing the suture patterns (U versus U + OS). This suggests a higher likelihood of reintervention in those with the U pattern, within 24 months after the procedure (time for stomach dilation due to deficient fibrosis, generally up to 12 months, plus the time required for the patient's decision to undergo a new suture). Furthermore, confirming the stomach fibrosis and tubularization process, chances of resuturing at 24 months were significantly lower than at 12 months—after fibrosis consolidation, the need for resuturing decreases.

Similarly, there was no significant difference in comparison of the suture pattern with resuturing after 24 months, which suggests that this data should also be interpreted based on the fact that, by this time, fibrosis of the sutured area has already occurred. Therefore, regardless of the suture pattern used, once fibrosis sets in, chances of the stomach dilating again become the same for both suture patterns.

Another additional finding of this research is that the number of bites (stitches) also had an influence on the ESG durability, since for each suture thread unit added the number of bites, patient's chance of having a tubularized stomach increases by 1.04 times. The central value in the number of bites for increased durability appears to be at the statistical cutoff of 98 bites.

A significant decrease in patient weight was observed from the initial measurements. At 6 months, when weight loss is fastest and most influenced by the procedure due to the adaptation period, patients had lost an average of 11.5 kg, whereas in the 48-month group, the average weight loss was 22.4 kg (sustained weight loss). As shown in literature on the subject [17, 18], the greatest weight loss typically occurs up to the 12th month (with the fastest weight loss occurring in the initial 6 months). That is further reinforced by the data from this research, which shows a significant difference in weight, with significant weight loss throughout the first year, with a tendency for weight stabilization after this time. This is, in fact, one of the great advantages of ESG, as it facilitates the maintenance of lost weight and reduces the weight regain index.

In the comparison of suture patterns, both the U and U + OS patterns showed greater TBWL reduction in the first 6 months and then up to the 12th month, with a tendency for patients with the U + OS pattern to have a higher TBWL than those with the U pattern. This means greater weight loss in the U + OS pattern, which may be due to the fact that when the suture is performed in U + OS pattern, the stomach usually has a smaller diameter (tighter) than the U pattern, which leads to greater restriction of food intake volume. This comparative variable of gastric diameter between the two suture patterns was not analyzed in this study. At 12 months, patients with a tubularized stomach had a higher %TBWL (more weight loss) than patients without a tubularized stomach (enlarged stomach with less restriction), confirming literature on the subject.

An interesting finding was the relationship between suture pattern and %EWL at 12 months. Patients with U + OS pattern had a lower %EWL than those with U pattern. However, this finding does not imply greater efficacy of the U pattern, as patients with the U + OS pattern had a higher initial excess weight than those with the U pattern.

Regarding the analysis of stomach tubularization at 12 months, %EWL was higher in patients with a tubularized stomach. In addition, in those in whom stomach tubularization was observed at 12 months (consolidated fibrosis), weight loss and %EWL were greater at all time intervals compared to those who did not have a tubularized stomach. This reinforces the hypothesis that the smaller diameter of the stomach directly influences weight loss.

5. Conclusions

The procedure proved to be safe in the short and medium term, without complications and with few intercurrences, which did not require new interventions. *The procedure proved to be effective for weight loss in the short term and for weight maintenance in the medium term, with 87.8% of patients achieving over 10% total body weight loss (%TBWL) and over 25% excess weight loss (%EWL).*

ESG also achieved good durability results, maintaining the tubularized stomach shape in the short and medium term. At 12 months, 85.1% of patients maintained a tubularized stomach with consolidated fibrosis between the gastric folds, which also influenced medium-term durability.

Analyzes demonstrated that the U + OS suture pattern ("Sander-Scarparo Technique") was more durable and more effective than the U pattern alone and proved to have better markers in other variables, such as weight reduction, % EWL and %TBWL and the need for resuturing.

Use of a greater number of threads and bites had a direct influence on the durability and effectiveness of the technique, nonetheless it increased the procedure execution time. Results suggest that the use of five or more threads, more than 98 bites, and the performance of oversuturing as a reinforcement to the U-suture pattern (U + OS) directly and positively influenced the consolidation of gastric fibrosis throughout the first-year post-procedure and the durability of ESG in the medium term, with a reduction in gastric diameter and maintenance of the tubular shape of the stomach.

Thus, ESG has been demonstrated to be durable, safe, and effective for short-term weight loss and medium-term weight loss maintenance, with sustained weight loss exceeding 20% of total initial body weight (%TBWL) and 70% of initial excess weight (%EWL), over a 48-month follow-up period.

Acknowledgements

Parts of this chapter were previously published in the doctoral thesis written in Portuguese by the co-author: Bruno Queiroz Sander. Title: "Evaluation of the Efficacy and Safety of Endoscopic Gastroplasty in the Management of Patients with Obesity in a Follow-up of 12 to 48 months". 2022. UFMG University (Universidade Federal de Minas Gerais). Available from: http://hdl.handle.net/1843/48466

Author details

Jimi Izaques Bifi Scarparo[1,2,3,4*] and Bruno Sander[1,2,3,5,6]

1 Brazilian Society of Digestive Endoscopy (SOBED), Brazil

2 Brazilian Society of Bariatric and Metabolic Surgery (SBCBM), Brazil

3 Brazilian Federation of Gastroenterology (FBG), Brazil

4 Scarparo Scopia Clinic and Day Hospital, São Paulo, Brazil

5 Federal University of Minas Gerais, Brazil

6 Sander Medical Center Day Hospital, Belo Horizonte, Brazil

*Address all correspondence to: drjimi@scarparoscopia.com

References

[1] De Moura DTH, Scarparo JIB, Souza TF, De Moura EGH. Gastroplastia endoscópica vertical ou endossutura gástrica (ESG – Endoscopic Sleeve Gastroplasty -(SOBED – Brazilian Society of Digestive Endoscopic) Como Eu Faço (The Way I Do). Editora dos editores. Brazil; 2021. ISBN: 978-65-86098-22-8(3)27-41

[2] Storm AC, Dayyeh BKA. Endoscopic sleeve gastroplasty for obesity: Defining the risk andreward after more than 1600 procedures. Gastrointestinal Endoscopy. 2019;**89**(6):1139-1140

[3] Barrichello S, de Moura DTH, de Moura EGH, Jirapinyo P, Hoff AC, Fittipaldi-Fernandez RJ, et al. Endoscopic sleeve gastroplasty in the management of overweight and obesity: An international multicenter study. Gastrointestinal Endoscopy. 2019;**90**(5):770-780

[4] Zorron R, Veltzke-Schlieker W, Adler A, Denecke C, Dziodzio T, Pratschke J, et al. Endoscopic sleeve gastroplasty using Apollo overstitch as a bridging procedure for superobese and high risk patients. Endoscopy. 2018;**41**(01):81-83

[5] Brunaldi VO, Jirapinyo P, Moura DTH, Okazaki O, Bernardo WM, et al. Endoscopic treatment of weight regain following roux-en-Y gastric bypass: A systematic review and meta-analysis. Obesity Surgery. 2018;**28**(1):266-276

[6] Lopez-Nava G, Asokkumar R, Negi A, Normand E, Bautista I. Re-suturing after primary endoscopic sleeve gastroplasty (ESG) for obesity. Surgical Endoscopy. 2021;**35**(6):2523-2530

[7] Marrache MK, Al-Sabban A, Itani MI, Sartoretto A, Kumbhari V. Endoscopic sleeve gastroplasty by use of a novel suturing pattern, which allays concerns for revisional bariatric surgery. Video GIE. 2020;**5**(4):133

[8] Bove V, Pontecorvi V, Matteo MV, Costamagna G, Boškoski I. Endoscopic sleeve gastroplasty is feasible after failed modified primary obesity surgery endoluminal procedure. Video GIE. 2021;**6**(9):410-412

[9] Lopez-Nava G, Galvão M, Bautista-Castaño I, Fernandez-Corbelle J, Trell M, Lopez N. Endoscopic sleeve gastroplasty for obesity treatment: Two years of experience. ABCD Arquivos Brasileiros de Cirurgia Digestiva (São Paulo). 2017;**30**(1):18-20

[10] Sullivan S, Edmundowicz S. Early experience with endoscopic sleeve gastroplasty and hints at mechanisms of action. Clinical Gastroenterology and Hepatology. 2017;**15**(1):44-45

[11] Lopez-Nava G, Bautista-Castaño I, Jimenez A, De Grado T, Fernandez-Corbelle JP. Endoscopic sleeve gastroplasty for the treatment of obesity. Endoscopy. 2015;**47**(05):449-452

[12] Sharaiha RZ, Kumta NA, Saumoy M, Desai AP, Sarkisian AM, Benevenuto A, et al. Endoscopic sleeve gastroplasty significantly reduces body mass index and metabolic complications in obese patients. Clinical Gastroenterology and Hepatology. 2017;**15**(4):504-510

[13] Sullivan S, Kumar N, Edmundowicz SA, Dayyeh BKA, Jonnalagadda SS, Larsen M, et al. ASGE position statement on endoscopic bariatric therapies in clinical practice. Gastrointestinal Endoscopy. 2015;**82**(5):767-772

[14] Li R, Veltzke-Schlieker W, Adler A, Specht M, Eskander W, Ismail M, et al. Endoscopic sleeve gastroplasty (ESG) for high-risk patients, high body mass index (> 50 kg/m^2): Patients, and contraindication to abdominal surgery. Obesity Surgery. 2021;**31**(8):3400-3409

[15] Lopez-Nava G, Laster J, Negi A, Fook-Chong S, Bautista-Castaño I, Asokkumar R. Endoscopic sleeve gastroplasty (ESG) for morbid obesity: How effective is it? Surgical Endoscopy. 2022;**36**(1):352-360

[16] Khan Z, Khan MA, Hajifathalian K, Shah S, Abdul M, Saumoy M, et al. Efficacy of endoscopic interventions for the management of obesity: A meta-analysis to compare endoscopic sleeve gastroplasty, AspireAssist, and primary obesity surgery endolumenal. Obesity Surgery. 2019;**29**(7):2287-2298

[17] Vargas EJ, Bazerbachi F, Rizk M, Rustagi T, Acosta A, Wilson EB, et al. Transoral outlet reduction with full thickness endoscopic suturing for weight regain after gastric bypass: A large multicenter international experience and meta-analysis. Surgical Endoscopy. 2018;**32**(1):252-259

[18] Sander BQ. Weight regain after bariactric surgery: Endoscopic suture with overstitch use for gastrointestinal anastomosis decrease - Inicial results: Brasilian multicenter study. Acta Scientific Gastrointestinal Disorders. 2020;**3**:2

Section 4

Complications after Bariatric Surgery

Chapter 13

Weight Regain after Bariatric and Metabolic Surgery: A Dreaded Complication

Asad Ullah, Muhammad Jamil and Johar Jamil

Abstract

The prevalence of obesity is increasing worldwide. It is a chronic relapsing disease. It requires a multifaceted treatment approach tailored to the individual's needs. Treatment options include lifestyle modifications, pharmacotherapy, and surgery. Bariatric metabolic surgery offers the best option to achieve sustained weight loss, alleviation of obesity-associated comorbidities, and improved quality of life. However, these benefits are dependent on compliance with long-term lifestyle changes. Unfortunately, some patients regain a significant amount of weight after the initial weight loss. The etiology of weight regain is not fully clear. Risk factors for weight regain after bariatric surgery include behavioral factors, lack of physical activity, loss of follow-up, hormonal changes, surgical factors, mental health, and psychological disorders. Ideally, management requires a multidisciplinary team approach. Non-invasive treatments include lifestyle modifications, behavioral therapy, exercise, and pharmacotherapy. Invasive options include endoscopic interventions and revisional surgery. Non-invasive options are utilized first. The decision about invasive therapy should be individualized due to the risk of complications. Future studies should aim for early identification of high-risk patients and managing them proactively. Moreover, clinical trials must test the safety and efficacy of existing and novel pharmacotherapies in managing weight regain.

Keywords: weight regain, suboptimal weight loss, bariatric surgery, obesity, revision surgery, lifestyle interventions, obesity pharmacotherapy

1. Introduction

Obesity is excessive or abnormal fat accumulation that poses a health risk [1]. It is a chronic and recurring condition [2]. Obesity is an important driver of chronic non-communicable diseases such as coronary artery disease (CAD), hypertension (HTN), type 2 diabetes mellitus (T2D), dyslipidemia, certain cancers (endometrial, breast, and colon), stroke, osteoarthritis, respiratory disorders, sleep apnea, non-alcoholic fatty liver disease (NAFLD), gall stones, certain gynecologic problems (infertility, abnormal menses, and polycystic ovary), and pseudotumor cerebri.

Modest intentional weight loss (5–10%) can significantly improve obesity-related morbidity and mortality. Weight loss is achieved via non-surgical and surgical approaches. The former include lifestyle modifications, psychiatric-behavior modification programs, and pharmacotherapy. Lifestyle modifications, which include nutritional therapy and physical activity, are hard to implement in primary care and have limited long-term efficacy due to non-adherence [3]. Pharmacotherapy could induce only a modest weight loss of 3–11% over 2 to 3 years [4]. Bariatric and metabolic surgery (BMS) can engender greater and sustainable weight loss in severe obesity than non-surgical treatments [5].

A certain degree of weight regain (WR) is natural after any intentional weight loss attempt; however, one of the long-term complications of BMS is significant WR [6]. The consequences are beyond gaining weight, resulting in recurrence or worsening of obesity-associated morbidities. WR could be an isolating and hopeless experience. Affected patients complain of emotional distress, anger, hopelessness, shame, discouragement, frustration, and depression [7]. Managing WR is costly [8].

It is critical to preemptively identify patients at risk of significant WR and intervene early.

2. Pathophysiology of weight regain

The pathophysiology of obesity is complex and multifactorial. Obesity is the outcome of the interaction between genetic and epigenetic factors [9]. This interaction is influenced by multiple factors such as environment, culture, food, physical activity, stress, sleep, and psychosocial factors. Inheritance explains 67% of the variability in body mass index (BMI). Approximately 40% of the total variability is attributable to the genes controlling food intake, 12% to metabolic rate, 5% to fat oxidation, and 10% to spontaneous physical activity [10–12].

The interplay of neuroendocrine, gastrointestinal, and adipose tissue plays a pivotal role in energy homeostasis.

The hypothalamus maintains energy and metabolic homeostasis by controlling hunger and satiety (**Figure 1**). It communicates reciprocally with other central and peripheral areas through neurotransmitters, afferent/efferent neurons, peptides, and hormones [14]. The Arcuate nucleus of the hypothalamus has two distinct neuronal populations with opposing effects on appetite. The orexigenic population stimulates appetite by releasing neuropeptide Y (NPY) and agouti-related peptide (AgRP). On the other hand, the anorexigenic neurons mediate satiety by releasing proopiomelanocortin (POMC) metabolites such as melanocyte-stimulating hormone (α-MSH), cocaine and amphetamine-regulated transcript (CART) [15]. Other central regions such as the nucleus of the solitary tract (NST) of the brain stem, paraventricular nucleus (PVN), lateral hypothalamic area (LHA) of the hypothalamus, and postrema area (PA) also play a role in energy homeostasis [16]. The reward control and stimulus perception areas influence energy intake.

The gastrointestinal tract releases peptide hormones in response to the presence or absence of nutrients. The X/A cells in the gastric fundus secrete ghrelin (an orexigenic hormone) during the fasting state. Ghrelin activates NPY/AgRP and orexigenic neurons in LHA [17]. The prokinetic action of ghrelin on the stomach reduces satiety by promoting gastric emptying. Food intake, on the other hand, generates mechanical and chemical stimuli, which leads to the release of anorexigenic peptides from the

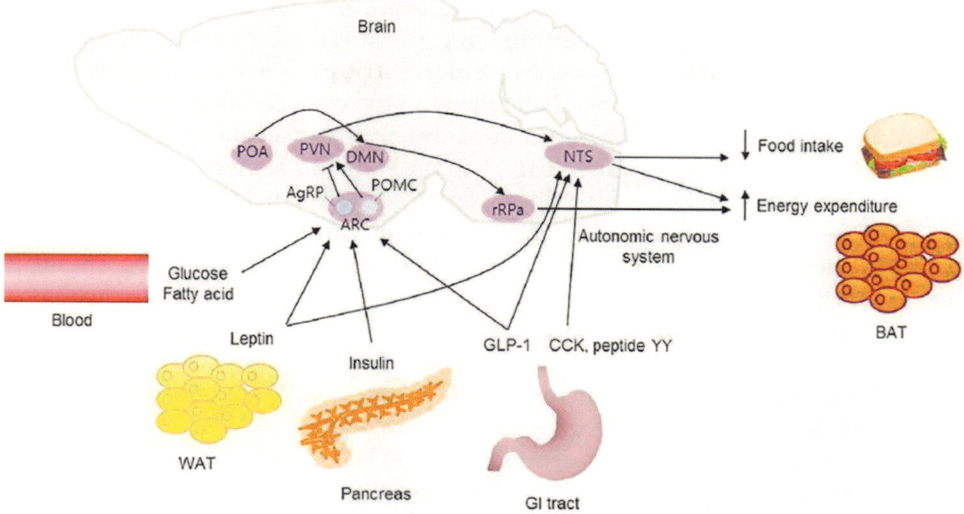

Figure 1.
Model of brain regulation of energy metabolism ["Copyright © Year Korean Endocrine Society from Endocrinol Metab. 2016, 31; 4: 520. Reprinted with permission from The Korean Endocrine Society." [13]].

gut. Cholecystokinin (CCK), peptide YY (PYY), and glucagon-like peptide-1 (GLP-1) are important hormones. They act either directly at the hypothalamus (PYY binding to Y2 receptors) or peripherally via mechanical satiety signals through the vagus nerve, which interacts with NST and AP (CCK) [18]. Furthermore, the gut hormones suppress the orexigenic pathways by activating serotonergic receptors (5HT-1b) in the subcortical area [19].

BMS counters some aspects of obesity pathophysiology but does not cure it; hence, the risk of recurrence of obesity remains after BMS. The energy balance regulates body weight. After BMS, energy intake diminishes, tilting the energy balance to negative. Both basal metabolic rate and resting energy expenditure decline. These changes stimulate increased energy intake and weight regain.

The pathophysiology of weight regain after BMS is poorly understood. Individuals who fail to achieve long-term weight loss have a higher level of orexigenic than anorexigenic hormones, resulting in increased appetite and energy intake [20]. After RYGB, PYY levels increase, and ghrelin levels decline, promoting weight loss [21]. Studies show that patients who do not lose adequate weight after RYGB have either no difference in pre- and post-surgery PYY and ghrelin levels or insignificant changes compared to those who achieved long-term weight loss [22, 23].

Gastro-gastric fistula (GGF) is a complication of RYGB and a common reason for weight regain. Ghrelin levels are high in GGF, which declines after correction of GGF and gastric stoma lengthening [24].

GLP-1 is an insulinotropic peptide secreted by enteroendocrine L cells in the small intestine and certain neurons in NST. It stimulates insulin secretion and inhibits glucagon secretion after food ingestion. After RYGB, GLP-1 levels increase, causing postprandial hypoglycemia (a feature of dumping syndrome) and rapid gastric emptying. These actions might contribute to weight regain by increasing energy intake [25].

The metabolic profile of adipose tissue changes with the caloric restriction after BMS, allowing adipogenesis and diminishing the adipocyte size and insulin sensitivity. These modifications increase glucose uptake by the adipose tissue, resulting in adipocyte hypertrophy, lipogenesis, and fat storage, a hallmark of obesity [26]. In other words, the abnormal adipose tissue in bariatric patients encourages weight regain via deflective endocrine metabolic signals. Moreover, the dysfunctional adipose tissue secretes pro-inflammatory adipokine leptin. It is an anorexigenic hormone and represents the amount of stored energy in the body [27]. Lower leptin levels are reported post-RYGB, compensating for the energy deficit state [28]. Low leptin levels initiate homeostatic activities, which promote energy conservation and weight gain. For example, it increases the production of endogenous endocannabinoids. These chemicals bind with CB1 receptors in adipose tissue and the hypothalamus, leading to lipogenesis and secretion of orexigenic factors [29]. It also lowers sympathetic and thyroid activity to save energy. Hypoleptinemia increases cortisol levels by stimulating PVN, which in turn causes appetite and fat storage [30]. Despite all these findings, the role of leptin in weight regain remains controversial.

Non-homeostatic mechanisms also contribute to WR. Functional imaging studies show that activating certain areas of the mesolimbic system in the brain promotes motivation and the desire to eat a high-calorie diet [31].

In summary, homeostatic and non-homeostatic compensatory mechanisms encourage individuals after BMS to relapse into high-energy intake patterns, promoting WR. Further research is required to understand the pathophysiology of WR after BMS.

3. How much weight regain is significant?

Despite its seriousness, there is no standard definition for WR. This dearth hinders our comprehension of the problem and interferes with timely intervention. **Table 1** illustrates frequently used definitions in the literature.

It is noteworthy that these definitions are arbitrary and lack association with clinical significance.

Insufficient weight loss (IWL) is defined as excess weight loss (EWL) of less than 50% 18 months after BMS [36]. IWL is different from WR. It is outside the scope of this chapter and has not been discussed further.

4. Risk factors for WR after BMS

The etiology of WR is multifactorial and overlapping. A systematic review of 25 studies categorized the causes of weight regain into five categories: dietary, genetic, psychiatric, temporal, and surgical or anatomic (**Table 2**) [37].

> 25% regain of excess weight loss (EWL) from nadir [32]
Weight gain of >10 kg from nadir [33]
>10% weight regain [34]
Increase in BMI of ≥5 kg/m^2 from nadir BMI [35]

Table 1.
Frequently reported weight regain definitions after BMS.

Patient related factors
Behavioral factors
• Maladaptive eating behavior
• Physical inactivity
• Processed food
• Liquid calories
Psychological factors
• Depression/Anxiety
• Alcohol & substance use
• Emotional eating
• Difficulty in adopting new habits
Physiological factors
• Genetic predisposition
• Muscle mass wasting
• Abnormal metabolism
Miscellaneous factors
• Lack of long term follow-up
• Medications
• Pre-operative features
Surgery related factors
• Stoma size
• Gastric volume
• Time after surgery
• Dysphagia & reflux

Table 2.
Risk factors for weight regain after BMS.

4.1 Patient-specific risk factors

4.1.1 Lifestyle and behavioral factors

Dietetic and nutritional advice is central to achieving meaningful results after BMS. Unfortunately, some patients fail to follow the dietary plan after BMS, resulting in suboptimal weight loss or WR [38]. WR is common in patients who continue high-calorie diets attributed to large amounts of high-fat food, sweets, junk food, and sugary drinks. Studies show a positive correlation between the Healthy Eating Index and WR (OR 0.95; $p = 0.04$) [38]. Eating large meals at night is associated with weight reacquisition [39].

Maladaptive eating behaviors such as binge eating disorder (BED), loss of control eating (LOCE), and grazing are frequent causes of WR after BMS. In a study, 23% of RYGB patients with inadequate weight loss and WR had maladaptive dietary habits [40].

The prevalence of BED is higher in patients undergoing BMS. A study reported BED in 40% of the cases, depending on the type of weight loss procedure, time after surgery, and method of BED assessment [41]. Furthermore, the prevalence of grazing increased from 26.3% pre-surgery to 38% after surgery. More than half of the BED cases switched to meet the criteria for grazing due to the inability to consume a large amount of food after BMS.

LOCE is defined as either the inability to resist food, stop eating, or be compelled to eat. It is associated with subjective distress [42] and WR after BMS [43].

Grazing is unplanned, repetitive, and uncontrolled eating between mealtimes. It is reported in 17–47% of the patients after BMS, depending on the assessment method and time after surgery [44]. In one study, grazing and LOCE were the two high-risk eating patterns linked with WR after BMS [45].

Dysphagia is common after BMS [46]. It is probably the outcome of time-dependent esophageal dysmotility after BMS. Dysphagia sways patients' choices to a soft or liquid diet, which is absorbed quickly and produces less satiety, resulting in increased calorie intake.

Macronutrients may contribute to WR. A meta-analysis showed diminished calorie [1050 kcal/day ($p < 0.001$)] and fat intake after BMS, but carbohydrate intake was not affected ($p = 0.006$) [47].

Although BMS improves mobility and reduces the burden of osteoarthritis, activity levels remain low in BMS patients compared to the general population (48 vs. 53%, respectively) [48]. In a study, only 10–26% of BMS patients met the minimal physical activity level [49]. It could be partly due to the physiologic reduction in energy expenditure and lean muscle mass associated with significant weight loss [50]. Maintaining adequate physical activity is an essential factor in sustaining weight after BMS [51]. Multiple studies have linked a sedentary lifestyle with WR after BMS [38, 52].

4.1.2 Neuropsychiatric and psychological factors

Mental health disorders (MHD) play an essential role in the causation of obesity and, hence, are prevalent in BMS patients. The frequency of a single mental health disorder was 40% in a study [53]. The prevalence of two or more MHDs was 33% in patients who underwent BMS in this study. Patients with two or more mental health disorders were at higher risk of WR (OR = 6.4, 95% CI = 1.3–12.4). Depression is the most common psychiatric disorder among BMS patients. It is linked with inadequate weight loss and weight regain, but the direction of the association is not clear [54].

Neuropsychiatric disorders promote WR by hindering adherence to the diet and behavioral interventions after BMS [55].

Alcohol use disorder (AUD) and substance use disorders (SUD) are associated with WR after BMS. Due to the diminished capacity for eating after BMS, some patients may seek relief from alcohol or substance abuse to satisfy the brain reward system [56]. A systematic review revealed a small but significant risk of new-onset alcohol use after BMS, especially RYGB [57]. The exact reason for this finding is not clear; however, some investigators have shown that the pharmacokinetics of alcohol change after RYGB and patients achieve higher blood alcohol levels after ingestion of a small amount of alcohol [58]. It is essential to assess the AUD and SUD pre- and post-bariatric surgery.

4.1.3 Endocrine and metabolic factors

Reactive hypoglycemia as part of the late dumping syndrome is common after esophageal and gastric surgery [59]. It is the consequence of insulin response to the rapid absorption of simple sugars from the small intestine. A study of 36 post-RYGB patients showed reactive hypoglycemia in 72% of the cases [25]. Of the 11 patients who regained >10% of their weight, 6 had reactive hypoglycemia. In another study, WR after BMS in 428 patients was associated with reactive hypoglycemia (OR = 1.66; 95% CI: 1.04–2.65) [60]. It could be concluded from these studies that reactive hypoglycemia might contribute to maladaptive eating disorder and WR.

Furthermore, as discussed in Section 2 of this chapter, other hormonal changes are involved in the pathophysiology of WR.

4.1.4 Lack of long-term support

Multidisciplinary support after BMS plays a pivotal role in achieving optimal results. The percentage of excess weight loss was 74% in patients who attended all follow-up visits for 4 years, compared to 56% in those who were lost to follow-up within a year after RYGB [61]. Among patients who stopped follow-up after 3 years of LSG, 75% gained 14% weight, compared to only 25% of those who continued follow-up for 5 to 6 years [62]. Patients who successfully maintained body weight 69 months after BMS held support from family, friends, and healthcare professionals responsible for achieving favorable outcomes [63].

4.1.5 Miscellaneous factors

Certain pre-operative characteristics may predispose to WR. For example, the risk of WR and surgical failure is high in the super-high BMI group [64]. Age, socioeconomic status, gender, time after surgery, and type II DM are linked with WR [65, 66].

Several medications promote WR, such as steroids, contraceptives, hypoglycemic agents, antipsychotics, tricyclic antidepressants, lithium, and valproic acid [67].

Individuals with certain genetic variations, e.g., LEPR Lys109Arg, LEPR Gln223Arg, LEPR Lys656Asn, and ADRB2 Gly16Arg and Gln27Glu, are prone to WR after BMS [68].

4.2 Surgery-related and anatomic factors

The prevalence of weight regain after BMS is poorly reported due to a lack of standardized definition and long-term follow-up. It depends on multiple factors, such as the surgical technique, time after the surgery, and the definition of weight regain. **Table 3** summarizes the prevalence of weight regain after commonly performed BMS.

Two common causes of WR after SG and RYGB are dilated gastric/gastrojejunal pouch and gastro-gastric fistula (GGF) [74]. Dilated gastrojejunal stoma (diameter > 2 cm) empties rapidly, causing lower satiety. In a retrospective study, dilated pouch and stoma after RYGB were observed in more patients with WR (71.2%) compared to 36.6% in those with successful weight loss [74]. A cohort study of 205 patients with WR after RYGB reported a dilated gastrojejunal pouch in 58.9%, an enlarged gastric pouch in 28%, and 12.3% had both these abnormalities [75].

GGF is an abnormal communication between the proximal gastric pouch and the remnant distal stomach. Food detours to the distal gastric remnant instead of the duodenum, increasing the gastric volume and available absorption area. These changes counter the purpose of BMS. GGF often requires revision of the surgery. A retrospective study of the endoscopic examination in 165 RYGB patients demonstrated an association between gastrojejunal stoma diameter and weight regain [8].

Surgical procedure	Weight regain prevalence (%)
RYGB	17% at 2 years [69] 22.5% at 3 years [70] 26.8% at 5 years [70] 3.9% between 3 and 7 years [71]
LSG	5.7% at 2 years [62] 39.5% at 5 years [72]
LAGB	38% at 10 years [73]

Table 3.
Prevalence of weight regain after BMS.

Every 10 mm increase in the size of gastrojejunal stoma was associated with an 8% increase in regaining the percentage of maximal weight loss. Interestingly, the length of the gastric pouch was not linked with weight regain.

The estimated weight regain after LSG is like RYGB. Procedure-specific causes of weight regain in LSG patients are sleeve dilation, residual gastric volume, retained gastric fundus, amount of antral resection, and size of bougie used [33, 76].

One study looked at the association of antral remnant length and weight regain after LSG [33]. Patients were divided into two groups, i.e., Group A with an antral remnant length of 6 cm from the pylorus and Group B with a shorter antral length of 2 cm. Weight regain was defined as >10 kg regain from the nadir weight. Weight regain was prevalent in group A compared to group B (22 vs. 4%). In another study, weight regain was related to the residual gastric volume using CT volumetry [76]. Gastric residual volume above 225 cc was associated with a failure rate of 80%.

5. Prevention and management of weight regain

The etiology of WR is multifactorial and, therefore, demands a multifaceted approach. Contemporary management options are lifestyle modifications, pharmacotherapy, endoscopic procedures, and surgical revision. Non-invasive options are employed initially. Surgical revision is the last resort due to the high complication rate [77].

5.1 Lifestyle modifications/behavioral therapy

The timely introduction of an exercise-based program combined with motivational support and dietary therapy showed promising results in a prospective controlled study [78]. Behavioral and physical outcomes improved with physical activity.

In a retrospective study, physical activity increased excess body weight loss (72.9 vs. 76.3%), fat-free mass, and health-related quality of life [79]. Mediterranean diet was associated with greater weight loss after BMS in a study [80].

Several studies have shown the efficacy of behavioral therapy in managing WR after BMS [81, 82].

A pilot study revealed the effectiveness of 10 weeks of Healthy Eating and Lifestyle Post-surgery (HELP) intervention in managing WR after BMS [83]. All patients were at least ≥1.5 years post-surgery. The intervention group experienced 5.1% weight loss within 3 months of the intervention. A retrospective study (n = 44) demonstrated a mean weight loss of 2.1 kg after 14.7 months of lifestyle intervention [84].

Other studies have refuted the success of lifestyle modifications claimed in some studies. A prospective study included 95 WR patients after RYGB (9 ± 4 years out of RYGB) divided into lifestyle intervention, Liraglutide, endosurgical Apollo's Overstitch system or implantation of Fobi-ring with pouch sizing [85]. Liraglutide and Fobi-ring achieved equal weight loss 24 months after the intervention (4.8 ± 2.9 kg/m2 and 5.5 ± 2.9 kg/m2, respectively). Patients in the lifestyle intervention experienced no weight loss, while the endosurgical procedure resulted in a weight loss of 1.0 ± 0.9 kg/m2. A randomized study in 3-year post-SG patients with WR compared intense exercise to the usual care group [86]. A mean weight loss of 1.2 kg occurred within 5 months of intervention. However, 2 months after the intervention, 1.1 kg weight was regained. Three small studies showed weight loss of 1.6 to 1.5% over 6–10 weeks [81–83].

5.2 Pharmacotherapy

Drugs are an essential part of AR management armamentarium. Before 2012, Orlistat and Phentermine were the only two drugs approved for obesity therapy [87]. However, the last few years have witnessed significant advancements in weight loss pharmacotherapy. There is no approved pharmacotherapy for post-BS cases. However, weight-reducing medications are used off-label to promote weight loss in case of AWL or WR.

GLP-1 analogues induce weight loss by reducing gastric emptying, increasing food ingestion-related insulin secretion, and inducing satiety via stimulating POMC/AgRP [88]. Liraglutide 3 mg for 7.6 ± 7.1 months achieved significant weight loss (−6.3 ± 7.7 kg, $P < .05$) regardless of the type of BMS [84]. Two other small studies reported similar results [89, 90]. Semaglutide, another GLP-1 analogue, reduced 6% weight in post-BMS patients who regained 12% of the weight in 1 year [91].

Metformin (1800 ± 350 mg/day) induced modest weight loss of 5% in post-BMS patients with WR when used as an adjuvant to an ad libitum low-carbohydrate, non-ketogenic, or high-protein diet. Fasting glucose, HbA1c, insulin resistance, and cholesterol levels improved [91].

Orlistat is a lipase inhibitor; it is used for long-term management. Phentermine is a sympathomimetic appetite suppressant and is recommended for short-term use. After 2012, a few other weight loss drugs were introduced to the market: Bupropion HCl-naltrexone HCl, Lorcaserin HCl, phentermine-topiramate, Liraglutide, and recently, Semaglutide was also added to the armamentarium. The first three medications are centrally acting appetite suppressants, while Liraglutide and Semaglutide are glucagon-like peptide-1 receptor agonists. They act peripherally and slow gastric emptying.

Few prospective trials have examined the efficacy or safety of these drugs after BS. Phentermine-fenfluramine induced EWL of 8–65% over 3 months in patients with WR after RYGB or biliopancreatic diversion [92]. In another study, Topiramate was used in patients with BED who had a premature weight plateau [93]. After 3 months of treatment, EWL increased from 20.4 to 34.1% without readjusting AGB.

Retrospective studies show favorable effects of weight loss pharmacotherapy in the BS population. A multi-center retrospective study reported >5% weight loss after RYGB/SG in half of the participants [94]. Fifteen different weight loss medications were used. Topiramate was the most frequently prescribed medicine. Patients on topiramate were twice as likely to lose 10% of their weight (odds ratio 1.9; P.018).

Some experts suggest better commencing weight loss drugs when the weight plateaus rather than at the weight regain stage [95].

Good-quality randomized studies of pharmacological agents are required in post-BMS patients with WR to determine their effective and safe use.

5.3 Endoscopic procedures

Various endoscopic interventions are used to manage WR after BMS. Transoral outlet reduction (TORe) proved to be safe and effective in dealing with WR after RYGB [96]. Patients lost 6.4 to 10.15 kg within 3–12 months of TORe. Other studies have confirmed these results, making it a promising option [97]. Two common suturing techniques are employed in TORe, i.e., full-thickness suture plus argon plasma mucosal coagulation (ft-TORe) and argon plus plasma mucosal coagulation alone (APMC-TORe). Both techniques have shown comparable results, though ft-TORe requires multiple endoscopies [98]. A modified endoscopic submucosal dissection (ESD) for TORe achieves higher weight loss when combined with the suturing after RYGB [99]. The ESD-TORe group experienced a total weight loss of 12.1 ± 9.3% versus 7.5 ± 3.3% for the traditional APMC-TORe with full-thickness suture.

5.4 Revisional surgery

If non-surgical therapies fail to achieve the desirable results, then revisional surgery could be considered as a last resort. Revisional procedures carry higher morbidity and mortality than primary surgery [100]. Therefore, it is vital to assess the risk-benefit ratio in each individual case, ideally by an experienced multidisciplinary team. As more BMS procedures are performed, the rate of revisional surgeries is also rising [101].

The indications for revisional surgery include enhancing the weight loss, reducing the side effects of the primary surgery, or completely reversing the original surgery. It could be restorative, e.g., in cases with gastric pouch dilatation or excess fundus post-LSG, or corrective, e.g., managing anastomotic stenosis or marginal ulcer or augmentation or conversion to another technique [102].

Revisional surgery is performed in approximately 10–20% of the individuals with WR who undergo revisional surgery [103].

Some patients with WR require revisional surgery or conversion to another type of weight loss surgery. Evidence shows that the prevalence of these procedures has increased recently. Contrary to previous studies, a meta-analysis reported the safety and efficacy of revisional surgeries [104]. In total, 94 individuals who either had inadequate weight loss or regained >20% of the weight lost >1 year after SG underwent revisional surgery [105]. Median BMI dropped significantly 1 year after revisional surgery (41.9 to 6.3 kg/m^2). Revisions included were re-sleeve, RYGB, single anastomosis duodenal switch, and biliopancreatic duodenal switch (BPD/DS). The highest total weight loss was seen with BPD/DS (21.8 kg) and the lowest (12 kg) with re-sleeve.

Some investigators support using silicon gastric rings again to manage WR after BMS. Although the short-term data is encouraging, studies with longer follow-up exploring less invasive options such as lifestyle modifications, behavioral therapies, pharmacotherapies, and invasive options are required.

6. Conclusion

Obesity and overweight are global public health problems. Traditional weight loss therapies, including lifestyle modifications, behavioral therapies, and pharmacotherapy, result in modest weight loss in the long run. Metabolic bariatric surgery is most efficacious in achieving significant and sustainable weight loss. Moreover, it improves and remits many obesity-related comorbidities, thus enhancing the quality of life. Contemporary surgical procedures include adjustable gastric banding, sleeve gastrectomy, Roux-en-Y gastric bypass, and biliopancreatic diversion with a duodenal switch.

Despite the numerous benefits of BMS, it has associated side effects and complications. Weight regain is one of the most dreaded long-term complications of BMS. It has a complex and multifactorial etiology. Therefore, it demands a multipronged management plan, including lifestyle changes, behavioral therapy, drugs, endoscopic procedures, and revisional surgery. Ideally, an experienced multidisciplinary team should deliver management. All the stakeholders need to contribute to the prevention and management of weight regain. For example, the surgeon has to perform a procedure that suits the patient. The patient must comply with post-operation recommendations for the diet and follow-up. Patient education, monitoring, and timely interventions must be considered for high-risk individuals. Further studies are required to elucidate the exact mechanisms involved in weight regain to establish an evidence-based management approach.

Acknowledgements

This work is not funded.

Conflict of interest

The authors declare no conflict of interest.

Notes/thanks/other declarations

I would like to express my gratitude to my parents, who always encouraged me to learn and flourish. I am thankful to my wife, Shama Rahman, who provided unwavering support through thick and thin. I would also like to thank my children (The late Hamdaan Jamil, Ayza Jamil, Azlaan Jamil, and Muhammad Jamil). I also acknowledge the support of my supervisors, Dr. Matthew Howes and Ida Ryland.

Abbreviations

AgRP	agouti-related peptide
APMC-TORe	argon plasma mucosal coagulation alone
ARC	arcuate nucleus
AT	adipose tissue
AUD	alcohol use disorder
BED	binge eating disorder
BMI	body mass index

BMS	bariatric metabolic surgery
BPD/DS	biliopancreatic duodenal switch
CAD	coronary artery disease
CART	amphetamine-regulated transcript
CCK	cholecystokinin
EWL	excess weight loss
f-TORe	argon plasma mucosal coagulation
GGF	gastro-gastric fistula
GLP-1	glucagon-like peptide-1
HELP	healthy eating and lifestyle post-surgery
HTN	hypertension
IWL	insufficient weight loss
LAGB	laparoscopic adjustable gastric banding
LHA	lateral hypothalamic area
LOCE	loss of control eating
LSG	laparoscopic sleeve gastrectomy
MHD	mental health disorders
NAFLD	non-alcoholic fatty liver disease
NPY	neuropeptide Y
NTS	nuclei of the solitary tract
POMC	proopiomelanocortin
PVN	paraventricular nucleus
PYY	peptide YY
RYGB	Roux-en-Y gastric bypass
SUD	substance use disorders
T2D	type 2 diabetes mellitus
TORe	trans oral outlet reduction
WHO	World Health Organization
WR	weight regain

Author details

Asad Ullah[1*], Muhammad Jamil[2] and Johar Jamil[3]

1 King Faisal Specialist Hospital Riyadh, Saudi Arabia

2 Retired General Practitioner, KPK, Pakistan

3 University of Swabi, KPK, Pakistan

*Address all correspondence to: drasadullah99@hotmail.com

References

[1] WHO. Obesity. Geneva, Switzerland: WHO; 2024

[2] WHO. Obesity and Overweight 2024. Geneva, Switzerland: WHO; 2024. Available from: https://www.who.int/news-room/fact-sheets/detail/obesity-and-overweight

[3] Dombrowski SU, Knittle K, Avenell A, Araújo-Soares V, Sniehotta FF. Long term maintenance of weight loss with non-surgical interventions in obese adults: Systematic review and meta-analyses of randomised controlled trials. BMJ. 2014;**348**:g2646

[4] Shi Q, Wang Y, Hao Q, Vandvik PO, Guyatt G, Li J, et al. Pharmacotherapy for adults with overweight and obesity: A systematic review and network meta-analysis of randomised controlled trials. Lancet. 2022;**399**(10321):259-269

[5] Maciejewski ML, Arterburn DE, Van Scoyoc L, Smith VA, Yancy WS Jr, Weidenbacher HJ, et al. Bariatric surgery and long-term durability of weight loss. JAMA Surgery. 2016;**151**(11):1046-1055

[6] Reis MG, Guimarães G, Moreira LF, de Siqueira Veloso Andrade Carvalho L, de Tianeze Castro C, Adrielle Lima Vieira R, et al. Weight regain after bariatric surgery: A systematic review and meta-analysis of observational studies. Obesity Medicine. 2024;**45**:100528

[7] Tolvanen L, Christenson A, Surkan PJ, Lagerros YT. Patients' experiences of weight regain after bariatric surgery. Obesity Surgery. 2022;**32**(5):1498-1507

[8] Abu Dayyeh BK, Lautz DB, Thompson CC. Gastrojejunal stoma diameter predicts weight regain after Roux-en-Y gastric bypass. Clinical Gastroenterology and Hepatology. 2011;**9**(3):228-233

[9] Flegal KM, Carroll MD, Kuczmarski RJ, Johnson CL. Overweight and obesity in the United States: Prevalence and trends, 1960-1994. International Journal of Obesity and Related Metabolic Disorders. 1998;**22**(1):39-47

[10] Stunkard AJ, Harris JR, Pedersen NL, McClearn GE. The body-mass index of twins who have been reared apart. The New England Journal of Medicine. 1990;**322**(21):1483-1487

[11] Price RA, Gottesman II. Body fat in identical twins reared apart: Roles for genes and environment. Behavior Genetics. 1991;**21**(1):1-7

[12] Allison DB, Kaprio J, Korkeila M, Koskenvuo M, Neale MC, Hayakawa K. The heritability of body mass index among an international sample of monozygotic twins reared apart. International Journal of Obesity and Related Metabolic Disorders. 1996;**20**(6):501-506

[13] Roh E, Kim MS. Brain regulation of energy metabolism. Endocrinology and Metabolism (Seoul). 2016;**31**(4):519-524

[14] Perry B, Wang Y. Appetite regulation and weight control: The role of gut hormones. Nutrition & Diabetes. 2012;**2**(1):e26

[15] Maclean PS, Bergouignan A, Cornier MA, Jackman MR. Biology's response to dieting: The impetus for weight regain. American Journal of Physiology. Regulatory, Integrative

and Comparative Physiology. 2011;**301**(3):R581-R600

[16] Kinasz KR, Ross DA, Cooper JJ. Eat to live or live to eat? The neurobiology of appetite regulation. Biological Psychiatry. 2017;**81**(9):e73-ee5

[17] Castañeda TR, Tong J, Datta R, Culler M, Tschöp MH. Ghrelin in the regulation of body weight and metabolism. Frontiers in Neuroendocrinology. 2010;**31**(1):44-60

[18] Owyang C, Heldsinger A. Vagal control of satiety and hormonal regulation of appetite. Journal of Neurogastroenterology and Motility. 2011;**17**(4):338-348

[19] Yabut JM, Crane JD, Green AE, Keating DJ, Khan WI, Steinberg GR. Emerging roles for serotonin in regulating metabolism: New implications for an ancient molecule. Endocrine Reviews. 2019;**40**(4):1092-1107

[20] Tamboli RA, Breitman I, Marks-Shulman PA, Jabbour K, Melvin W, Williams B, et al. Early weight regain after gastric bypass does not affect insulin sensitivity but is associated with elevated ghrelin. Obesity (Silver Spring). 2014;**22**(7):1617-1622

[21] Tsouristakis AI, Febres G, McMahon DJ, Tchang B, Conwell IM, Tsang AJ, et al. Long-term modulation of appetitive hormones and sweet cravings after adjustable gastric banding and Roux-en-Y gastric bypass. Obesity Surgery. 2019;**29**(11):3698-3705

[22] Meguid MM, Glade MJ, Middleton FA. Weight regain after Roux-en-Y: A significant 20% complication related to PYY. Nutrition. 2008;**24**(9):832-842

[23] Santo MA, Riccioppo D, Pajecki D, Kawamoto F, de Cleva R, Antonangelo L, et al. Weight regain after gastric bypass: Influence of gut hormones. Obesity Surgery. 2016;**26**(5):919-925

[24] O'Brien CS, Wang G, McGinty J, Agénor KK, Dutia R, Colarusso A, et al. Effects of gastrogastric fistula repair on weight loss and gut hormone levels. Obesity Surgery. 2013;**23**(8):1294-1301

[25] Roslin M, Damani T, Oren J, Andrews R, Yatco E, Shah P. Abnormal glucose tolerance testing following gastric bypass demonstrates reactive hypoglycemia. Surgical Endoscopy. 2011;**25**(6):1926-1932

[26] MacLean PS, Higgins JA, Giles ED, Sherk VD, Jackman MR. The role for adipose tissue in weight regain after weight loss. Obesity Reviews. 2015;**16**(Suppl. 1):45-54

[27] Farr OM, Gavrieli A, Mantzoros CS. Leptin applications in 2015: What have we learned about leptin and obesity? Current Opinion in Endocrinology, Diabetes, and Obesity. 2015;**22**(5):353-359

[28] Korner J, Inabnet W, Febres G, Conwell IM, McMahon DJ, Salas R, et al. Prospective study of gut hormone and metabolic changes after adjustable gastric banding and Roux-en-Y gastric bypass. International Journal of Obesity. 2009;**33**(7):786-795

[29] Matias I, Bisogno T, Di Marzo V. Endogenous cannabinoids in the brain and peripheral tissues: Regulation of their levels and control of food intake. International Journal of Obesity. 2006;**30**(Suppl. 1):S7-s12

[30] Blomain ES, Dirhan DA, Valentino MA, Kim GW, Waldman SA. Mechanisms of weight regain following weight loss. ISRN Obesity. 2013;**2013**:210524

[31] Rosenbaum M, Sy M, Pavlovich K, Leibel RL, Hirsch J. Leptin reverses weight loss-induced changes in regional neural activity responses to visual food stimuli. The Journal of Clinical Investigation. 2008;**118**(7):2583-2591

[32] Homan J, Betzel B, Aarts EO, van Laarhoven KJ, Janssen IM, Berends FJ. Secondary surgery after sleeve gastrectomy: Roux-en-Y gastric bypass or biliopancreatic diversion with duodenal switch. Surgery for Obesity and Related Diseases. 2015;**11**(4):771-777

[33] Obeidat F, Shanti H, Mismar A, Albsoul N, Al-Qudah M. The magnitude of antral resection in laparoscopic sleeve gastrectomy and its relationship to excess weight loss. Obesity Surgery. 2015;**25**(10):1928-1932

[34] Voorwinde V, Steenhuis IHM, Janssen IMC, Monpellier VM, van Stralen MM. Definitions of long-term weight regain and their associations with clinical outcomes. Obesity Surgery. 2020;**30**(2):527-536

[35] Brethauer SA, Aminian A, Romero-Talamás H, Batayyah E, Mackey J, Kennedy L, et al. Can diabetes be surgically cured? Long-term metabolic effects of bariatric surgery in obese patients with type 2 diabetes mellitus. Annals of Surgery. 2013;**258**(4):628-636; discussion 36-7

[36] Nedelcu M, Khwaja HA, Rogula TG. Weight regain after bariatric surgery-how should it be defined? Surgery for Obesity and Related Diseases. 2016;**12**(5):1129-1130

[37] Athanasiadis DI, Martin A, Kapsampelis P, Monfared S, Stefanidis D. Factors associated with weight regain post-bariatric surgery: A systematic review. Surgical Endoscopy. 2021;**35**(8):4069-4084

[38] Freire RH, Borges MC, Alvarez-Leite JI, Correia TD, MI. Food quality, physical activity, and nutritional follow-up as determinant of weight regain after Roux-en-Y gastric bypass. Nutrition. 2012;**28**(1):53-58

[39] Zalesin KC, Franklin BA, Miller WM, Nori Janosz KE, Veri S, Odom J, et al. Preventing weight regain after bariatric surgery: An overview of lifestyle and psychosocial modulators. American Journal of Lifestyle Medicine. 2010;**4**(2):113-120

[40] Rusch MD, Andris D. Maladaptive eating patterns after weight-loss surgery. Nutrition in Clinical Practice. 2007;**22**(1):41-49

[41] Kalarchian MA, Marcus MD, Wilson GT, Labouvie EW, Brolin RE, LaMarca LB. Binge eating among gastric bypass patients at long-term follow-up. Obesity Surgery. 2002;**12**(2):270-275

[42] Latner JD, Mond JM, Kelly MC, Haynes SN, Hay PJ. The loss of control over eating scale: Development and psychometric evaluation. The International Journal of Eating Disorders. 2014;**47**(6):647-659

[43] Smith KE, Orcutt M, Steffen KJ, Crosby RD, Cao L, Garcia L, et al. Loss of control eating and binge eating in the 7 years following bariatric surgery. Obesity Surgery. 2019;**29**(6):1773-1780

[44] Pizato N, Botelho PB, Gonçalves VSS, Dutra ES, de Carvalho KMB. Effect of grazing behavior on weight regain post-bariatric surgery: A systematic review. Nutrients. 2017;**9**(12):1322

[45] Colles SL, Dixon JB, O'Brien PE. Grazing and loss of control related to eating: Two high-risk factors following bariatric surgery. Obesity. 2008;**16**(3):615-622

[46] Miller AT, Matar R, Abu Dayyeh BK, Beran A, Vela MF, Lacy BE, et al. Postobesity surgery esophageal dysfunction: A combined cross-sectional prevalence study and retrospective analysis. The American Journal of Gastroenterology. 2020;**115**(10):1669-1680

[47] Janmohammadi P, Sajadi F, Alizadeh S, Daneshzad E. Comparison of energy and food intake between gastric bypass and sleeve gastrectomy: A meta-analysis and systematic review. Obesity Surgery. 2019;**29**(3):1040-1048

[48] Colley RC, Garriguet D, Janssen I, Craig CL, Clarke J, Tremblay MS. Physical activity of Canadian adults: Accelerometer results from the 2007 to 2009 Canadian health measures survey. Health Reports. 2011;**22**(1):7-14

[49] Rosenberger PH, Henderson KE, White MA, Masheb RM, Grilo CM. Physical activity in gastric bypass patients: Associations with weight loss and psychosocial functioning at 12-month follow-up. Obesity Surgery. 2011;**21**(10):1564-1569

[50] Tam CS, Redman LM, Greenway F, LeBlanc KA, Haussmann MG, Ravussin E. Energy metabolic adaptation and cardiometabolic improvements one year after gastric bypass, sleeve gastrectomy, and gastric band. The Journal of Clinical Endocrinology and Metabolism. 2016;**101**(10):3755-3764

[51] Livhits M, Mercado C, Yermilov I, Parikh JA, Dutson E, Mehran A, et al. Exercise following bariatric surgery: Systematic review. Obesity Surgery. 2010;**20**(5):657-665

[52] Amundsen T, Strømmen M, Martins C. Suboptimal weight loss and weight regain after gastric bypass surgery-postoperative status of energy intake, eating behavior, physical activity, and psychometrics. Obesity Surgery. 2017;**27**(5):1316-1323

[53] Rutledge T, Groesz LM, Savu M. Psychiatric factors and weight loss patterns following gastric bypass surgery in a veteran population. Obesity Surgery. 2011;**21**(1):29-35

[54] Sheets CS, Peat CM, Berg KC, White EK, Bocchieri-Ricciardi L, Chen EY, et al. Post-operative psychosocial predictors of outcome in bariatric surgery. Obesity Surgery. 2015;**25**(2):330-345

[55] Kofman MD, Lent MR, Swencionis C. Maladaptive eating patterns, quality of life, and weight outcomes following gastric bypass: Results of an internet survey. Obesity (Silver Spring). 2010;**18**(10):1938-1943

[56] Lindgren E, Gray K, Miller G, Tyler R, Wiers CE, Volkow ND, et al. Food addiction: A common neurobiological mechanism with drug abuse. Frontiers in Bioscience (Landmark Ed). 2018;**23**(5):811-836

[57] Kenkre JS, Gesell S, Keller A, Milani RM, Scholtz S, Barley EA. Alcohol misuse post metabolic and bariatric surgery: A systematic review of longer-term studies with focus on new onset alcohol use disorder and differences between surgery types. Current Obesity Reports. 2024:596-616

[58] Engel SG, Schaefer LM, Kerver GA, Leone LM, Smith G, Mitchell JE, et al. The rewarding effects of alcohol after bariatric surgery: Do they change and are they associated with pharmacokinetic changes? Surgery for Obesity and Related Diseases. 2022;**18**(2):190-195

[59] Hui C, Bauza GJ. Dumping Syndrome. In: StatPearls [Internet]. Treasure Island (FL): StatPearls Publishing; 2025. PMID: 29261889

[60] Varma S, Clark JM, Schweitzer M, Magnuson T, Brown TT, Lee CJ. Weight regain in patients with symptoms of post-bariatric surgery hypoglycemia. Surgery for Obesity and Related Diseases. 2017;**13**(10):1728-1734

[61] Gould JC, Beverstein G, Reinhardt S, Garren MJ. Impact of routine and long-term follow-up on weight loss after laparoscopic gastric bypass. Surgery for Obesity and Related Diseases. 2007;**3**(6):627-630; discussion 30

[62] Lauti M, Kularatna M, Hill AG, MacCormick AD. Weight regain following sleeve gastrectomy-a systematic review. Obesity Surgery. 2016;**26**(6):1326-1334

[63] Liebl L, Barnason S, Brage HD. Awakening: A qualitative study on maintaining weight loss after bariatric surgery. Journal of Clinical Nursing. 2016;**25**(7-8):951-961

[64] Magro DO, Geloneze B, Delfini R, Pareja BC, Callejas F, Pareja JC. Long-term weight regain after gastric bypass: A 5-year prospective study. Obesity Surgery. 2008;**18**(6):648-651

[65] Al-Khyatt W, Ryall R, Leeder P, Ahmed J, Awad S. Predictors of inadequate weight loss after laparoscopic gastric bypass for morbid obesity. Obesity Surgery. 2017;**27**(6):1446-1452

[66] Keith CJ Jr, Gullick AA, Feng K, Richman J, Stahl R, Grams J. Predictive factors of weight regain following laparoscopic Roux-en-Y gastric bypass. Surgical Endoscopy. 2018;**32**(5):2232-2238

[67] Sepúlveda-Lizcano L, Arenas-Villamizar VV, Jaimes-Duarte EB, García-Pacheco H, Paredes CS, Bermúdez V, et al. Metabolic adverse effects of psychotropic drug therapy: A systematic review. European Journal of Investigation in Health, Psychology and Education. 2023;**13**(8):1505-1520

[68] Salazar J, Duran P, Garrido B, Parra H, Hernández M, Cano C, et al. Weight regain after metabolic surgery: Beyond the surgical failure. Journal of Clinical Medicine. 2024;**13**(4):1322

[69] Shantavasinkul PC, Omotosho P, Corsino L, Portenier D, Torquati A. Predictors of weight regain in patients who underwent Roux-en-Y gastric bypass surgery. Surgery for Obesity and Related Diseases. 2016;**12**(9):1640-1645

[70] King WC, Hinerman AS, Belle SH, Wahed AS, Courcoulas AP. Comparison of the performance of common measures of weight regain after bariatric surgery for association with clinical outcomes. Journal of the American Medical Association. 2018;**320**(15):1560-1569

[71] Courcoulas AP, King WC, Belle SH, Berk P, Flum DR, Garcia L, et al. Seven-year weight trajectories and health outcomes in the longitudinal assessment of bariatric surgery (LABS) study. JAMA Surgery. 2018;**153**(5):427-434

[72] Braghetto I, Csendes A, Lanzarini E, Papapietro K, Cárcamo C, Molina JC. Is laparoscopic sleeve gastrectomy an acceptable primary bariatric procedure in obese patients? Early and 5-year postoperative results. Surgical Laparoscopy, Endoscopy & Percutaneous Techniques. 2012;**22**(6):479-486

[73] Sjöström L, Lindroos AK, Peltonen M, Torgerson J, Bouchard C, Carlsson B, et al. Lifestyle, diabetes, and cardiovascular risk factors 10 years after bariatric surgery. The New England Journal of Medicine. 2004;**351**(26):2683-2693

[74] Heneghan HM, Yimcharoen P, Brethauer SA, Kroh M, Chand B.

Influence of pouch and stoma size on weight loss after gastric bypass. Surgery for Obesity and Related Diseases. 2012;**8**(4):408-415

[75] Yimcharoen P, Heneghan HM, Singh M, Brethauer S, Schauer P, Rogula T, et al. Endoscopic findings and outcomes of revisional procedures for patients with weight recidivism after gastric bypass. Surgical Endoscopy. 2011;**25**(10):3345-3352

[76] Deguines JB, Verhaeghe P, Yzet T, Robert B, Cosse C, Regimbeau JM. Is the residual gastric volume after laparoscopic sleeve gastrectomy an objective criterion for adapting the treatment strategy after failure? Surgery for Obesity and Related Diseases. 2013;**9**(5):660-666

[77] Patel S, Szomstein S, Rosenthal RJ. Reasons and outcomes of reoperative bariatric surgery for failed and complicated procedures (excluding adjustable gastric banding). Obesity Surgery. 2011;**21**(8):1209-1219

[78] Gallé F, Marte G, Cirella A, Di Dio M, Miele A, Ricchiuti R, et al. An exercise-based educational and motivational intervention after surgery can improve behaviors, physical fitness and quality of life in bariatric patients. PLoS One. 2020;**15**(10):e0241336

[79] Nuijten MAH, Tettero OM, Wolf RJ, Bakker EA, Eijsvogels TMH, Monpellier VM, et al. Changes in physical activity in relation to body composition, fitness and quality of life after primary bariatric surgery: A two-year follow-up study. Obesity Surgery. 2021;**31**(3):1120-1128

[80] Gils Contreras A, Bonada Sanjaume A, Becerra-Tomás N, Salas-Salvadó J. Adherence to Mediterranean diet or physical activity after bariatric surgery and its effects on weight loss, quality of life, and food tolerance. Obesity Surgery. 2020;**30**(2):687-696

[81] Bradley L, Forman E, Kerrigan S, Butryn M, Herbert J, Sarwer D. A pilot study of an acceptance-based behavioral intervention for weight regain after bariatric surgery. Obesity Surgery. 2016;**26**:2433-2441

[82] Himes SM, Grothe KB, Clark MM, Swain JM, Collazo-Clavell ML, Sarr MG. Stop regain: A pilot psychological intervention for bariatric patients experiencing weight regain. Obesity Surgery. 2015;**25**(5):922-927

[83] Bradley LE, Forman EM, Kerrigan SG, Goldstein SP, Butryn ML, Thomas JG, et al. Project HELP: A remotely delivered behavioral intervention for weight regain after bariatric surgery. Obesity Surgery. 2017;**27**(3):586-598

[84] Wharton S, Kuk JL, Luszczynski M, Kamran E, Christensen RAG. Liraglutide 3.0 mg for the management of insufficient weight loss or excessive weight regain post-bariatric surgery. Clinical obesity. 2019;**9**(4):e12323

[85] Horber FF, Steffen R. Reversal of long-term weight regain after Roux-en-Y gastric bypass using liraglutide or surgical revision. A prospective study. Obesity Surgery. 2021;**31**(1):93-100

[86] Marc-Hernández A, Ruiz-Tovar J, Aracil A, Guillén S, Moya-Ramón M. Effects of a high-intensity exercise program on weight regain and cardio-metabolic profile after 3 years of bariatric surgery: A randomized trial. Scientific Reports. 2020;**10**(1):3123

[87] Guerciolini R. Mode of action of orlistat. International Journal of Obesity and Related Metabolic Disorders. 1997;**21**(Suppl. 3):S12-S23

[88] Kaineder K, Birngruber T, Rauter G, Obermüller B, Eichler J, Münzker J, et al. Chronic intrahypothalamic rather than subcutaneous liraglutide treatment reduces body weight gain and stimulates the melanocortin receptor system. International Journal of Obesity. 2017;**41**(8):1263-1270

[89] Rye P, Modi R, Cawsey S, Sharma AM. Efficacy of high-dose liraglutide as an adjunct for weight loss in patients with prior bariatric surgery. Obesity Surgery. 2018;**28**(11):3553-3558

[90] Pajecki D, Halpern A, Cercato C, Mancini M, de Cleva R, Santo MA. Short-term use of liraglutide in the management of patients with weight regain after bariatric surgery. Revista do Colégio Brasileiro de Cirurgiões. 2013;**40**(3):191-195

[91] Lautenbach A, Wernecke M, Huber TB, Stoll F, Wagner J, Meyhöfer SM, et al. The potential of semaglutide once-weekly in patients without type 2 diabetes with weight regain or insufficient weight loss after bariatric surgery—A retrospective analysis. Obesity Surgery. 2022;**32**(10):3280-3288

[92] Jester L, Wittgrove AC, Clark W. Adjunctive use of appetite suppressant medications for improved weight management in bariatric surgical patients. Obesity Surgery. 1996;**6**(5):412-415

[93] Zilberstein B, Pajecki D, Garcia de Brito AC, Gallafrio ST, Eshkenazy R, Andrade CG. Topiramate after adjustable gastric banding in patients with binge eating and difficulty losing weight. Obesity Surgery. 2004;**14**(6):802-805

[94] Stanford FC, Alfaris N, Gomez G, Ricks ET, Shukla AP, Corey KE, et al. The utility of weight loss medications after bariatric surgery for weight regain or inadequate weight loss: A multi-center study. Surgery for Obesity and Related Diseases. 2017;**13**(3):491-500

[95] Nor Hanipah Z, Nasr EC, Bucak E, Schauer PR, Aminian A, Brethauer SA, et al. Efficacy of adjuvant weight loss medication after bariatric surgery. Surgery for Obesity and Related Diseases. 2018;**14**(1):93-98

[96] Dhindsa BS, Saghir SM, Naga Y, Dhaliwal A, Ramai D, Cross C, et al. Efficacy of transoral outlet reduction in Roux-en-Y gastric bypass patients to promote weight loss: A systematic review and meta-analysis. Endoscopy International Open. 2020;**8**(10):E1332-E1e40

[97] Vargas EJ, Bazerbachi F, Rizk M, Rustagi T, Acosta A, Wilson EB, et al. Transoral outlet reduction with full thickness endoscopic suturing for weight regain after gastric bypass: A large multicenter international experience and meta-analysis. Surgical Endoscopy. 2018;**32**(1):252-259

[98] Jaruvongvanich V, Vantanasiri K, Laoveeravat P, Matar RH, Vargas EJ, Maselli DB, et al. Endoscopic full-thickness suturing plus argon plasma mucosal coagulation versus argon plasma mucosal coagulation alone for weight regain after gastric bypass: A systematic review and meta-analysis. Gastrointestinal Endoscopy. 2020;**92**(6):1164-75.e6

[99] Jirapinyo P, de Moura DTH, Thompson CC. Endoscopic submucosal dissection with suturing for the treatment of weight regain after gastric bypass: Outcomes and comparison with traditional transoral outlet reduction (with video). Gastrointestinal Endoscopy. 2020;**91**(6):1282-1288

[100] Brethauer SA, Kothari S, Sudan R, Williams B, English WJ, Brengman M, et al. Systematic review on reoperative bariatric surgery: American society for metabolic and bariatric surgery revision task force. Surgery for Obesity and Related Diseases. 2014;**10**(5):952-972

[101] Li S, Jiao S, Zhang S, Zhou J. Revisional surgeries of laparoscopic sleeve gastrectomy. Diabetes, Metabolic Syndrome and Obesity. 2021;**14**:575-588

[102] Ma P, Reddy S, Higa KD. Revisional bariatric/metabolic surgery: What dictates its indications? Current Atherosclerosis Reports. 2016;**18**(7):42

[103] Noel P, Nedelcu M, Eddbali I, Manos T, Gagner M. What are the long-term results 8 years after sleeve gastrectomy? Surgery for Obesity and Related Diseases. 2017;**13**(7):1110-1115

[104] Kermansaravi M, Davarpanah Jazi AH, Shahabi Shahmiri S, Eghbali F, Valizadeh R, Rezvani M. Revision procedures after initial Roux-en-Y gastric bypass, treatment of weight regain: A systematic review and meta-analysis. Updates in Surgery. 2021;**73**(2):663-678

[105] Andalib A, Alamri H, Almuhanna Y, Bouchard P, Demyttenaere S, Court O. Short-term outcomes of revisional surgery after sleeve gastrectomy: A comparative analysis of re-sleeve, Roux en-Y gastric bypass, duodenal switch (Roux en-Y and single-anastomosis). Surgical Endoscopy. 2021;**35**(8):4644-4652

Chapter 14

Causes of Intestinal Obstructions after Roux-En-Y Gastric Bypass

Mónica Angulo Trejo, Bonifacio García Ramos, José Antonio Angulo Trejo and Víctor García Ramos

Abstract

Obesity is a global pandemic and bariatric surgery is one of the fastest-growing surgical procedures performed worldwide. Roux-en-Y gastric bypass (RYGB) remains one of the most commonly performed bariatric procedures, with more than 480,000 procedures performed in 2022. The RYGB is characterized by a small proximal gastric pouch that is divided and separated from the distal stomach and anastomosed to an alimentary limb of the small intestine, thus bypassing a large portion of the small intestine preventing the absorption of nutrients. Small bowel obstruction after gastric bypass is not uncommon; the internal hernia is the most common etiology followed by postoperative adhesions, although there are less common causes. Diagnosis can be challenging due to the altered anatomy of the gastrointestinal tract; CT imaging is frequently used to establish the diagnosis. Since an internal hernia can be a life-threatening situation, early treatment is critical. The management of internal hernias after RYGB remains surgical. The urgency of surgical intervention depends on the clinical condition of the patient. Surgery should be attempted laparoscopically first if possible.

Keywords: bariatric surgery, internal hernia, intestinal obstruction, obesity, gastric bypass, roux-en-y

1. Introduction

Obesity is a worldwide pandemic, nearly every country in the world is affected by it and its increased prevalence shows no significant signs of slowing down any time soon. It is estimated that over 4 billion people may be affected by overweight and obesity by 2035, compared to over 2.6 billion in 2020 [1]. This reflects an increase from 38% of the world's population in 2020 to over 50% by 2035 [2].

The World Health Organization (WHO) defines overweight and obesity as excessive fat accumulation that may impair health [3]. A broader definition of obesity would encompass a chronic, systemic, multi-organ, metabolic, and inflammatory disease expressed phenotypically by an excess of body fat.

Overweight and obesity are well-known risk factors for other diseases like diabetes mellitus, cardiovascular disease, and several types of cancers [4] including breast, colon, endometrial, and prostate cancer [5]. Other major comorbidities include degenerative joint disease, obstructive sleep apnea, and cholesterol gallstone disease [6], all of which have a major bearing on life expectancy, quality of life, and mental health on an individual level, and detriment in work productivity and healthcare costs at a population level.

2. Bariatric surgery

Bariatric surgery is a medical specialty dedicated to the surgical treatment of obesity and its comorbidities. It is one of the fastest-growing operative procedures performed worldwide, with an estimated >480,000 operations performed by 24 countries in 2022 according to the 8th Global Registry Report of the International Federation for the Surgery of Obesity and Metabolic Disorders (IFSO) [7].

In 1991, the U.S. National Institutes of Health (NIH) created a Consensus Conference that established the patient selection criteria for undergoing bariatric surgery [8]:

- BMI >40 kg/m2
- Or BMI >35 kg/m2 with comorbidities related to obesity.
- ≥18 years of age

Thirty years later, in 2022, with evidence of good outcomes, a decrease in morbi-mortality, improvements in patient safety, and development of laparoscopic techniques, the IFSO wrote major updates to the 1991 guidelines [9]:

- BMI >35 kg/m2 regardless of presence, absence, or severity of comorbidities.
- Metabolic disease and BMI of 30–34.9 kg/m2
- Appropriately selected children and adolescents should be considered for surgery

The physiology of digestion and nutrient absorption must be comprehended in order to understand the fundamentals of bariatric surgery. As the chime passes through the duodenum, pancreatic enzymes break down peptides and carbohydrates, and lipids are degraded by the pancreatic lipase and bile. Those nutrients are absorbed by the enterocytes and transported to the liver. More than 75% of carbohydrates, proteins, and fats are normally absorbed within 70 cm of the small intestine [10].

Bariatric malabsorptive procedures divert the flow of bile and pancreatic enzymes from food, thereby avoiding digestion of nutrients in the most proximal part of the GI tract where absorption is greater, resulting in reduced caloric intake.

Restrictive procedures, on the other hand, reduce the size or storage capacity of the stomach to induce satiety with less food, therefore reducing calorie consumption.

Malabsorptive/restrictive (mixed) procedures use both mechanisms: a restrictive component to initiate rapid weight loss, combined with a malabsorptive component to ensure long-lasting effects.

According to IFSO [7], the sleeve gastrectomy is the most commonly performed primary procedure (defined as the first procedure a person with obesity undertakes as a treatment for their obesity) in the majority of reporting countries, accounting for 63.3% of the total number of registered procedures. With 28.8% of procedures, Roux-en-Y gastric bypass (RYGB) was the second most common primary procedure. In contrast, Roux-en-Y gastric bypass is the most commonly performed revisional metabolic bariatric procedure. The revisional procedures are those performed to change one type of bariatric procedure to another bariatric procedure, most often secondary to a failure of the primary procedure either due to weight gain, side effects of the initial procedure, or recurrence of metabolic disorders [11]. Nearly half of the revisional procedures correspond to RYGB.

3. Roux-en-Y gastric bypass

As discussed above, RYGB is the second most common bariatric procedure performed today and has long been considered the "gold standard" of bariatric surgery. Although originally performed as an open procedure, it is now almost exclusively performed using a laparoscopic approach.

It is important for the non-surgical healthcare professional to have a basic understanding of the surgical technique involved in creating a gastric bypass, as altering the gastrointestinal (GI) anatomy can lead to potentially serious complications that may be life-threatening to the patient.

RYGB is a restrictive-malabsorptive (mixed) procedure that creates a small gastric pouch that connects directly to the small intestine. **Figure 1**. This pouch is created by dividing the stomach into two parts. The first one is the most proximal and receives up to 30 ml of food, the second is the remaining stomach and does not receive food. The surgery also involves dividing the small intestine at a distance of 50 to 150 cm distal to the ligament of Treitz. The division of the small intestine creates two limbs, the first one is the "biliopancreatic limb" which transports the secretions of the gastric

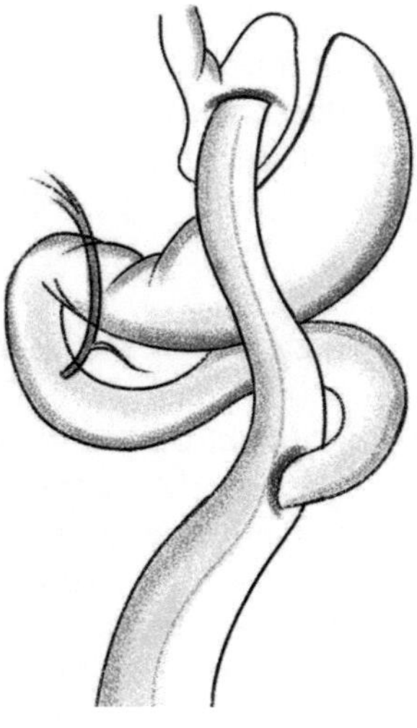

Figure 1.
Schematic representation of a Roux-en-Y gastric bypass. The gastric pouch is anastomosed to the alimentary limb. The digestive juices of the remaining stomach and biliopancreatic secretions are carried through the biliopancreatic limb. Note the site where the two limbs join. Swallowed food bypassed a portion of the small intestine.

remnant, liver, and pancreas; and the second limb or "alimentary limb" which is anastomosed at one end to the gastric pouch and the biliopancreatic limb at the other end. The distance between the two anastomoses is generally 75 to 150 cm. The connection of the biliopancreatic and alimentary limbs forms a common duct where pancreatic enzymes and bile mix with ingested food.

The surgical technique has two variations depending on the passage of the alimentary limb. In the retrocolic technique, the limb is passed through a mesocolic window (creating the Petersen's defect), whereas in the anterocolic approach, the limb is localized anterior to the colon. As discussed below, this difference in surgical technique creates more or less mesenteric defects that may result in a higher incidence of complications.

In summary, RYGB creates a small gastric pouch that restricts food intake and connects it to another distant portion of the intestine, which bypasses a large portion of the small intestine preventing the absorption of nutrients until they reach the distal part of the intestine where the "common duct" connects the two limbs.

In addition to promoting weight loss through a restrictive and malabsorptive mechanism, RYGB induces other physiologic changes in GI hormone secretion, intestinal bacterial colonization, bile acid metabolism, and epigenetic changes [10].

The restriction of food passage through the duodenum and jejunum in RYGB is thought to induce changes in postprandial gut hormone secretion [12]. For example, there is a decrease in the levels of gastrin, a peptide hormone that stimulates the secretion of gastric acid and aids in gastric motility. The appetite-stimulating hormone ghrelin is also suppressed postoperatively, as is cholecystokinin, which slows gastric emptying and suppresses hunger.

The vast majority of bile acids are reabsorbed in the terminal ileum and reused by the liver, forming the "enterohepatic circulation". In patients with RYGB, the biliopancreatic limb shortens the route for bile acids to reach the ileum, resulting in more active bile acid reabsorption [13]. This increased luminal bile acid concentration has antibacterial effects, killing certain strains of bacteria and allowing others to survive, although the contribution of the gut microbiota to the metabolic benefits after bariatric surgery has not been elucidated [14].

Finally, epigenetic markers are chemical modifications mediated by DNA enzymes that regulate genomic functions. Several studies have shown DNA methylation in adipose or muscle tissue after RYGB [15], which may explain the changes in physiology and metabolism after bariatric surgery.

4. RYGB complications that produce intestinal obstruction

RYGB is a procedure with a mortality of 0.5% and a morbidity of 7 to 14% [16]. It is not uncommon for patients to present to the emergency department with abdominal pain after RYGB, so the general practitioner must be aware of the unique complications of this type of surgery in order to make a prompt diagnosis and avoid delaying treatment with potentially fatal consequences.

Small bowel obstruction (SBO) is a common complication of RYGB with a lifetime incidence of 6 to 9.6 percent [17] and is one of the most feared complications since it can become a life-threatening situation.

The etiology of SBO has numerous causes which makes differential diagnosis particularly difficult. Among the diverse etiologies, the most frequent are internal hernia, postoperative adhesions, anastomotic stricture, incisional hernia, and intussusception. 60% of SBO after a RYGB is due to an internal hernia [18].

4.1 Roux-en-O misconstruction

One cause of SBO early after surgery (<30 days postoperative) may be the misidentification of the alimentary and biliopancreatic limbs during surgery, resulting in a loop obstruction as the distal jejunum of the biliopancreatic limb is anastomosed to the gastric pouch. A condition known as "Roux-en-O misconstruction" requires a second surgical intervention to correct the mistake.

The clinical presentation encompasses abdominal pain, nausea, and bilious vomiting. It is an extremely difficult diagnosis to make, as radiological modalities may appear normal.

4.2 Internal hernia

An internal hernia (IH) is the protrusion of the bowel through the mesenteric defects created by the division of the small bowel to form de biliopancreatic and alimentary limbs or the defect in the mesocolon when a retro colic roux limb technique is used. The incidence of IH is higher in the laparoscopic technique rather than in the open approach due to lesser postoperative adhesions.

The IH is the most common long-term complication after Roux-en-Y gastric bypass with an incidence of 12% without routine closure of the mesenteric defects [19] and between 0.9% and 4.5% [20] when mesenteric defects are closed with non-absorbable sutures. It often presents as a late complication (>30 days postoperative) of surgery.

There are three potential spaces for internal hernia formation in an RYGB depending upon the surgical technique used, as illustrated in **Figure 2**. When an antecolic RYGB is performed, only two spaces are created: a mesenteric defect at the jejuno-jejunostomy (also known as Brolin's space) and a space between the transverse mesocolon and Roux limb mesentery (Petersen's defect). If a retro colic roux limb technique is used, another space is added: a defect in the transverse mesocolon [21]. The incidences of IH in each space vary among studies.

The clinical presentation of late SBO is variable, ranging from mild digestive symptoms to acute abdomen. The reducibility of the hernia, the presence or absence of strangulation, and incarceration all influence the severity of the symptoms. Abdominal pain is the most common complaint [22], often described as deep, continuous, and gradual onset, with the majority of patients localizing the pain in the left upper quadrant of the abdomen. Few patients report changes in bowel frequency.

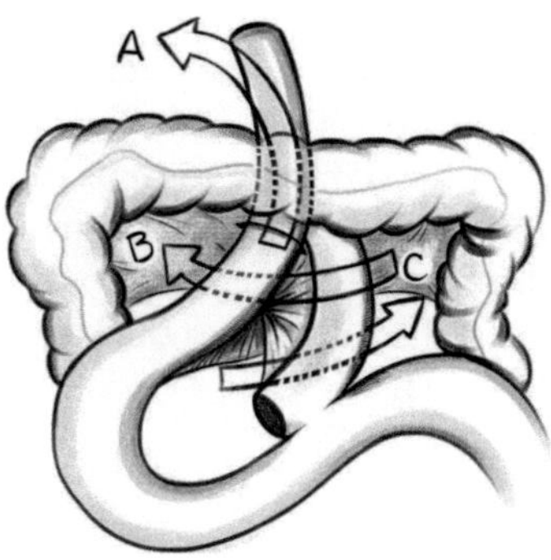

Figure 2.
Schematic representation of potential sites for internal hernia formation. (A) Defect in the transverse mesocolon, (B) Petersen's space, and (C) Brolin's space.

Nausea and vomiting are less common, with less than half of patients experiencing these symptoms [23], due to lack of involvement of the alimentary limb.

Because clinical diagnosis is difficult, imaging studies play an important role in the evaluation of patients with high clinical suspicion. Abdominal computed tomography (CT) is the preferred imaging modality for the diagnosis of IH prior to surgery, as its sensitivity and specificity has been reported to exceed 80% [24]. Traditionally, three signs have been described [25] with variable diagnostic sensitivity and specificity. The "swirl sign", which is considered the best predictor of IH, consists of the twisted appearance of vessels and fat at the mesenteric root; abnormal clustered loops; and the "mushroom sign", which is formed by the herniated mesenteric root in a mushroom shape with mesenteric vessel stretching.

Other authors have proposed additional signs such as the small bowel (other than duodenum) posterior to the superior mesenteric artery and right-sided location of the distal jejunal anastomosis [26], or the "superior mesenteric vein (SMV) beaking" [27] which consists of decreased caliber of the SMV. Although no sign alone is pathognomonic of IH, prompt interpretation of CT may lead to an early diagnosis and prompt treatment of a potentially serious complication like ischemia, necrosis, or perforation of the involved intestinal segment. However, diagnostic laparoscopy should be performed immediately if there is any doubt in the imaging studies or if the patient is critically ill.

Surgical exploration is recommended for bariatric patients suspected of having IH. Either open or laparoscopic exploration can be performed, although the latter can be technically challenging due to bowel dilatation which increases the risk of injury during trocar placement and also decreased working space.

In both cases, the recommended first step of the procedure is to identify the ileocecal valve and explore the terminal ileum (the common channel) toward the ligament of Treitz until the jejuno-jejunostomy is reached [28]. The potential mesenteric gap at the jejuno-jejunostomy is then explored. The biliopancreatic and alimentary limbs are identified and explored, as well as Petersen's space and the gap between the transverse mesocolon (in cases where the retrocolic technique was used). All the intestine trapped within the hernia defect should be carefully reduced with atraumatic forceps to avoid iatrogenic injury. Once all the herniated bowel has been reduced, it should be carefully examined to determine perfusion. If perfusion is compromised or frank necrosis is encountered, resection with primary anastomosis is required [21].

It is very important that all mesenteric defects are carefully examined and closed with non-absorbable sutures if found open, as there is a 14% risk of recurrence of IH in the untreated mesenteric gaps [29]. As for the rates of IH in the antecolic vs. retrocolic technique, the latter have a lower incidence (1.3% vs. 2.3%), since there is a smaller number of mesenteric defects [30].

Because IH is a relatively common complication of RYGB, a single anastomosis procedure called open gastric bypass (OAGB) has been developed to reduce the incidence of IH. The OAGB eliminates the mesenteric defect in Brolin's space due to the absence of the jejuno-jejunostomy, although the risk of Petersen's hernia remains, with an incidence of IH of 2.8% [31].

4.3 Intussusception

Intussusception after RYGB is a rare late complication of RYGB, with an incidence ranging from 0.15 to 4.7% [32]. It is thought to originate from motility disorders in the divided small intestine, secondary to the disruption of the natural intestinal pacemakers in the duodenum, and allows for the formation of ectopic pacemakers in the alimentary limb [33].

Most intussusceptions after RYGB occur at the jejuno-jejunostomy site and are retrograde (antiperistaltic) [34], telescoping the distal bowel segment into the proximal segment. If left untreated, it may progress to bowel ischemia and wall necrosis.

Clinical presentation includes abdominal pain, constipation, nausea, and vomiting, with or without signs of acute abdomen. The most useful diagnostic tool is the CT, which shows the classic "target sign" (concentric rings) [35].

Most patients require surgical intervention. If exploration of the jejuno-jejunostomy reveals ischemic bowel or perforation, bowel resection is mandatory. If the exploration reveals no complications, it can be treated with a reduction of the bowel segment without resection, although this approach has a risk of recurrence, so some authors suggest that the invaginated segment should be resected whether it is viable or not [36].

4.4 Bezoars

A bezoar is a combination of ingested materials that cannot be digested and are therefore retained in the GI tract. They are classified according to their composition, with phytobezoars (composed of plant fibers) being the most common type [37]. They are a rare etiology of bowel obstruction after RYGB, accounting for <1% of cases [38].

Most patients have a history of gastro-duodenal surgery [39] resulting in altered GI anatomy and/or motility. Bariatric surgery may promote bezoar formation due to small gastric pouches, decreased gastric motility and acidity, and narrow stomas at anastomoses [40]. The most common location of bezoars is the stomach, although the bezoar may migrate to the small or large intestine [41].

Reported sites of intestinal obstruction after RYGB include the gastric pouch, the gastrojejunostomy, the alimentary or biliopancreatic limb, or, extremely rarely, the jejuno-jejuno anastomosis [42].

Clinical presentation varies depending on the location of the bezoar but often includes nausea, vomiting, and/or symptoms of gastric outlet obstruction. If complicated by GI bleeding from ulcer or wall necrosis (secondary to increased intraluminal pressure), they may present with anemia, bloody stools, or hematemesis [43]. If perforation is present, the patient will develop signs of acute abdomen.

Diagnosis requires a high index of suspicion. Plain radiographs may show radiotranslucents, ultrasound can show the presence of an intraluminal mass with a hyperechoic surface and prominent acoustic shadow, CT can show a round intraluminal mass in the GI tract with retained air bubbles inside, endoscopy is the preferred method as it allows direct visualization of the bezoar and allows therapeutic applications [40, 42, 43].

Current treatment options include chemical dissolution of the bezoar (in the absence of SBO) with Coca-Cola [37] or papain [44], an enzyme extracted from the Carica papaya plant and used in some meat tenderizing products. Endoscopic fragmentation and removal are also possible. In the case of SBO or ileus due to bezoar, surgical removal is indicated via enterotomy [43] or the milking technique, which consists of pushing the bezoar toward the stomach or through the ileocecal valve, a technique that is not without complications [45].

Nutritional counseling is essential to prevent bezoar formation and recurrence, which has a 14% risk of recurrence [46]. Dietary counseling should include eating small meals, increasing fluid intake, chewing slowly and carefully, and avoiding high-fiber foods [40].

4.5 Anastomotic stricture (stenosis)

The stenosis at the gastrojejunostomy after RYGB occurs in up to 27% of patients [47]. The etiology is multifactorial, proposed mechanisms involved in the formation of stenosis include stomal ulcer, reflux, ischemia of the suture, or an inadequate surgical technique (size of circular staple anastomoses, or the initial size of the anastomosis) [48].

The gastroenterostomy constructed during an RYBG is made deliberately small to archive the restrictive effect of gastric bypass, with an optimal size between 10 and 12 mm [49]. It has been proposed that clinical manifestations occur when the anastomosis narrows to a diameter of <10 mm [50].

Symptoms include dysphagia, nausea, vomiting, and abdominal pain. Diagnosis is usually made by endoscopy, which also allows therapeutic treatment with endoscopic dilatation. To reduce the likelihood of recurrence, many authors advocate the use of through-the-scope (TTS) balloon catheters and dilatation to at least 15 mm [51]. If no improvement is achieved after four consecutive endoscopic dilations, surgical revision with reconstructive surgery may be indicated.

5. Conclusions

Bariatric surgery is growing in popularity worldwide as the prevalence of obesity increases. As the number of postoperative patients increases, so does the incidence of postoperative complications.

Postoperative bariatric surgery patients may seek urgent care at any emergency department, so in order to suspect and make a timely diagnosis, emergency physicians and general surgeons should have a basic knowledge of bariatric procedures and their potential complications.

Frequently, some of the complications of RYGB manifest as SBO. These include internal hernia, intussusception, bezoar formation, and anastomotic stenosis. The altered anatomy of the gastrointestinal tract secondary to the creation of a Roux-en-Y gastric bypass makes the symptoms very vague and different from classic bowel obstruction, making the diagnosis challenging. Misdiagnosis could result in inappropriate attempts at non-operative management with delays in surgical consultation and treatment with potentially fatal consequences.

Conflict of interest

The authors declare no conflict of interest.

Author details

Mónica Angulo Trejo[1]*, Bonifacio García Ramos[1], José Antonio Angulo Trejo[2] and Víctor García Ramos[3]

1 Mexican Institute of Social Security, Monterrey, Mexico

2 Mexican Institute of Social Security, Querétaro, Mexico

3 Mexican Institute of Social Security, Veracruz, Mexico

*Address all correspondence to: angulo.t.monica@gmail.com

References

[1] World Obesity Federation. World Obesity Atlas 2023 [Internet]. 2023. Available from: https://data.worldobesity.org/publications/?cat=19 [Accessed: January 11, 2024]

[2] World Health Organization. Fact sheet: Obesity and Overweight [Internet]. 2015. Available from: https://www.who.int/news-room/fact-sheets/detail/obesity-and-overweight [Accessed: January 4, 2024]

[3] Scully T, Ettela A, LeRoith D. Obesity, type 2 diabetes, and cancer risk. Frontiers in Oncology. 2021;**10**:615375. DOI: 10.3389/fonc.2020.615375

[4] Redinger RN. The pathophysiology of obesity and its clinical manifestations. Gastroenterology & Hepatology. 2007;**3**:856-863

[5] Pi-Sunyer FX. Comorbidities of overweight and obesity: Current evidence and research issues. Medicine & Science in Sports & Exercise. 1999;**31**:S602-S608. DOI: 10.1097/00005768-199911001-00019

[6] Fontaine KR, Redden DT, Wang C. Years of life lost due to obesity. Journal of the American Medical Association. 2003;**289**:187-193. DOI: 10.1001/jama.289.2.187

[7] International Federation for the Surgery of Obesity and Metabolic Disorders. Eighth Global Registry Report [Internet]. 2023. Available from: https://www.ifso.com/pdf/8th-ifso-registry-report-2023.pdf [Accessed: January 4, 2024]

[8] Brolin RE. Update: NIH consensus conference. Gastrointestinal surgery for severe obesity. Nutrition. 1996;**12**:403-404. DOI: 10.1016/s0899-9007(96)00154-2

[9] Eisenberg D, Shikora SA, Aarts E. 2022 American Society for Metabolic and Bariatric Surgery (ASMBS) and International Federation for the Surgery of obesity and metabolic disorders (IFSO): Indications for metabolic and bariatric surgery. Surgery for Obesity and Related Diseases. 2022;**18**:1345-1356. DOI: 10.1016/j.soard.2022.08.013

[10] Billeter AT, Fischer L, Wekerle AL. Malabsorption as a therapeutic approach in bariatric surgery. Viszeralmedizin. 2014;**30**:198-204. DOI: 10.1159/000363480

[11] Switzer NJ, Karmali S, Gill RS. Revisional bariatric surgery. Surgical Clinics of North America. 2016;**96**:827-842. DOI: 10.1016/j.suc.2016.03.004

[12] Dimitriadis GK, Randeva MS, Miras AD. Potential hormone mechanisms of bariatric surgery. Current obesity reports. 2017;**6**:253-265. DOI: 10.1007/s13679-017-0276-5

[13] Wang W, Cheng Z, Wang Y. Role of bile acids in bariatric surgery. Frontiers in Physiology. 2019;**10**:374. DOI: 10.3389/fphys.2019.00374

[14] Ulker İ, Yildiran H. The effects of bariatric surgery on gut microbiota in patients with obesity: A review of the literature. Bioscience of microbiota, food and health. 2019;**38**:3-9. DOI: 10.12938/bmfh.18-018

[15] Izquierdo AG, Crujeiras AB. Obesity-related epigenetic changes after bariatric surgery. Frontiers in endocrinology. 2019;**10**:232. DOI: 10.3389/fendo.2019.00232

[16] Sakran N, Assalia A, Sternberg A. Smaller staple height for circular stapled gastrojejunostomy in laparoscopic gastric bypass: Early results in 1,074 morbidly obese patients. Obesity Surgery. 2011;**21**:238-243. DOI: 10.1007/s11695-010-0308-7

[17] Elms L, Moon RC, Varnadore S. Causes of small bowel obstruction after roux-en-Y gastric bypass: A review of 2,395 cases at a single institution. Surgical Endoscopy. 2014;**28**:1624-1628. DOI: 10.1007/s00464-013-3361-1

[18] Geubbels N, Lijftogt N, Fiocco M. Meta-analysis of internal herniation after gastric bypass surgery. British Journal of Surgery. 2015;**102**:451-460. DOI: 10.1002/bjs.9738

[19] Collard MK, Torcivia A, Genser L. Laparoscopic management of internal hernia after roux-en-Y-gastric bypass. Journal of Visceral Surgery. 2020;**157**:423-427. DOI: 10.1016/j.jviscsurg.2020.08.013

[20] Madan AK, Lo Menzo E, Dhawan N. Internal hernias and nonclosure of mesenteric defects during laparoscopic roux-en-Y gastric bypass. Obesity Surgery. 2008;**19**:549-552. DOI: 10.1007/s11695-008-9722-5

[21] Pokala B, Giannopoulos S, Stefanidis D. Prevention and management of internal hernias after bariatric surgery: An expert review. Mini-invasive Surgery. 2022;**6**:23. DOI: 10.20517/2574-1225.2021.136

[22] Tartamella F, Ziccarelli A, Cecchini S. Abdominal pain and internal hernias after roux-en-Y gastric bypass: Are we dealing with the tip of an iceberg? Acta bio-medica. 2019;**90**:251-258. DOI: 10.23750/abm.v90i2.7145

[23] Husain S, Ahmed AR, Johnson J. Small-bowel obstruction after laparoscopic roux-en-Y gastric bypass. Archives of Surgery. 2007;**142**:988-993. DOI: 10.1001/archsurg.142.10.988

[24] Nawas MA, Oor JE, Goense L. The diagnostic accuracy of abdominal computed tomography in diagnosing internal herniation following roux-en-Y gastric bypass surgery. Annals of Surgery. 2021;**275**:856-863. DOI: 10.1097/SLA.0000000000005247

[25] Bordonaro V, Brizi MG, Lanza F. Role of CT imaging in discriminating internal hernia from aspecific abdominal pain following roux-en-Y gastric bypass: A single high-volume Centre experience. Updates in Surgery. 2020;**72**:1115-1124. DOI: 10.1007/s13304-020-00767-w

[26] Lockhart ME, Tessler FN, Canon CL. Internal hernia after gastric bypass: Sensitivity and specificity of seven CT signs with surgical correlation and controls. American journal of roentgenology. 2007;**188**:745-750. DOI: 10.2214/AJR.06.0541

[27] Maier J, Herrasti Gallego A, Floyd AK. Compression of the superior mesenteric vein—A sign of acute internal herniation in patients with antecolic laparoscopic roux-en-Y gastric bypass. European Radiology. 2016;**27**:1733-1739. DOI: 10.1007/s00330-016-4526-9

[28] Kollmann L, Lock JF, Kollmann C. Surgical treatment of internal hernia after roux–en-Y gastric bypass — Impact of institutional standards and surgical approach. Langenbeck's Archives of Surgery. 2023;**408**:318. DOI: 10.1007/s00423-023-03049-2

[29] Zaigham H, Ekelund M, Regnér S. Long-term follow-up and risk of recurrence of internal herniation after roux-en-Y gastric bypass. Obesity Surgery. 2023;**33**:2311-2316. DOI: 10.1007/s11695-023-06653-9

[30] Harakeh A, Kallies KJ, Borgert AJ. Bowel obstruction rates in antecolic/antegastric versus retrocolic/retrogastric roux limb gastric bypass: A meta-analysis. Surgery for Obesity and Related Diseases. 2016;**12**:194-198. DOI: 10.1016/j.soard.2015.02.004

[31] Petrucciani N, Martini F, Kassir R. Internal hernia after one anastomosis gastric bypass (OAGB): Lessons learned from a retrospective series of 3368 consecutive patients undergoing OAGB with a biliopancreatic limb of 150 cm. Obesity Surgery. 2021;**31**:2537-2544. DOI: 10.1007/s11695-021-05269-1

[32] Oor JE, Goense L, Wiezer MJ. Incidence and treatment of intussusception following roux-en-Y gastric bypass: A systematic review and meta-analysis. Surgery for Obesity and Related Diseases. 2021;**17**:1017-1028. DOI: 10.1016/j.soard.2021.01.006

[33] Kumar A, Ogbonda S, Persaud P. Retrograde intussusception after roux-en-Y gastric bypass. Cureus. 2020;**12**:e8825. DOI: 10.7759/cureus.8825

[34] Simper SC, Erzinger JM, McKinlay RD. Retrograde (reverse) jejunal intussusception might not be such a rare problem: A single group's experience of 23 cases. Surgery for Obesity and Related Diseases. 2008;**4**:77-83. DOI: 10.1016/j.soard.2007.12.004

[35] Singla S, Guenthart BA, May L. Intussusception after laparoscopic gastric bypass surgery: An Underrecognized complication. Minimally Invasive Surgery. 2012;**2012**:1-8. DOI: 10.1155/2012/464853

[36] Daellenbach L, Suter M. Jejunojejunal Intussusception After Roux-en-Y Gastric Bypass: A Review. 2011;**21**:253-263. DOI: 10.1007/s11695-010-0298-5

[37] Iwamuro M, Okada H, Matsueda K. Review of the diagnosis and management of gastrointestinal bezoars. World Journal of Gastrointestinal Endoscopy. 2015;**7**:336-345. DOI: 10.4253/wjge.v7.i4.336

[38] Roy M, Fendrich I, Li J. Treatment option in patient presenting with small bowel obstruction from Phytobezoar at the Jejunojejunal anastomosis after roux-en-Y gastric bypass. Surgical Laparoscopy Endoscopy & Percutaneous Techniques. 2012;**22**:e243-e245. DOI: 10.1097/SLE.0b013e31825d6c07

[39] Ertugrul I, Tardum Tardu A, Tolan K. Gastric bezoar after roux-en-Y gastric bypass for morbid obesity: A case report. International Journal of Surgery. 2016;**23**:112-115. DOI: 10.1016/j.ijscr.2016.04.008

[40] Ben-Porat T, Sherf Dagan S, Goldenshluger A. Gastrointestinal phytobezoar following bariatric surgery: Systematic review. Surgery for Obesity and Related Diseases. 2016;**12**:1747-1754. DOI: 10.1016/j.soard.2016.09.003

[41] Dikicier E, Altintoprak F, Ozkan OV. Intestinal obstruction due to phytobezoars: An update. World Journal of Clinical Cases. 2015;**3**:721-726. DOI: 10.12998/wjcc.v3.i8.721

[42] Rodríguez J, Kobus V, Téllez I. Obstrucción intestinal por fitobezoar en una paciente con bypass gástrico laparoscópico en Y de Roux: Reporte de un caso. Revista de cirugía. 2019;**71**:330-334. DOI: 10.4067/S2452-45492019000400330

[43] Paschos KA, Chatzigeorgiadis A. Pathophysiological and clinical aspects of the diagnosis and treatment of bezoars. Annals of Gastroenterology. 2019;**32**:224-232. DOI: 10.20524/aog.2019.0370

[44] Dwivedi AJ, Chahin F, Agrawal S. Gastric phytobezoar: Treatment using meat tenderizer. Digestive Diseases and Sciences. 2001;**46**:1013-1015. DOI: 10.1023/a:1010701809950

[45] Yakan S, Sirinocak A, Telciler KE. A rare cause of acute abdomen: Small bowel obstruction due to phytobezoar. Turkish journal of trauma & emergency surgery. 2010;**16**:459-463

[46] Kanwar P, Cheung D, Verma S. Bezoars: A rare, late complication of roux-en-Y gastric bypass and a novel endoscopic technique for treatment. American Journal of Gastroenterology. 2016;**111**:S1098-S1099

[47] Nguyen NT, Stevens CM, Wolfe BM. Incidence and outcome of anastomotic stricture after laparoscopic gastric bypass. Journal of Gastrointestinal Surgery. 2003;7:997-1003. DOI: 10.1016/j.gassur.2003.09.016

[48] Espinel J, Pinedo E. Stenosis in gastric bypass: Endoscopic management. World Journal of Gastrointestinal Endoscopy. 2012;**4**:290-295. DOI: 10.4253/wjge.v4.i7.290

[49] Schwartz ML, Drew RL, Roiger RW. Stenosis of the Gastroenterostomy after laparoscopic gastric bypass. Obesity Surgery. 2004;**14**:484-491. DOI: 10.1381/096089204323013460

[50] Ukleja A, Afonso BB, Pimentel R. Outcome of endoscopic balloon dilation of strictures after laparoscopic gastric bypass. Surgical Endoscopy. 2008;**22**:1746-1750. DOI: 10.1007/s00464-008-9788-0

[51] Huang CS. The role of the endoscopist in a multidisciplinary obesity center. Gastrointestinal Endoscopy. 2009;**70**:763-767. DOI: 10.1016/j.gie.2009.01.009